Praise for *Health Care Choices for Today's Consumer*

"*Health Care Choices for Today's Consumer* is a comprehensive guide to help you and your family ensure that you receive the best and most affordable health care. It comes to you from Families USA, an organization that is a thoughtful and effective advocate for the American health care consumer."

—Hillary Rodham Clinton

"Parents, as consumers, deserve to have information available to them to make informed decisions about the medical treatment of their children. *Health Care Choices for Today's Consumer* provides an excellent resource of information for parents."

—Joe M. Sanders Jr.
Executive Director, American Academy of Pediatrics

"*Health Care Choices for Today's Consumer* provides readers with a wealth of information about the various aspects of making health care choices. It will be a valuable resource for consumers with questions about how to make the best decisions about their health care and how to be in control of their choices."

—Arthur S. Flemming
Secretary of Health, Education and Welfare under President Eisenhower

"With great clarity, *Health Care Choices for Today's Consumer* helps to demystify a health care system that can be utterly confusing. Families USA has come to our aid by showing us what to look for—and what to look out for—in a health care provider."

—Ben Cohen
Founder and Chairman, Ben & Jerry's Homemade, Inc.

"*Health Care Choices for Today's Consumer* is a remarkable book that serves as a detailed road map—helping the consumer navigate in today's complex health care system—and an encyclopedia of useful information about specific health issues. For those moving into a new community or a new stage of life, for those facing unfamiliar health-related problems, or for those simply seeking to reevaluate the treatment they have been getting, it will be a very valuable resource."

—Jean A. Dowdall
President, Simmons College

"This book is a veritable treasure of essential, user-friendly information for the health care consumer. I enthusiastically recommend it as an important part of the education of those who are or will be faced with health care decisions—which includes us all. Elders and families—professionals and nonprofessionals alike—should get and read a copy now."

—John R. Delfs, M.D.
Associate Medical Director for Medicare Programs
Harvard/Pilgrim Health Care

"There is a need . . . for sensible manuals for patients, guides to choosing and using medical care in this complicated new world. This new book is an admirable contributor, clearly written, well organized, superbly printed to make reading easy and helpful."

—Washington Post

"If ever there was a time when guidance [to health care options] was needed, that time is now, and if ever there was a book that provided such guidance, that book is *Health Care Choices for Today's Consumer*. . . . While other books have covered some of these topics . . . none has come close to this one in terms of clarity of purpose and style. Essential for every library serving health care consumers and indeed for every consumer."

—Library Journal

"Here's a candidate for a permanent position on your medical reference shelf. . . . This no-nonsense guide covers topics ranging from women's health issues to choosing health insurance, selecting and working with doctors, and learning about alternative medicine. The book tells you what the medical establishment, insurance companies, and hospitals probably won't: What are your rights? What are the most important questions to ask before making decisions? How can you control costs? Where can you get more information?"

—Fitness Magazine

"For soup-to-nuts advice on a wide range of health topics, pick up a copy of *Health Care Choices for Today's Consumer*. . . . The book's strong consumer-advocacy slant emphasizes how you can take charge of your health care—and its costs."

—Kiplinger's Personal Finance Magazine

Health Care Choices for Today's Consumer

Revised and Expanded

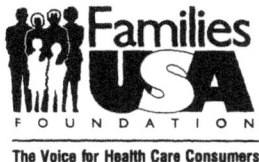

Families USA FOUNDATION
The Voice for Health Care Consumers

Guide to Quality and Cost

Edited by Marc S. Miller, Ph.D.

A ROBERT L. BERNSTEIN BOOK

John Wiley & Sons, Inc.
New York ■ Chichester ■ Weinheim ■ Brisbane ■ Singapore ■ Toronto

To S. P., A. L., W. G., and K. P.,
for keeping me healthy through the years.

This text is printed on acid-free paper.

First published in the United States by Living Planet Press
First John Wiley & Sons, Inc., paperback edition 1997

Published by John Wiley & Sons, Inc.

The information contained in this book is not intended to serve as a replacement for professional medical advice or professional psychological counseling. Any use of the information in this book is at the reader's discretion. The publisher specifically disclaims any and
all liability arising directly or indirectly from the use or application of any information contained in this book. The appropriate professional should be consulted regarding your specific condition.

Grateful acknowledgment is made for permission to use the following material:
"Home Care," copyright © 1994 by United Seniors Health Cooperative.
"Environmental Causes of Medical Problems," copyright © 1981 by American Medical Asso-
ciation Center for the Study of Services for materials on eye and dental care.

Library of Congress Cataloging-in-Publication Data

Health care choices for today's consumer: Families USA guide to
   quality and cost / Marc S. Miller, editor.
      p.   cm.
   Includes bibliographical references and index.
   ISBN 978-1-62045-688-0
   1. Medical care. 2. Consumer education.   I. Miller, Marc S.
II. Families United for Senior Action Foundation.
RA410.5.H396   1997
362.1—dc20   96-35919

10 9 8 7 6 5 4 3 2 1

Contents

Part One: Getting Started   1

Part Two: The Heart of the Matter   **39**

Contents

Part Five: For Everyone's Health   397

Foreword:
A Message From
Families USA

Since its founding in 1981, Families USA Foundation has focused its resources and attention on the U.S. health care system and how to improve it. As the voice of health care consumers, it has worked hard to bring about the day when every American receives high-quality, affordable health care and long term care.

We at Families USA believe that the United States will attain this long-awaited goal in the foreseeable future. But even then, you and your family will require, as you do today, solid information on which to base a wide variety of critical decisions about health care. That's why Families USA decided to initiate the Health Care Choices project: to provide you with information every consumer needs—but that is rarely available in a form you can easily understand and *apply* to your own life.

The fact is that most Americans encounter the health care system as a kind of jungle in which anyone can easily get lost. All of us must adapt to bewildering changes in that system, sometimes for the better, too often not. At the top of the list of transformations, managed care has come to dominate the market. Meanwhile, local, state, and federal authorities are constantly revising regulations, services, and laws, and employers are shifting the health care options they offer to their employees.

Consumers say they are more troubled and confused than ever. As you seek to travel and unravel this maze, you and your family will benefit from taking to heart the information and advice in *Health Care Choices for Today's Consumer.*

We at Families USA see the Health Care Choices books, including this volume and a series of companion regional guides, as one of our contributions to the health and well-being of our 185,000 members and of all Americans. Besides helping you *now,* these books can act as a powerful incentive for the health care industry to serve you and your neighbors well *in the future.* We expect the next edition of *Health Care Choices for Today's Consumer* will report that providers and policymakers are meeting your needs better than they do today—in response to increased pressure from informed consumers like you.

To help us design an even more effective consumer weapon, we invite your suggestions for improving future editions of *Health Care Choices for Today's Consumer.* Send your comments directly to my attention: Philippe Villers, President, Families USA, 97 Lowell Road, Concord, MA 01742.

Thank you.

—Philippe Villers, President

Philippe Villers and his wife, Katherine S. Villers, founded Families USA Foundation in 1981.

Acknowledgments

Literally countless people contributed to *Health Care Choices for Today's Consumer*. First on the list are my colleagues in the Health Care Choices project: project associates Martha S. Grover and Rebecca Derby, and Philippe Villers, president and founder of Families USA Foundation and the guiding light for this project.

In addition, two groups of people have been invaluable: the authors and the project advisory board. The members of both groups contributed far and beyond their "official" roles. For example, many authors provided critical insight for chapters by other people, as well as guidance for the project as a whole. The advisory board, chaired by Mr. Villers, consists of J. Larry Brown, Michael Crump, Thomas Delbanco, M.D., Barbara Ferrer, Norbert Goldfield, M.D., Suzanne Mercure, Joseph Restuccia, D.Ph., Richard Rockefeller, M.D., Richard Rowe, Michael Segal, Rina Spence, and Harriet Tolpin. Richard Rowe deserves special mention for contributing the initial *idea* that Families USA Foundation issue a consumer's guide to health care.

Several colleagues at Families USA Foundation borrowed time from the intense demands of their jobs to assist this project, in particular Executive Director Ron Pollack and Kate Villers, director of the Massachusetts office. Many others at Families USA contributed as well, including board members Robert Kuttner, who played a major role in fleshing out the original concept, Robert Crittendon, and Velvet Miller. My apologies for not naming the entire organization.

Interns have been indispensable. Special thanks to Katrina Avila, Doreen Balbuena, Chanza Baytop, Sherrylyn Cotaco, David Cuttino, Joshua Dyckman, Susan Han, Shulamit Lewin, Kathryn McKinney, Nonkosi Mzamane, Jason Reblando, Deepika Reddy, Rita Rhone, Magda Elise Schaler, Alison Sherwat, Laura Shimberg, and Raghuveer Vallabhaneni for volunteering their time and skills.

In preparing metropolitan-area editions in the Health Care Choices series, Families USA collaborated with several state-based advocacy groups, and their contributions played a major role in ensuring that all these books serve consumers. Thanks to Health Care For All in Boston, especially Kim Shellenberger and Rob Restuccia; Jim Duffet of the Illinois Campaign for Better Health Care and Margie Schaps and Linda Diamond Shapiro of the Chicago-based Health and Medicine Policy Research Group; Bruce Livingston and Jennifer Greene of Health Access Foundation in California; and Miranda Bayne and David West of Washington Citizen Action.

Many other individuals and organizations contributed time and expertise to *Health Care Choices for Today's Consumer.* In roughly alphabetical order, they are Myron Allukian (Boston Department of Health and Hospitals); Diane Archer (Medicare Beneficiaries Defense Fund); Elaine Barkley and Dan Bevins (Wheaton Regional Library); Charles Bell, Joel Gurin, and Rhoda Karpatkin (Consumers Union); James Bentley, Peter Kralovic, and Richard Wade (American Hospital Association); Robert Blendon and John Benson (Harvard School of Public Health); Stan Butler (Gay and Lesbian Advocates and Defenders); Center for Health Care Rights; Frank Coldiron and Andrew Dreyfus (Massachusetts Hospital Association); Linda deBenedictis and Ann Mueller (New England Patient Rights Group); John Delfs and Alan Raymond (Harvard-Pilgrim Health Care); Cathy Dunham (Robert Wood Johnson Foundation); Maria Durham; Susan Edgman-Levitan, Margaret Gerteis, and Jan Walker (Picker-Commonwealth Program for Patient-Centered Care); Roz Feldberg (Massachusetts Nurses Association); Barbara Giloth; Jennifer Frost and Rachel Benson Gold (Alan Guttmacher Institute); Suzanne Gordon; Group Health Association of America; Jeffrey Kichen (Massachusetts Medical Association); Martha Kleinerman and Alice Verhoeven (Planned Parenthood Clinic of Greater Boston); Edward Madara (American Self-Help Clearinghouse); Medirisk, Inc.; National Association of Community Health Centers; National Women's Health Network; National Women's Health Resource Center; Judith Norsigian and Norma Swenson (Boston Women's Health Book Collective); Margaret O'Kane and Linda Shelton (National Committee for Quality Assurance); Patrick O'Reilly (Massachusetts Peer Review Organization); Lee Phenner; Barbara Popper (Children in Hospitals); Anne Read; Gail Ross; Judith Schindul-Rothschild; Martin Schneider (*Health Pages* magazine); Terry Shannon (Agency for Health Care Policy and Research); Gary Snyderman and Doug Steel (Joint Commission for the Accreditation of Health Care Organizations); Gillian Thomas (American Medical Women's Association);

United Seniors Health Cooperative; Women's Educational and Industrial Union; Karen Wong (Hobbamock Design); Richard Wurman; and Arnold Zide.

Finally, special thanks to Lotus Development Corporation and the Nathan Cummings Foundation for major support for the Health Care Choices project, to Jesse Gruman of the Center for the Advancement of Health for helping us expand this edition's coverage of wellness, and to our editors at Wiley, PJ Dempsey and Tom Miller.

—Marc S. Miller
Jamaica Plain, Massachusetts

Part One

Getting Started

1

A User's Guide to *Health Care Choices for Today's Consumer*

Marc S. Miller, Ph.D.

Marc S. Miller, director of Families USA's Health Care Choices project, is the author of *Irony of Victory* (University of Illinois Press, 1988). He is the editor of *State of the Peoples: A Global Human Rights Report on Societies in Danger* (Beacon Press, 1993) and *Working Lives* (Pantheon, 1981).

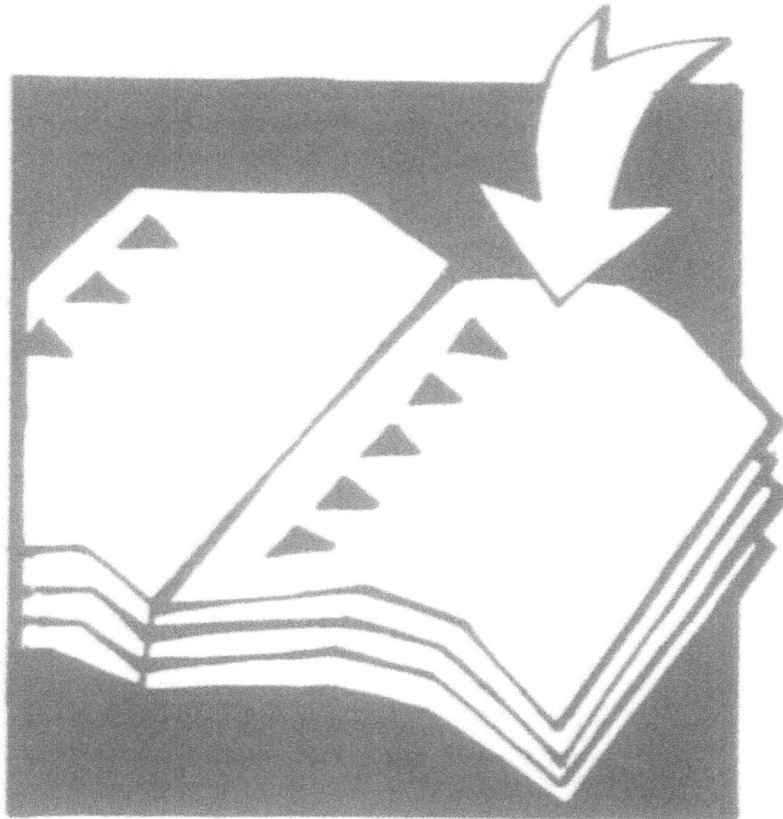

Once upon a time, doctors spoke and patients obeyed. Doctors told you what to do and how to do it—when to stay in bed, how often to take medicine, what hospital to use.

As both doctors and patients now know, this approach to medicine fails you as well as the professionals you entrust with your health. And today that view of health care is undergoing a multifaceted revolution:

■ First, even as new and better treatments for physical and mental conditions appear at a breathtaking pace, health care has come to mean treating people—both the well and the ill—as whole human beings with emotional, mental, and social needs, not just medical problems.

■ Second, hospitals are merging, HMOs are multiplying, and health care bills are soaring—leaving consumers more confused each day as they face the intricacies of access and quality. In particular, the sudden displacement of traditional forms of health insurance by large managed care companies has thrown American consumers into unfamiliar—and sometimes hazardous—territory.

■ Third and most important, more and more consumers recognize that quality care goes far deeper than tending to the sick and injured—and that medical professionals aren't the only ones responsible for health. You, too, are central to the pursuit of a healthy life for yourself and your family.

The good news is that this revolution *can* benefit you. But there are risks as well: Uninformed and passive consumers will lose—in terms of their health, their happiness, and their bank balances. Americans are finding that they must either learn to be better consumers or do without possibly essential care. The bottom line is that you play the starring role in your own health care. It's a role millions of Americans must learn to play to the fullest, day in and day out, in sickness *and* in health.

Health Care Choices will help you play that role with skill. Its theme is information: The aware consumer is a healthier consumer. According to researchers at New England Medical Center, patients with chronic diseases who communicate well with doctors benefit both medically *and* emotionally. They are physically healthier, recover faster, and can tolerate pain and handle stress better.

The informed health care consumer also saves money. For example, Dartmouth Medical School researchers report that men who receive thorough, unbiased explanations of all the reasonable treatments for prostate cancer feel safer in *not* choosing expensive surgery. Instead, more men choose "watchful waiting," which is often more appropriate than facing the risks associated with surgery.

Use *Health Care Choices* to . . .

- Become an active partner with health care professionals.
- Find the answers to key health care questions.
- Negotiate your path through the health care maze.
- Make sure you receive high-quality health care.
- Invest your health care dollars wisely.

Follow the Icons

As you read and use *Health Care Choices,* the icons will point you to particular types of guidance:

The heart icons guide you to choices and services that will help you receive better care.

The dollar icons suggest ways to invest your health care dollars wisely.

The check-mark icons highlight *lists* of questions to ask and steps to get quality care.

The consumer alert icons are a warning, helping you avoid pitfalls in the health care system.

Partnerships and Good Health

The premise of *Health Care Choices* is that the aware consumer benefits from a full partnership with professional caregivers—and that you could suffer if you fail to accept this responsibility. In other words, *Health Care Choices* works best for the person who:

- Asks questions about treatment options and costs
- Makes his or her own medical decisions, *and*
- Demands evidence of quality and expertise

A strong partnership between you and health care professionals rests on a number of principles. We invite you, as an aware health care consumer, to keep these in mind as you read on:

TIP

Find It Faster

- To locate a chapter quickly, use the tabs on every right-hand page.

- Follow the "for more information" triangle signposts that direct you to related sections in *Health Care Choices.*

- Record your own notes as you read *Health Care Choices,* using the blank space in the margins on each page.

1

■ Learn what you can do for yourself, what professionals can do for you—and what you can do together.

■ Plan ahead. Get care while you're healthy—and prepare for the time when you'll need professional assistance.

■ Ignorance isn't bliss. A true partner in care accepts and deals with both bad news and good.

■ Health care is both an art and a science, with few cut-and-dried "right" answers. Only you can decide among the many possible options for your own situation.

■ Health care is also personal. No one plan of care works best for everybody.

■ The vast majority of health care professionals are competent and can serve you well—*if* you do your part.

■ The health care system contains some second-rate facilities and uninformed providers, as well as a few seedy characters. Know how to recognize and deal with them.

Consumer Alert: Raising a New Standard

Aware consumers improve care for themselves—and for others. From hospitals to insurance plans to nursing homes to doctors, health care providers are now ready to work closely with the informed consumer, resulting in better health care for all.

On the other hand, some providers try to attract consumers in less commendable ways. Learn to recognize a good provider—and when to ignore slick advertisements and fast talkers.

Ask Questions

A New England Medical Center team reports that patients ask an average of only four questions in a fifteen-minute visit, including those such as "Will you validate my parking?" The typical man asks zero questions. But the price of this passivity is poorer health.

A Look Ahead

Like the health care system itself, *Health Care Choices* will serve you best if you know how to use it. That's the thinking behind the unique format and writing style of this book. The authors purposely avoid fancy phrases and scientific jargon in favor of plain English and straightforward facts and advice. You'll find that the information is succinct and easy to understand and apply.

Throughout, *Health Care Choices* directs you to your first steps. You probably won't sit down and read the entire book immediately (although you'll benefit if you do). Instead, thumb through the whole book today, and return to the parts you need when you need them. Pay special attention to the bulleted items, which represent points to keep in mind and steps to take. And don't skip the fast-action "Tips" in every chapter or the sidebars that look deeper at individual topics.

Right now, read the two other chapters in Part One, "Getting Started." You'll benefit each and every day from knowing your health care rights and how you and health care providers can work together to keep you well.

Before your next encounter with the health care system, read Part Two, "The Heart of the Matter." This part begins with your first choice as a consumer: an insurance or health plan for you and your family. A wise health care consumer assembles a personal and family health care system *now* to provide and finance comprehensive care over the years. Part of doing that well centers around understanding the basic components of health care: primary care, hospitals, and medications.

Find the time soon to study one or more of the chapters in Part Three, "Focusing on You." You'll find chapters here that address the particular concerns of men, women, parents and children, seniors, and workers.

As specific needs arise, examine the chapters in Part Four, "The Complete Package." However, take the time soon to skim these chapters to get a sense of how the diverse pieces of the health care system can fit together.

Finally, *Health Care Choices* intentionally focuses on *first* steps. Part Five, "For Everyone's Health," guides you deeper, both for your own care and for improving the system for all.

For a brief summary of every chapter, consult the table of contents. For specific questions, turn to the comprehensive index that begins on page 449.

The Unaware Majority

Failing to make a choice about your own care is a choice in itself. But it's a choice you make to the detriment of your health.

Unfortunately, four out of five Americans don't know enough about medical concepts to make intelligent choices about their own health care. That's the conclusion of a study by the International Center for the Advancement of Science Literacy.

To help Families USA Foundation correct this situation, send in your suggestions for improving this book. Write to Health Care Choices, Families USA Foundation, 30 Winter St., Boston, MA 02108.

2 Healthy Living

Rena Convissor and Audrey Chang

Rena Convissor, M.P. H., is deputy director of the Center for the Advancement of Health. The center promotes widespread acceptance and application of an expanded view of health that recognizes psychological, social, behavioral, economic, and environmental factors.

Audrey Chang is communications coordinator for the Center for the Advancement of Health.

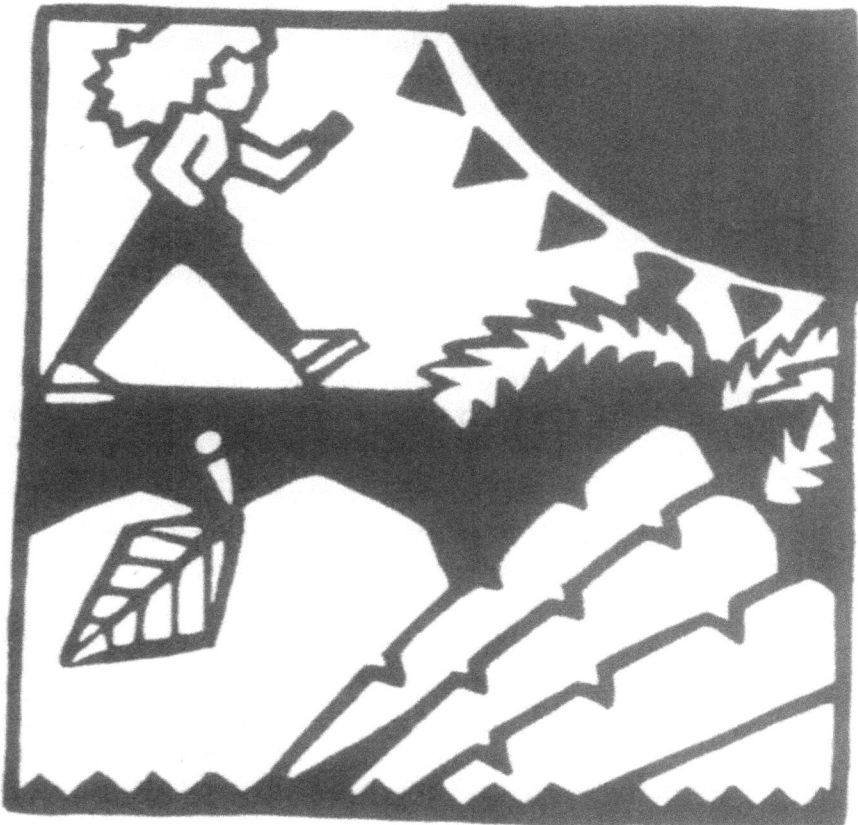

Jay started smoking when he was thirteen. His friends encouraged him to take up cigarettes, and he didn't see much harm in it. After all, his parents and his older sister smoked. Three years later, he's smoking a pack a day, and one of his favorite hobbies is collecting T-shirts, posters, hats, and other items adorned with the logo of his favorite cigarette brand.

Jane is forty pounds overweight. She has an incredible sweet tooth and loves to snack on ice cream, cakes, and cookies, so much so that she has dessert with every meal—even breakfast. She feels sluggish all the time. A voice in the back of her mind tells her she has to lose weight, but she doesn't know how to go about it.

Eleanor turned eighty-three recently and has been widowed for several years. Her children live far away, and many of her friends have either moved into nursing homes or died. She feels lonely and a bit isolated in her apartment. She used to go to the nearby market once or twice a week, but she just broke her hip and can't get out now. She has few opportunities for social contact, and her children worry about her health.

Like Jay, Jane, and Eleanor, many Americans are thinking and talking a lot about their health these days. How can we eat more nutritious food? How much alcohol can we safely consume? Is it safe to get a suntan? How *can* we act to stay as healthy as possible for as long as possible?

Americans also have many individual reasons for seeking to learn about and follow health-promoting behaviors. Some people want to feel better and look better. Others are interested in healthy living and preventing disease because sickness can be very expensive—not just in the direct costs for care but also in terms of missed work, school, and other opportunities.

These are not just tasks for yourself. In 1990 the U.S. government established a set of national health goals for the year 2000. Known as *Healthy People 2000,* these objectives identify opportunities for improved health for all Americans. The broad goals for the nation are to:

1. Help people live for as long and as well as possible.
2. Narrow the gaps in health status across income, race, and education levels.
3. Improve access to preventive services.

To achieve these goals, the report presents three main categories of actions that you and others in the health care system and your community can take: health promotion, health protection, and preventive services.

Health promotion goals relate to physical activity, fitness, nutrition, tobacco, alcohol and other drug use, family planning, mental health, violent and abusive behavior, and education and community-based programs.

Health protection refers to injuries, occupational safety and health, environmental health, food and drug safety, and oral health.

Preventive services refers to maternal and infant health, heart disease and stroke, cancer, chronic and disabling conditions, HIV and other sexually transmitted diseases, clinical preventive services, and immunization.

As an introduction to *Health Care Choices* and your quest for the best health care, this chapter focuses primarily on health promotion in general. That is, it will introduce you to ways that can help you and your family be as healthy and active as possible. And as you read on in *Health Care Choices,* you'll gather guidance and resources for achieving other year 2000—and personal—goals as a health care consumer.

Healthy People 2000: The Book

You can order a copy of *Healthy People 2000,* which describes specific targets for improving the overall health of the American public, from the National Health Information Center, P.O. Box 1133, Washington, DC 20012-1133, tel. (301) 565-4167. Send $25.75, plus $4 for shipping and handling.

Practicing Good Health

On a day-to-day level, you can do many things to practice good behaviors and live full and healthy lives. In particular, a 1978 study by researchers at the University of California, Los Angeles, identified for the first time seven key habits practiced by healthy people that keep them healthier. The study found that healthy people:

1. Eat moderately.
2. Eat regularly—three meals a day.
3. Eat breakfast.
4. Don't smoke cigarettes.
5. Drink alcohol moderately or not at all.
6. Exercise at least moderately.
7. Sleep seven to eight hours each night.

Healthy Fashions?

You've heard many stories that the way to longer, healthier living is to give up some of your favorite foods such as butter and eggs, and to take up others such as oat bran. But it also seems that the next day another study reveals that butter is better than margarine, eggs are a good source of protein, and oat bran may not be all it's cracked up to be.

How can you sort through all these conflicting research studies? How can you know what each new study *really* means for you?

Start by keeping a few points in mind as you evaluate the latest health findings:

■ Although the jury may still be out on a specific issue, common sense and a knowledge of basic healthy living are a good guide when reading the latest findings. For example, the link between high-fat diets and breast cancer isn't proven definitely, but you can expect your health to suffer generally if you eat a high-fat diet.

■ The basics of healthy living *are* proven. New research usually points to small changes in the knowledge of what

On average, the physical health of people who practiced all seven good health habits was consistently about the same as those thirty years younger who followed few or none of these practices. In other words, a sixty-year-old man who practiced good habits could enjoy the health status of a man half his age who didn't.

These seven basic healthy behaviors still hold true, but the list has grown more specific since the 1970s, based on new research and advances in medicine and technology. For example, in addition to eating moderately and regularly, it's now known that it's important for you to eat at least five servings of fruits and vegetables each day. In addition, moderate exercise now means engaging in some physical activity at least three times a week for thirty minutes. This can range from going on a brisk walk in your neighborhood to doing heavy housecleaning to playing ball with your kids; you don't have to join a gym or start using fancy equipment.

Since 1978, the list of healthy behaviors has lengthened as well. For example, with the advent of HIV/AIDS, practicing safe sex is more vital than ever for maintaining good health. Moreover, as the incidence of skin cancers rises, we are beginning to realize that a healthy tan may not be so healthy after all. And seat belts and motorcycle and bicycle helmets can go a long way toward protecting you and your children from injuries on the road.

In addition to building on the basic steps of healthy living, research has also shown that paying attention to other aspects of your life can protect you from getting sick and help you if you do become sick. Maintaining relationships with friends, loved ones, and neighbors is important for good health. People who have strong social networks report better health and live longer.

On the other hand, stress and anger can seriously damage your health. Stress is associated with a number of health conditions. These include headaches; diarrhea, constipation, and other stomach disorders; and high blood pressure, diabetes, and other chronic conditions. In fact, one of the healthiest actions you can take is to lessen the stress in your life. Learning to manage stress and anger can result in not just healthier but also more enjoyable lives.

For more information on ways to reduce stress, turn to chapter 10.

Prevention Principles

Modifying your behavior by following good health habits will improve your health and the quality of your life. In other words, *prevention works.*

That fact shouldn't surprise you. Actually, there are very few things you can do for yourself that you wouldn't guess are important based on your own experience, what you read in magazines, and what you hear on TV. Most of the principles underlying healthy practices are just simple common sense:

■ No magic pill will keep you healthy, no vaccine will ward off the body's natural aging process, no vitamin will promise a disease-free life, and no operation can cure stress and anxiety. There *are* a series of small steps that you can take each day that over time, build your reserves and give you the strength and support you need to ward off ill health, minimize illness if and when it comes, and participate as fully as possible at home, at work, at school, and with your friends.

■ The guidelines for healthy living provide a basic map for maintaining good health, but as with any map, it only provides directions. You have to do the rest and follow those directions carefully and consistently.

■ You probably won't see the results of your behavior change overnight. You may not reap the benefits of eating right, protecting yourself from too much sun, and getting your teeth cleaned until years later—when you don't develop heart disease, skin cancer, or gum disease.

healthy living means, but these findings very rarely alter the fundamentals: A reasonable diet matters. Regular exercise counts. And above all, moderation is the key.

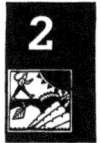

2

One Step at a Time

When you are trying to make healthy changes for you and your family and you face multiple options, remember that practicing good health requires common sense! If you have never exercised before, don't sign up to run a marathon—take a more moderate first step such as walking three times a week. In a few years you'll be ready to run that marathon, and in the meantime you'll be developing good health habits.

Challenges across the Life Span

You'll want to "customize" the list of basic healthy practices to fit the different needs and situation of you and your family. For example, caring for your diabetes requires different skills than remembering to get a prostate exam. Most important, each age group needs to focus on a particular subset of behaviors and activities to maintain health. Here are a few of the basic challenges at each age. Other chapters in *Health Care Choices* provide details on solutions and the resources you can draw on to meet these challenges.

Unhealthy Burdens

■ People who are isolated—because they live alone, don't have family or friends, or don't participate in activities—are two to three times more likely to die prematurely than people with strong social ties.

■ Tobacco addiction, the single most serious medical problem in the United States, affects 30 percent of all Americans. It causes 420,000 premature deaths a year and costs $2 in medical expenses for every package of cigarettes sold.

■ Poor diet and insufficient exercise are associated with perhaps 30 percent of cardiovascular deaths, 30 percent of cancer deaths, and 80 percent of the cases of adults getting diabetes.

■ Alcohol accounts for 100,000 deaths a year at a cost of $99 billion. About 25 percent of Americans are either risky drinkers or alcoholics.

■ Illicit drug use, perhaps a major transmitter of HIV, hepatitis, and tuberculosis, causes 20,000 deaths a year at a cost to society of $67 billion.

■ By 1994, AIDS was the leading cause of

Childhood

Childhood is the time each person establishes the basic patterns of healthy behavior; it's also when many people develop unhealthy habits that are extremely difficult to break later.

On one important level, parents provide health insurance for their children, take their sons and daughters to the doctor, and care for them when they're sick. Just as important, families teach their children what is healthy and how to care for themselves, not only directly but also as the most important role model in shaping health habits. For example, if you are active—both physically and by involving yourself in your community—your daughters and sons will be more likely to follow in your footsteps. Conversely, you can't teach your children that smoking is dangerous if you smoke.

Children also learn from other role models around them, and parents have other sources to draw on as health mentors. These mentors and models include teachers and siblings, as well as the formal health care system, which is a great place for you to get information and help in preparing your children with good health habits. The pediatrician, nurse, or other health care providers can be great partners in helping you solve problems and find effective ways to work with your children.

Your community is also a valuable resource. For example, many schools provide some health care services, such as annual sports checkups and immunizations. Clubs such as the Boy Scouts and Girl Scouts, community centers, and religious education classes all encourage the social involvement and participation that are necessary for good health at any age.

For more information on children, turn to chapter 8.

Adolescence

Teenagers have a different set of needs than younger kids do. It is a time of life when the human body undergoes incredible transformations—and the brain works overtime to catch up to the physical changes. It's also a period during which young people begin to establish their independence and personal beliefs, separate from their parents.

Another hallmark of adolescence is that teenagers believe they will live forever, with no permanent consequences from their actions. In the teen years, peer pressure can lead to such harmful behaviors as smoking, using alcohol and other drugs, driving without a seat belt, or taking unnecessary risks. Adolescents are especially vulnerable to depression because of the changes occurring in their lives and the impact these changes can have on their self-esteem. And it's a time when many people become sexually active, making it all the more important that teens learn about contraception and ways to prevent sexually transmitted diseases.

For people this age, it's important that they receive the information about what to do, how to do it, and why it's so important to develop healthy habits *now*. One key to this is making sure your teenager has a health care provider that she or he can talk with confidentially. This may be the time to leave the pediatrician and find a physician with whom your teenager can talk comfortably. As a parent, it's important for you to support your teenager in developing good health habits.

death among people between the ages of twenty-five and forty-four. Changing behavior remains the only method of preventing AIDS.

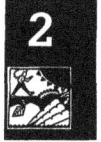

2

Healthy Schools

Schools provide many resources that can help your teenager. For example, the school nurse or health center may have information or drop-in programs led by counselors who can help foster self-esteem and self-confidence and answer questions about the physical changes that are occurring. Talk to your children's teachers about the available health resources in schools.

For more information on adolescents, turn to chapter 8.

Adulthood

By the time you are an adult, your health behaviors have become ingrained, and it may take a special effort to change any bad habits you first acquired as a child. Losing weight, starting an exercise program, quitting smoking, and joining a civic organization all take time, initiative, and encouragement.

Changing your behavior is especially difficult if the results only show up years later, but a number of steps can make it more likely you'll adopt a healthier lifestyle and practice prevention:

■ ***Think ahead.*** Learn to recognize when the benefits of change outweigh the costs. For example, reducing the risk of losing your teeth probably outweighs the inconvenience of flossing each night. The costs and benefits are going to be different for each person and different depending on the perceived health risk. To help you make the right decisions, obtain all the information you can about particular behaviors by talking with health care providers and family members.

Care Credits

Maintaining independence is difficult for many seniors, as well as for people with disabilities. Shopping, visiting the doctor, or even doing the laundry can be overwhelming tasks. Yet accepting help poses different but equally difficult challenges.

One solution is the concept of "care credits." Participants in such programs acquire care credits by providing volunteer services, such as friendly visits, transportation, financial counseling, and much more. Volunteers can use the credits to get help when they need it, or they can donate their credits to a cooperating organization or another person in the program.

One model care-credit program, the Cooperative Caring Network of the United Seniors Health Cooperative, serves people in the Washington, D.C., metropolitan area. It links generations and increases opportunities for independence. Similarly, some HMOs across the country have established care-credit programs that match volunteer caregivers with HMO members who need assistance.

■ *Find out if you are especially likely to develop a particular disease or condition.* It's easier to remember to get an annual mammogram and practice breast self-examination if someone in your family had breast cancer. Find out what you can do to reduce your health risks, given your age, your lifestyle, and your family's health history. But remember, prevention is always a good idea, no matter what your family history.

■ *Acquire the skills and information needed to get you started and keep you on track.* For example, if you are accustomed to fast food and eating on the run, you could enroll in a class to learn to cook healthy foods. Alternatively, if you have a particular health condition, there are literally thousands of local mutual-help groups that can help you with this task.

For more information on mutual-help groups, turn to chapter 22.

■ *Cultivate a strong social support network.* This will make it easier to change your health habits and provide a source of strength and encouragement throughout your life. For example, having a partner to accompany you on an evening walk will keep both of you committed to your exercise plan. You can find and nurture support networks among current friends and family, of course, but your health will also benefit if you are active in civic associations such as the PTA or the Elks Club, join a church or synagogue, or participate in a bowling league or other group sports.

Primary Prevention

At every age, prevention is one of the central goals of primary care. And one of your greatest assets in practicing prevention is your primary care provider.

For more information on primary care, turn to chapter 5.

Old Age

People are living longer: By the year 2020, more than one in six Americans will be sixty-five or over, compared with one in eight now, according to the U.S. Census Bureau. And not only are people living longer, they are staying more active and involved than the previous generation.

As you get older, it's particularly important to focus on activities that build your physical and psychological reserves—exercising, eating right, getting enough sleep, and maintaining your intellectual life. There is also an increased need for preventive and supportive services that can help you remain independent, avoid inappropriate uses of the medical care system, and avert medical emergencies. These things will help to manage the impact that aging has on the body and the mind and keep you strong and active.

While you are paying attention to your health needs as an older person, recognize that your life may be changing in profound ways. Retiring from work can have a enormous impact on how you feel about yourself, structure your day, and interact with other people. It's important to stay intellectually challenged and physically active after you retire.

In addition, the death of a spouse or close friends can be devastating and put you at increased risk for depression. Learn how to distinguish the signs of depression as opposed to feeling sad and lonely. Try to talk openly with your health care providers about how you are feeling and the emotions you are experiencing; in many cases, they can help you get the support you need.

For more information on seniors, turn to chapter 11.

For more information on depression, turn to chapter 14.

For more information on the Cooperative Caring Network, contact the United Seniors Health Cooperative, 1331 H Street, N.W., Washington, DC 20005, tel. (202) 393-6222.

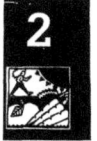

Chronic Conditions

No matter who you are, quitting smoking, eating healthier, exercising regularly, and changing other health-related behaviors can improve your life and reduce your risk of suffering a wide variety of chronic diseases and conditions, including diabetes, asthma, arthritis, hypertension, and coronary heart disease, among many other serious long term illnesses. In fact, perhaps half of deaths from the ten leading causes are linked to lifestyle; heart disease and cancer alone account for 56 percent of all deaths.

Modifying health-related behavior is especially important if you are one of the millions of people who *already* suffer from a chronic disease. Not only will this result in fewer complications associated with an illness, it can also lower your health care bills. And among other significant benefits, changing your behavior can reduce the time you miss from work and improve your day-to-day functioning and quality of life.

Changing Behavior

While it's difficult to predict who will develop a particular chronic illness or when chronic illness will occur, almost everyone will suffer from a sig-

The Informal Health Care System

With people staying in the hospital for fewer days or having procedures done on an outpatient basis, services that used to be delivered at the hospital, such as health education or physical therapy, now take place in the home and the community. Schools, religious organizations, and neighborhood groups often offer critical resources for health and prevention. For their part, employers can distribute health-education materials, and they can also support healthy behaviors by banning smoking in the work environment or reducing the quantity of dangerous substances used or stored in the workplace.

Community-based agencies organize, coordinate, and maintain a wide variety of social and health support services. And communities can provide a critical sense of connection and belonging that supports people and their families.

Each of the following services is an example of health care you can find outside a medical office:

- Free blood-pressure screenings in the office cafeteria

nificant chronic or ongoing illness at some time in his or her lifetime. Whether its effects are limited and manageable or uncomfortable and long-lasting depends on how serious your condition is, what financial and social resources you have, the support and availability of friends and family, and how well you understand the illness.

Most people with a chronic illness would agree that the medical treatments they receive are necessary but not enough. While medical treatments may reduce fatigue or nausea, they don't minimize the impact of the illness on work and family life. Each day of their life, people with chronic illness experience pain and emotional distress and most confront decisions about lifestyle changes.

While every person differs in the ability to persist with long-term medical treatments or make changes in lifestyle, all need support from the health care system to achieve both goals. Fortunately, a number of health care services can support the ability of you and your family to manage chronic conditions and live a fuller life. This means services that help you to:

- Engage in activities that promote health and build strength and stamina—for example, exercise, eating right, being socially active, and getting enough sleep.

- Maintain effective communications with health care providers in following treatment plans.

- Keep track of your own physical and emotional health and make appropriate lifestyle decisions based on how you feel.

- Adjust to how your illness affects emotions, self-esteem, and relationships with family, friends, and co-workers.

Changing your health habits can be a difficult assignment under the best of circumstances, but it's especially challenging for people who are coping with a chronic condition. Nevertheless, adopting healthy lifestyles is even more important in such instances. To live as long and as well as possible with a chronic condition, people must learn to care for themselves.

Support Groups and Chronic Illness

Educational programs are widely available to help people with chronic conditions learn how to change their behavior and adjust to an illness. In particular, national organizations such as the American Cancer Society and the Arthritis Foundation offer these through local affiliates. In addition, certain health plans offer programs; ask the member services department of your health plan.

For a list of national organizations that provide community-based services to people with chronic conditions, turn to chapter 22.

Taking Charge of Your Health

Until recently, people went to the doctor only when they were sick. The doctor would diagnose the complaint, prescribe medicine or give a few words of advice, and send you back home. But fewer and fewer people—patients and health care professionals alike—accept that course as a complete approach to health care any longer. Today, doctors and other health care providers interact with their patients in complex ways, with consumers taking an increasingly active role and working closely with health care providers.

The new standard for care is a shared responsibility between you and the health care system. Many health professionals—from doctors and nurses to dietitians to physical therapists—will now collaborate with you specifically to *change* the way you live day to day. Along with health insurers, doctors now recognize the need to give consumers the knowledge they need to prevent diseases and accidents in the first place and to live longer and better if and when they develop serious and long term conditions.

Increasingly, the community and the health care system work together to support positive changes in health. Schools, communities, and workplaces *can* play an important and vital role in prevention and in encouraging healthy behaviors. The family *can* support and encourage healthy behavior changes and provide a positive social support.

Managing Your Own Care

Health care consumers are gaining a better and better understanding of how to play a more integral role in caring for themselves and practicing preventive behavior. Whether it's by getting rid of an existing behavior—that second drink before dinner—or learning to manage an existing condition, such as following an exercise regimen to help your arthritis, you can shift the balance of health care to make the system more responsive to your needs.

You won't have to do this alone. In particular, more than ever before, primary care providers are offering patients more information and help in changing high-risk behaviors. They are also becoming more comfort-

- Hot meals delivered to homebound people with AIDS

- Immunizations delivered in schools to children and their parents

- Annual physical exams at school or work

- A volunteer program to deliver medication or provide companionship

For more information on many community-based services, turn to chapters 15 and 16.

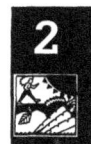

Take Charge

If your health care providers don't ask you about your health habits, take the initiative and bring up the subject of lifestyle yourself. According to recent studies, only 60 percent of current smokers report that their doctors ever advised them to quit smoking. Only 19 percent of family physicians asked their patients about diet and nutrition and physical exercise, and only 39 percent inquired about alcohol use.

Unfortunately, fewer than half of traditional health plans cover routine examinations, which afford the best opportunity for you to learn about healthy behavior and receive preventive care. But the spread of managed care plans, which sometimes cover regular checkups and may even *insist* that you sign up with a primary care provider, could make it easier to forge a health care partnership. In some cases, a primary care provider might even enroll you in a smoking-cessation class right at his or her clinic, which would make it clear that stopping smoking is part of your health care.

able discussing lifestyle changes and supporting their patients' improved health habits. And they are increasingly willing to help their patients learn the skills needed to manage and control chronic conditions.

The key, however, is to assume responsibility for your own care. As a consumer, you can improve and maintain your own health and that of your family by actively seeking information from physicians, from others in the health care system, and from people and organizations in your community. No matter where you live, learn about and draw on the countless services and programs that can strengthen and support your efforts to improve health and quality of life.

That's what has helped the three people in this chapter's introduction:

Jay took a physical exam at school when he tried out for the soccer team. The school doctor realized that Jay smoked from the smell of his clothes and hair. The doctor asked him how long he had been smoking, how much he smoked, and if it interfered with his ability to run up and down the soccer field. As a result of their conversation, the doctor referred Jay to a smoking-cessation program targeted specifically for teenagers. Jay went to the class after school and learned about the dangers of smoking. He even signed his older sister up for the same class.

Jane's sister saw an ad for a walking group at a local shopping mall. She thought the exercise might help her sister lose weight. Jane would also benefit from talking to other people instead of sitting at home alone and eating ice cream. After only a few weeks in the club, Jane lost several pounds; just as important, she values the company and social support that comes from the group and is determined to stick with the program.

Eleanor's doctor assigned a volunteer from his clinic to visit Eleanor twice a week, bring books from the library, and help prepare her meals. Within a few months, Eleanor could walk with assistance, and she now goes to a nearby community center to play cards and spend the afternoon with other people her age. Her mood has improved, and she's less lonely.

Resources

Organizations

American Self-Help Clearinghouse
St. Clares-Riverside Medical Center
25 Pocono Road
Denville, NJ 07834
(800) 367-6274 (New Jersey only)

(201) 625-7101
(201) 625-9053 TDD
Call to locate local self-help groups or to receive help starting your own self-help group if a similar type doesn't already exist. For a copy of *The Self-Help Sourcebook: Finding and Forming*

Mutual Aid Self-Help Groups, a national directory of self-help groups, send $10.

National Self-Help Clearinghouse
CUNY Graduate School
25 West 43rd Street
New York, NY 10036
(212) 354-8525
Call for assistance with starting a self-help group and referrals to regional clearinghouses and groups around the country. Send a stamped, self-addressed envelope for a list of support group information. The clearinghouse publishes a quarterly newsletter, *The Self-Help Reporter* ($10 for one year).

Publications

ACSM Fitness Book, by the American College of Sports Medicine (Human Kinetics Publishers, 1992), $13.95. A step-by-step guide to physical fitness by a major exercise-science organization, this book can help you start an exercise program.

The American Way of Life Need Not Be Hazardous to Your Health, by John W. Farquhar (Addison-Wesley, 1987), $12. With a focus on preventing heart disease, this book demystifies medicine with a practical, proven approach to preventing chronic disease and disabilities.

Arthritis Helpbook, by Kate Lorig and James Fries (Addison-Wesley, 1990), $14. A valuable resource with many practical suggestions for self-management, used in the Arthritis Self-Help Course.

Diabetes 101, by Betty Brackenridge; edited by Donna Hoel (Chronimed, 1989), $9.95. A general guide to diabetes and its treatment, written for patients.

The D.O.'s: Osteopathic Medicine in America, by Norman Gevitz (The Johns Hopkins University Press, 1982), $16.95.

The Exercise Habit, by James Gavin (Leisure Press, 1992), $14.95. Addresses personality and lifestyle issues and ways to make exercise a lifelong habit.

Full Catastrophe Living: Using the Wisdom of Your Body and Mind to Face Stress, Pain, and Illness (Delacorte Press, 1990) and *Wherever You Go, There You Are* (Hyperion Press, 1994), both by Jon Kabat-Zinn, each $19.95. Meditation navigational charts for people facing physical or emotional pain or feeling the effects of too much stress.

Harvard Health Letter ($24 per year), *Harvard Mental Health Letter* ($48), and *Harvard Women's Health Letter* ($24). To order any of these Harvard Medical School Publications, call (800) 829-9080.

Healing and the Mind with Bill Moyers, video ($129.95 for the five-part set; $29.95 per part) and book ($25). To order the video, call PBS Video at (800) 328-7271. The book is available at bookstores.

The Healthy Brain, by David Sobel (Simon & Schuster, 1987), $10.95.

The Healthy Mind, Healthy Body Handbook, by David Sobel and Robert Ornstein, $16.95. Available from DRx, P.O. Box 176, Los Altos, CA 94023; tel. (415) 948-6293.

Healthy Pleasures, by Robert Ornstein and David Sobel (Addison-Wesley, 1989), $11. Presents evidence that positive experiences are especially important in health maintenance.

Living a Healthy Life with Chronic Conditions, by Kate Lorig et al. (Bull Publishing, 1994), $14.95.

Living Beyond Limits, by David Spiegel (Random House, 1993), $23. Discusses the current research on mind-body interaction.

Medicine at the Crossroad, $149.95. An eight-part film series that sorts through the promises and troubling questions associated with scientific breakthroughs. To order the video, call PBS Video at (800) 328-7271.

Mind/Body Health Newsletter (formerly *Mental Medicine Update*), $10 per year. Order from Center for Health Services, c/o ISHK Book Service, P.O. Box 381062, Cambridge, MA 02238-1062; tel. (800) 222-4745.

Mind Body Medicine: How to Use Your Mind for Better Health, edited by Daniel Goleman and Joel Gurin (Consumer Reports, 1995), $14.95. Sorts out the facts from the growing body of medical mythology surrounding the mind's role in health.

Nutrition Action Newsletter, $24 per year. To order, call the Center for Science in the Public Interest, (202) 332-9110.

Relief from IBS, by Elaine F. Shimberg (Ballantine, 1991), $5.99. A self-help guide concerning Irritable Bowel Syndrome, written by someone with the disorder, including a detailed discussion of the role of stress and suggestions for controlling it.

The Savvy Patient: How to Be an Active Participant in Your Medical Care, by David Stutz and Bernard Feder (Consumer Reports Books, 1990), $13.95. Advice on communicating with your doctor and getting the best possible care in hospitals.

Sound Mind, Sound Body, by Ken R. Pelletier. (Simon & Schuster, 1994), $23. Explores how personal health practices and a sense of meaningful purpose play a major role in the health, inner fulfillment, and success of fifty-one prominent men and women.

The Wellness Encyclopedia of Food and Nutrition: How to Buy, Store, and Prepare Every Fresh Food, by the editors of the University of California at Berkeley *Wellness Letter* (Random House, 1992), $29.95.

Wellness Letter, University of California at Berkeley, 12 issues for $24. Features stories and advice on health and wellness, including buying guides on food and exercise programs. Call or write for a one-year subscription: Subscription Department, P.O. Box 420163, Palm Coast, FL 32142; tel. (904) 445-4662.

What You Can Do About Asthma, by Nathaniel Altman (Dell, 1991), $4.99. A guide to understanding the nature of asthma, with a focus on specific forms of treatment.

Your Gut Feelings: A Complete Guide to Living Better with Intestinal Problems, by Henry D. Janowitz (Oxford University Press, 1989), $11.95. Written by a gastroenterologist, this book describes the most common diseases of the large intestine and diagnostic tests doctors may perform for bowel symptoms; especially useful for preparing for a visit to the physician.

3 Consumer Rights

George J. Annas

George J. Annas is the Edward R. Utley Professor of Health Law at the Boston University School of Medicine and head of the Health Law Department at the Boston University School of Public Health. He is the author of *The Rights of Patients* (Southern Illinois University Press, 1989) and *Standard of Care: The Law of American Bioethics* (Oxford University Press, 1993). He writes a regular feature on law in the *New England Journal of Medicine*.

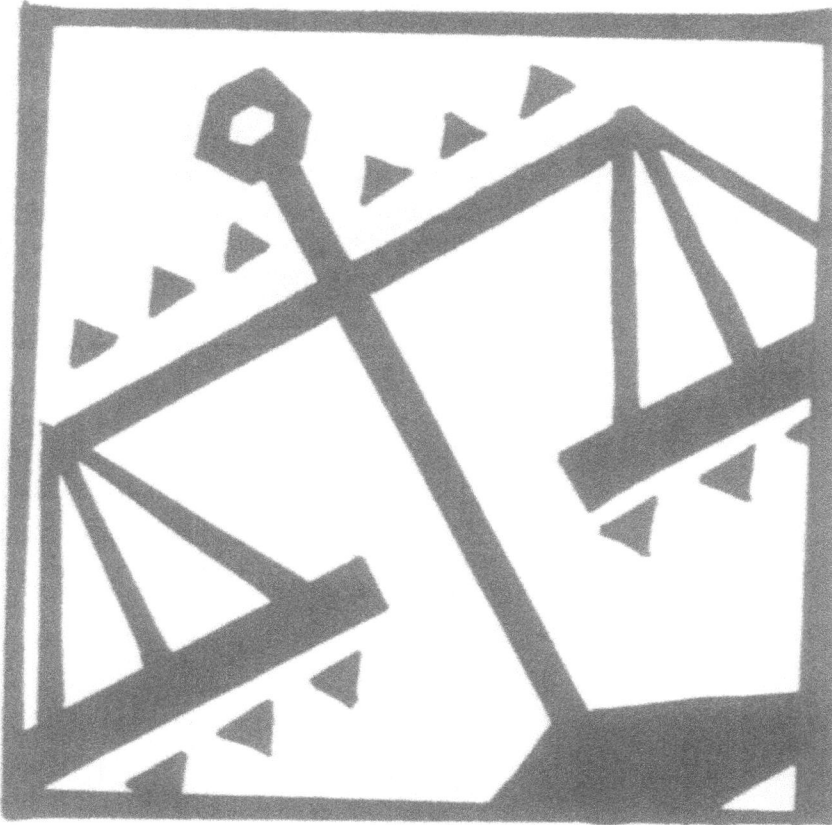

One of the most powerful forces shaping the practice of modern medicine is the recognition that patients have rights. Respect for these rights can transform the doctor-patient relationship into a partnership dramatically improving the quality of medical care.

Patients have only recently begun to reject medical paternalism and to assert their rights. Unlike virtually all other groups that have proclaimed or discovered their rights, patients are often sick, and thus "not themselves." Moreover, they hope to quickly become nonpatients and are usually far less concerned about exercising their rights than about getting better.

Nonetheless, it's critical that you and your family know your rights when you see health care providers and make decisions about your care. Most important is your *right to decide* about your treatment. You also have the *right to information* about all reasonable treatment alternatives and the *right to decide* among all the options available, although you may have to go outside your health plan if you choose certain ones. And all competent adults have the *right to refuse* any treatment, even if such a refusal means you will likely get sicker or even die.

Consumer Alert: Saying No

The description of what treatment options *exist* is medical, but the decision to *undergo* treatment is personal—only you can make it.

Physicians *can* treat you in an emergency without consent, but if the emergency can be anticipated and you refuse to consent in advance, no one has the right to impose any procedure on you.

Technology and Rights

Medical technology tends to distance health care staff from patients and turn hospitals into alien and alienating places. The recognition of patient rights, on the other hand, humanizes both hospitals and encounters with health care professionals.

Informed Consent

As the words *informed consent* imply, unless you are legally declared incompetent, no one can treat or even touch you until you make an educated decision to accept or reject treatment. Health care providers must supply the information you need to make this decision, and they must do so in language you can understand. Many court decisions support your right to information, which rests on common sense: Because you have to live with the consequences of treatment, you have the greatest interest in deciding how your body will be treated.

These principles underlie the doctrine of informed consent, which is founded on two fundamental propositions:

1. It's your body—you should be able to decide what is done with it. This idea is sometimes referred to as self-determination.
2. You are likely to make a better decision about what is done with your body if you are provided with information on which to base a decision.

When providers and patients take informed consent seriously, their relationship can be a true partnership, with shared authority, decision making, and responsibility.

As part of that partnership, physicians have obligations that ordinary business people don't have to their customers because they possess special knowledge, and because patients trust them. These obligations include providing patients with at least the following information:

- A description of the recommended treatment or procedure
- A description of the risks and benefits of the recommended procedure, with a special emphasis on the risk of death or serious disability
- A description of alternative treatments and procedures, together with the risks and benefits of each
- The likely results if you refuse any treatment
- The probability of success, and what the physician means by success
- The major problems anticipated in recuperation, and how long it will be until you can resume your normal activities, *and*

- Any other information patients in your situation generally receive, such as cost and how much of the cost your health plan will cover

There is nothing profound or mysterious about this list. It's what you need to know to decide whether to accept or question a recommended treatment plan.

Some physicians have argued that it's difficult to determine what risks to disclose. In general, physicians must tell you about *material* risks—those that might lead you or another reasonable person like you to reject a recommendation, choose an alternative, or decide on no treatment at all.

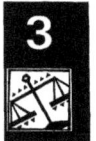

A Test for Competence

✔ No magic formula proves competence, but a person who can understand the answers to these questions generally passes the test:

■ What is your present physical condition?

■ What treatment is being recommended for you?

■ What do you and your doctor think might happen if you accept the treatment?

■ What do you and your doctor think might happen if you reject it?

■ What alternatives are available? What are the probable consequences of each option—including no treatment?

One way to think about the importance of a risk is to multiply its probability of occurring by its magnitude if it occurs. For example, a physician must tell you about even a small risk of death, but not necessarily about the possibility of a two-hour headache.

Wake-Up Call

A patient who took a sleeping pill was awakened in the middle of the night and asked to sign a consent form. Later, the patient couldn't remember the event. His consent wasn't valid. Memory isn't a measure of valid consent, but the circumstances in which consent is requested can make it invalid.

Consent Must Be Competent and Voluntary

The idea of *voluntary* consent is simple. You must not be medicated, intoxicated, threatened by the physician, or under extreme duress. Obviously, consent is involuntary if someone holds a gun to your head and says, "Sign!"

Competence is more complex. The key point is that the law presumes that every adult is competent. A person who tries to take away your right to decide must prove that you are "incompetent," and this usually must be done in a courtroom unless you are unconscious or incapable of communicating your decision. If you are a competent adult, only you can consent to medical care. It is both unnecessary and inappropriate for your family—or anyone else—to give consent.

If you are under eighteen, your parent or legal guardian usually makes decisions about your medical care. Mature minors may legally make health care decisions on their own.

For more information about the rights of children, turn to chapter 8.

Another important point is that you can't be labeled incompetent simply because you refuse treatment or disagree with your physician. Otherwise, informed consent would collapse into the "right" to agree with the doctor.

In health care, *you are competent if you understand the information needed to give informed consent for a proposed treatment.* Only a judge can *legally* declare you "incompetent" and appoint a guardian to act for you. Guardians must act in a way that is consistent with your best interests, and courts usually defer to your family's judgment. Thus, rarely does anyone gain by having a legal guardian appointed, a process that is time-consuming and expensive.

Because competence ultimately rests on your ability to understand the nature and consequences of your decisions, it's appropriate for health care providers to conduct a basic informed-consent discussion with you. In such discussions, medical personnel carefully explain the proposed treatment, its likely risks and benefits, the alternatives, their risks and benefits, and the likely consequences of refusing treatment.

Ideally, the discussion determines if you understand this basic information *before* you are asked to consent. Making that determination beforehand avoids the *outcome approach* pitfall—that is, labeling a person incompetent solely based on a refusal to undergo a recommended treatment.

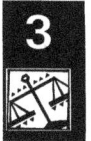

When Your Consent Isn't Possible

By custom, health care personnel defer to the next of kin to speak for incompetent patients. By consenting to a treatment, relatives effectively waive their rights to sue a physician for failure to obtain consent.

Their consent also demonstrates that the doctor consulted someone likely to know the patient well and be concerned about his or her best interests. This will probably persuade a patient who recovers not to sue a doctor for failing to obtain consent.

The Consent Form

Consent is *not* a form, but doctors and hospitals usually want to put your consent in writing for the same reason most contracts are written down: to preserve the exact terms in case of future disagreement. If you later sue a doctor alleging lack of informed consent, the doctor can present the form as evidence.

To be useful evidence of your informed consent, the written form must contain everything you need to know to grant consent: a description of the proposed procedure, its risks and benefits, the alternatives and their risks and benefits, the risks of nontreatment, success rates, problems of recuperation, and so on. In general, the form contains the names of the physicians involved, and it may also deal with such topics as the disposition and use of removed tissues, organs, and body parts.

You can limit a doctor's authority in the consent form. However, a surgeon, for example, who believes the limitations are too strict to proceed with an operation safely might reasonably decide not to go ahead with it. The surgeon could also reasonably note in the medical record the

The Informed Consent Checklist

Before you sign a consent form, make sure you completely understand everything about the proposed treatment:

■ Know the name and nature of your injury, illness, or disability, as well as the dangers or disadvantages of not treating it.

■ Understand the nature of the specific procedure recommended to deal with your problem.

■ Know if there are other ways of treating the problem and their associated risks and benefits. Feel confident that the procedure proposed is the best one. *List the alternatives.*

■ Know the advantages, risks, and side effects of this procedure. *List these if you can.*

■ Know the probability of success. *What is it? What is meant by success?*

■ Know the likely result if you aren't treated. *What is it?*

■ Understand all you've been told and explain it in your own words. *Try to explain it to your closest friend or relative.*

■ Make sure that your doctor has answered all

limitations you have placed on his or her authority, together with the fact that you understand and consent to the associated risks.

You can withdraw your consent at any time. First, tell the physician about your change of mind. Then, either obtain and destroy the original consent form or write a "nonconsent form," noting on it the date and time of day you are withdrawing consent. This is the rule, but there are practical limitations. For example, if you're under general anesthesia and on the operating table, it's obviously too late to change your mind.

Very few situations *legally* require a written consent form. The most common situation requiring a form is when you consent to be a research subject.

Your Right to Emergency Treatment

If you have a medical emergency or are in labor, any hospital with emergency facilities must treat you if it can. If it can't, it must refer you elsewhere. An emergency is an injury or acute medical condition likely to cause death, disability, or serious illness if not attended to very quickly.

The physician's role is central. First, the physician has a duty to determine if an emergency exists. If an emergency exists, law and medical ethics require the physician to treat you or to find someone who can.

Conditions that require the immediate attention of a physician include:

■ Heavy bleeding
■ Heart stoppage
■ Breathing stoppage
■ Profound shock from any cause
■ Ingestion or exposure to a rapidly acting poison
■ Labor
■ Severe head injuries
■ Sudden and complete changes in personality
■ Anaphylactic reactions (allergic response)

An emergency can be less serious, however. It could include broken bones, fevers, and cuts that require stitches.

The Hospital Emergency Department

You have a legal right to be screened by competent personnel, and they must examine you within a reasonable time. *If* they determine that a medical emergency exists, you have a right to be examined by a physician. Both the federal government, in the Medicare Conditions of Participation, and the American College of Surgeons, in its Standards for Emergency Departments in Hospitals, go further and specify that a physician should see every applicant for treatment.

Usually a nurse does the screening, but occasionally it's done by a clerk. He or she determines your need for immediate care and decides how long you can reasonably wait to see a physician. A hospital must continue to treat you until it can transfer or discharge you safely.

For more information about your rights in the hospital, turn to chapter 6.

Your Right to Your Medical Records

The *information* in your medical record is *your* information. Nonetheless, in general, the owner of the paper, computer file, or photographic film that contains the information owns the physical record itself, and thus has custody of the information in them.

In most states, you have an explicit legal right to see and copy your medical records. In other states, you probably have this legal right even though no specific law exists on the subject. Regardless of the law, you deserve routine access to your medical record. You may need the information to decide on treatment, determine if and when to change physicians or health plans, and prepare for your future.

In some states, you only have legal access to your hospital records after leaving the hospital. Some states also limit access to psychiatric records, while others limit the types of records that are open to you. For example, some laws exclude access to lab reports, X rays, prescriptions, and other technical information. A few states require you to show *good cause* before you can read the record, but this term is virtually meaningless because almost any reason you have fulfills that requirement. Other states either provide for access under specific circumstances or require you to go through an attorney, physician, or relative; these outmoded requirements should be rescinded. Physicians and health facilities can charge you a reasonable fee for making a copy of your medical record, but this should not exceed the cost of duplication.

Getting Your Medical Records

Despite the laws, obtaining your records is often a long and difficult process. To lessen delays, it's a good idea to request the records as your

your questions openly and offered to discuss any additional concerns with you. *Get satisfactory answers to your questions before you sign the consent form.*

■ Understand the meaning of all the words in the consent form. *If you don't, have them explained.*

■ Carefully read the consent form and add new requirements or cross out points you disagree with. Make sure your doctor is aware of these changes. *If you don't agree to everything in the form, don't sign it.*

■ Know the identity and qualifications of the people who will perform this procedure. *If you don't know, find out who they are or cross out the words "or designee."*

■ Have a clear head and an alert mind. Make sure you aren't too anxious to feel that this decision isn't your own free choice.

■ Feel confident that the benefits to you of this procedure outweigh the risks. *If not, reconsider your decision.*

■ Know that you don't have to consent to this procedure.

The Right to Emergency Treatment

The leading court case explicitly dealing with the right to emergency care involved a four-month-old baby with diarrhea. The family physician prescribed medication by phone on the second day of the illness and saw the child on the third day. The child didn't sleep that night, so the parents took the child to the emergency room in the morning, knowing the doctor wasn't in his office.

The nurse on duty refused to examine the child, saying the hospital couldn't treat anyone under a doctor's care without contacting the doctor first. The parents took the child home and made an appointment with their doctor for that night, but the child died of bronchial pneumonia in the afternoon.

The court ruled that the parents could recover damages from the hospital for refusal to treat an "unmistakable emergency" if the nurse should have been able to spot the child's emergency condition.

treatment progresses, rather than at the end of your illness or when you change doctors. It's also important to specify which records you want to see, such as lab reports, X rays, prescriptions, and other technical information. Keep a file at home with your own copy of all your records.

Medical Records: Getting Yours, by Bruce Samuels and Sidney M. Wolfe is a comprehensive guide to state-by-state rules. To order, send $10 ($20 for businesses) plus $2 for postage and handling to Public Citizen, Publications Dept., 2000 P Street, N.W., Washington, DC 20036.

For help in obtaining your medical record, contact the American Health Information Management Association, 919 N. Michigan Avenue, Chicago, IL 60611; tel. (800) 335-5535. Send $1.35 for the pamphlet, "Your Health Information Belongs to You."

Medical Records and Insurance

Health insurance companies often report the contents of medical records to national databanks, such as the Medical Information Bureau. The largest such private databank in the United States, MIB holds records on more than 12 million Americans and Canadians. It releases data to its members—mostly insurance companies—to control fraud.

Check with MIB to see if it has a file on you. Because it affects your insurance claims, make sure that any information about you in the databank is accurate. The bureau will answer your request and may correct errors you report at no charge. MIB reports that errors occur in fewer than 1 percent of the files.

For a free brochure, contact the MIB, P.O. Box 105, Essex Station, Boston, MA 02112; tel. (617) 426-3660.

What Your Record *Shouldn't* Contain

It's inappropriate for your medical record to include personal criticisms, such as "This patient is fat and sloppy." Nor should it contain offhand comments, such as "I love her perfume." Statements like these unfairly color the attitudes of others who read the record. They can also lead health care providers to try to conceal the record from you out of fear of embarrassing the person who wrote the remarks.

Health care providers should record *facts* about a patient (for example, "speech slurred, eyes bloodshot") rather than conclusions that may not be true ("patient is an alcoholic").

Why Read Your Medical Record?

The primary reason to read your medical record is to better understand your health condition and cooperate in improving it. Other reasons include:

- To check the accuracy of family and personal histories
- To be informed about diagnoses and options when asked to consent to any procedures
- To understand the role of the physician and others in treatment
- To make sure you aren't unfairly denied insurance benefits
- To help prevent a recurrence of a disease or condition in the future

Your medical record can be a powerful means of health education, of benefit to you both in a hospital and outside it. In one study, for example, a pregnant patient noted an incorrect blood typing in her record. In another study, half the patients found at least one factual error in their records.

The (Limited) Right to Privacy

All health care practitioners have an ethical and legal duty to maintain confidentiality about you. The Hippocratic Oath sets out this duty: "Whatsoever things I see or hear concerning the life of man, in any attendance on the sick or even apart therefrom, which ought not to be noised about, I will keep silent thereon, counting such things to be professional secrets."

The American Medical Association Principles of Ethics reinterprets this oath: "A physician shall respect the rights of patients, of colleagues, and of other health professionals, and shall safeguard patient confidences within the constraints of the law."

The American Osteopathic Association Code of Ethics states, "The physician shall keep in confidence whatever he may learn about a patient in the discharge of his professional duties."

The American Nurses Association Code provides that: "The nurse safeguards the client's right to privacy by judiciously protecting information of a confidential nature."

These rules arise from the fact that health care providers often must know the most personal details of your life in order to help you. You are unlikely to speak freely unless you know that no one not directly involved in your care will learn of the information you provide.

TIP

Be Selective

When asking for copies of your medical record, try to review the entire record first and order only the pages you need. You may have little interest in lab reports and many other parts of the record, which could cover hundreds of pages.

3

TIP

On the Move

If you move out of town or go on a long trip, consider taking along a copy of your medical record or at least the discharge summary of your most recent hospital visit.

How Can Health Care Facilities Enhance Patient Rights?

Every health care facility should adopt a simple five-point agenda to greatly enhance patient rights:

1. *Eliminate "routine" procedures:* Health care personnel commonly answer the question "Why are you doing this?" with "Don't worry, it's routine." This isn't acceptable. Procedures are acceptable only if they are *specifically* indicated for the patient.

2. *Open access to medical records:* Patient access to medical records remains difficult, despite many federal and state laws and regulations. A patient often asserts the right to see the record at the peril of being labeled a troublemaker.

3. *Provide 24-hour-a-day visitor rights:* At least one person of the patient's choosing needs unlimited access to the patient's room at any time of day or night. This person also needs the right to stay with the patient during any procedure as long

Nevertheless, it isn't realistic to expect medical information to remain secret: Information about you goes into your medical record so that it can be shared with others. The general rule is that everyone in the hospital—including you—has access. Information exchange in a hospital is essential to the "team" approach to health care. Moreover, medical records are central to education, financial decisions, and quality monitoring.

Thus, even on a "need-to-know" basis many people have access to your medical record. That's why it's reasonable to fear that very sensitive information about you, such as a psychiatric diagnosis or an HIV infection, is included in the record. This information could spread rapidly in the hospital and change the way members of the hospital staff treat you. It could also leak from the hospital, affecting your housing, employment, and insurance.

Who Sees Your Record

Physician Mark Siegler decided to find out how many people might read the medical record of one of his patients. As Siegler wrote in the *New England Journal of Medicine,* among the many people at the hospital with a *legitimate* need were six attending physicians, twelve house officers, twenty nurses, six respiratory therapists, three nutritionists, two pharmacologists, four secretaries, fifteen students, four financial officers, and four chart reviewers.

And that's only in the hospital. Insurers will see your record as well.

Enforcing Your Rights

The ideal standard for the doctor-patient relationship is a *partnership.* When the relationship doesn't meet this standard, you need an advocate for your rights and dignity.

The Patient-Rights Advocate

The job of a patient-rights advocate is to help you exercise your rights within the health care system, whether these are outlined in state or federal law, an institution's Patient Bill of Rights, or simple common sense.

The employer of the advocate may be a health care facility, health plan, insurance company, government agency, consumer group, or you. The critical factor is loyalty: *The advocate must represent you, the patient.* The goal of a true patient-rights advocate is to enhance your ability to make decisions, not to encourage you to "behave."

More than three thousand hospitals and health plans employ at least one person with the job title "patient representative." Unfortunately, this title can be misleading, and true *patient* advocates are difficult to find in many health care settings. Often their real assignment is to represent their employer, not you, but some patient representatives do an excellent job on behalf of patients.

Ask the nurse how to get in touch with the patient advocate or patient representative, or call the hospital switchboard. Give the representative a fair chance to help you, but explore other avenues of redress immediately if it becomes clear that he or she is more concerned with protecting the institution. If a hospital or other health care facility doesn't supply you with a real advocate, find your own: a friend, lawyer, physician, nurse, social worker, or relative.

Unfortunately, few health care institutions have a *formal* advocate system, despite the potential benefit to patients. Formal advocates would have direct access to the hospital staff, administration, and relevant committees in the hospital structure, which would help them develop credibility as problem solvers.

Advocates of patients' rights serve four main goals:

1. They protect patients, especially those at a disadvantage. This includes patients who are young, severely handicapped, poor, without relatives, or unable to speak English well.

2. They enable patients and health care personnel to work as partners.

3. They place medical technology and pharmaceutical advances in perspective by confronting the exaggerated expectations of some health care consumers.

4. They explain the health-sickness continuum and assert the humanness of death as a natural and inevitable reality.

For information on finding advocates that can help you obtain your rights, turn to chapters 21 and 22.

Complaining to the Licensing Board

All physicians and nurses, and most other health care providers, are licensed by an agency of the state government, usually called a licensing board or board of registration. If you believe your health care provider has acted unethically or negligently in your care, you can *and should* file a written complaint with this board. You should receive a written response, which is likely to include a request to see your medical records covering the care about which you are complaining.

as this doesn't interfere with the care of other patients.

4. *Require full disclosure of practitioners' experience before procedures are performed:* Despite the almost universal acknowledgment of the need for informed consent, an important fact is still routinely withheld: the experience of the person doing the procedure. Patients have a right to know if the person asking permission to draw blood, do a bonemarrow aspiration, or do a spinal tap—to list just a few examples—has performed the procedure before, and if so, the rate of adverse effects. This applies to medical students and board-certified surgeons alike.

5. *Implement an effective patient-rights advocate program:* This would include a patient-centered bill of rights.

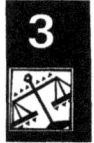

3

TIP

Keep a Record

If you file a complaint against a hospital, physician, HMO, or any other health care provider, keep copies of all letters and other materials you send and receive that pertain to the complaint. Keep notes on phone conversations as well.

A Bill of Rights for Hospital Patients

The American Hospital Association, of which most hospitals are members, has adopted the following Hospital Patient's Bill of Rights. It's a welcome move, but don't feel limited by this statement: It's the hospital's—not a consumer's—view of your rights. In addition, rights are only as good as a health care facility's enforcement mechanism. In most cases, protecting your rights is up to you and your family.

Also, note that the AHA has prepared this "short version" of your rights. To get a copy of the full version, expanding on these points, call the AHA at (312) 280-6263.

We consider you to be a partner in your hospital care. When you are well informed, participate in treatment decisions, and communicate openly with your doctor and other

The board should investigate your complaint. It may take action against the health care provider, including reprimanding him or her, suspending the license to practice, or even revoking the license.

Even if the board finds your complaint was correct, you won't get any money. However, you'll be helping other patients by alerting the health care practitioner and those responsible for licensing him or her. This may help prevent future injury.

For more information on registering a complaint about a physician, turn to chapter 13.

Medical Malpractice and Informed Consent

Taking informed consent and shared decision making seriously enhances the doctor-patient partnership and goes a long way toward preventing unhappy surprises. This requires both patients and physicians to acknowledge uncertainty in medicine. However, you may have the misfortune to encounter a situation in which you suspect medical malpractice may have occurred.

The term *medical malpractice* denotes the basis for a lawsuit for injuries you suffer due to a health care provider's negligence or carelessness. A trial or other adversary proceeding determines if the health care provider is at fault. Usually a jury makes that decision; and if the provider is found negligent, how much the provider should pay you as compensation.

Many malpractice lawsuits against doctors arise not from poor quality of care or medical negligence but rather from poor physician-patient communication. In other words, informed consent is central to *preventing* malpractice from occurring. Unrealistic expectations on the part of patients—and ritualistic silence or demands for blind faith on the part of physicians—only lead to more malpractice suits.

Arbitration, mediation, and other possible alternatives to a malpractice lawsuit deserve consideration, but all should serve three primary goals:

1. Compensate victims for injury.
2. Foster quality.
3. Respond to consumers' needs to have their grievances fairly heard.

Only changes in the malpractice system that enhance these goals deserve serious consideration as an alternative to your right to sue unprofessional health care personnel.

The Few Who Sue

About 1 percent of all hospitalized patients are treated negligently in a way that results in injury to them. However, a recent study published in the *Journal of the American Medical Association* showed that less than 3 percent of hospitalized patients who suffer injury due to negligence or their families initiate a malpractice claim.

The reasons aren't well understood, but many injured patients may not know their injury results from the physician's mistake rather than their underlying illness or injury. Others may want to avoid litigation or may have difficulty finding a lawyer to take their case.

Proving Malpractice

To win a malpractice claim against a health care provider, you must prove four things: duty, breach, damages, and causation.

1. The health care provider had a *duty* toward you. Duty is defined by the standard of care: What would a reasonably prudent practitioner do under the same or similar circumstances?

2. The practitioner—by action or inaction—*breached* that duty.

3. The breach of duty resulted in actual *damages,* usually physical harm. These are measured in monetary terms.

4. The breach of duty was the act that specifically *caused* the harm.

Ordinarily, an expert medical witness must testify that the health care provider failed to fulfill his or her duty, resulting in an injury to you. In most cases, only a physician with "expert" knowledge can legally establish that fact (because a jury of lay people doesn't know what constitutes good medical practice). The witness explains what the health care community recognizes as the standard of care in the particular situation and gives an opinion on whether the defendant's conduct met that standard.

It can be at least as hard to find a lawyer as it is to find a physician you can work with effectively. Probably the best way to start is to ask your friends and associates if they have used a lawyer for a malpractice suit, what happened, and whether they would recommend that person. If you can't locate a lawyer this way, you can call the local bar association or use a lawyer referral service.

health professionals, you help make your care as effective as possible. The hospital encourages respect for the personal preferences and values of each individual.

While you are a patient in the hospital, your rights include the following:

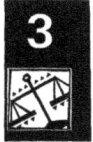

■ You have the right to considerate and respectful care.

■ You have the right to be well informed about your illness, possible treatments, and likely outcomes and to discuss this information with your doctor. You have the right to know the names and roles of people treating you.

■ You have the right to consent to or refuse a treatment, as permitted by law, throughout your hospital stay. If you refuse a recommended treatment, you will receive other needed and available care.

■ You have the right to have an advance directive, such as a living will or health care proxy. These documents express your choices about your future care or name someone to decide if you cannot speak for yourself. If you have a written advance directive, you should provide a copy to the hospital, your family, and your doctor.

(continues)

■ You have the right to privacy. The hospital, your doctor, and others caring for you will protect your privacy as much as possible.

■ You have the right to expect that treatment records are confidential unless you have given permission to release information or reporting is required or permitted by law. When the hospital releases records to others, such as insurers, it emphasizes that the records are confidential.

■ You have the right to review your medical records and to have the information explained, except when restricted by law.

■ You have the right to expect that the hospital will give you necessary health services to the best of its ability. Treatment, referral, or transfer may be recommended. If transfer is recommended or requested, you will be informed of risks, benefits, and alternatives. You will not be transferred until the other institution agrees to accept you.

■ You have the right to know if this hospital has relationships with outside parties that may influence your treatment and care. These relationships may be with educational institutions, other health care providers, or insurers.

If you try to find a lawyer without the benefit of a personal reference, try to interview at least three candidates before making a final choice. There should be no charge for the initial interview, although some lawyers will charge for an independent assessment of your medical records before deciding whether to take your case. After that, malpractice lawyers work on a *contingency-fee* basis: You pay the lawyer a portion of any monetary recovery for their service (usually about one-third). If your case is unsuccessful, you don't pay for the lawyer's time.

Resources

Organizations

American Civil Liberties Union
132 West 43rd Street
New York, NY 10036
(212) 944-9800
This national organization and its state affiliates and local chapters actively protect people's constitutional rights. In the health field, the ACLU is most concerned about the right to privacy, confidentiality, access to records, and equal access to care. The ACLU may help you find legal assistance in exercising your rights.

Campaign for Quality and Choice in Managed Health Care
c/o NY Health Care Campaign
94 Central Avenue
Albany, NY 12206
(518) 465-4600
Contact the campaign for a copy of a model bill of rights for managed care members.

National Center for Patient Rights
666 Broadway
New York, NY 10012
(212) 979-6670
Contact this support and advocacy organization if you believe you may be a victim of medical malpractice.

People's Medical Society
462 Walnut Street
Allentown, PA 18102
(800) 624-8773
(215) 770-1670 in Pennsylvania
Call or write for information on a variety of issues regarding patient rights, including *Your Medical Rights: How to Be an Empowered Consumer* ($14.95; $12.95 for members) and *Your Complete Medical Record* ($12.95; $11.95 for members).

Public Citizen Health Research Group
2000 P Street, N.W.
Washington, DC 20036
(202) 588-1000
This consumer-advocacy group is a good source of basic information about medical care, drug safety, medical-device safety, physician competence, and health issues in general. It prepares many publications, offers testimony before Congress and regulatory agencies, participates in lawsuits on patient-rights issues, and publishes "Health Letter" monthly.

Publications

The Consumer's Legal Guide to Today's Health Care: Your Medical Rights and How to Assert Them, by Stephen Isaacs and Ava Swartz (Houghton Mifflin, 1992), $12.70.

Patient Power: How to Have a Say During Your Hospital Stay, by Iris Sneider (Betterway, 1986), available in many libraries.

"Putting Patients First." This pamphlet summarizes twenty rights and responsibilities for members of managed care plans, endorsed by over one hundred national health organizations. For a free copy, contact National Health Council, 1730 M Street, N.W., #500, Washington, DC 20036-4505.

The Rights of Patients, by George J. Annas (Southern Illinois University Press, 1989), $8.95.

Take This Book to the Hospital with You: A Consumer Guide to Surviving Your Hospital Stay, by Charles B. Inlander and Ed Weiner (Outlet Book Co., 1993), $7.99.

■ You have the right to consent or decline to take part in research affecting your care. If you choose not to take part, you will receive the most effective care the hospital otherwise provides.

■ You have the right to be told of realistic care alternatives when hospital care is no longer appropriate.

■ You have the right to know about hospital rules that affect you and your treatment and about charges and payment methods. You have the right to know about hospital resources, such as patient representatives or ethics committees, that can help you resolve problems and questions about your hospital stay and care.

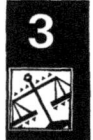

Part Two

The Heart
of the
Matter

4

Health Insurance: Managing Managed Care

Nancy Turnbull

Nancy Turnbull is an instructor in health policy and management at the Harvard School of Public Health. As a former first deputy commissioner of insurance for the Massachusetts Division of Insurance, her responsibilities included regulating HMOs and other health plans. She also worked for five years for the Blue Cross Blue Shield system. After fifteen years of dealing with the private insurance system, she's a big fan of the single-payer approach to health care.

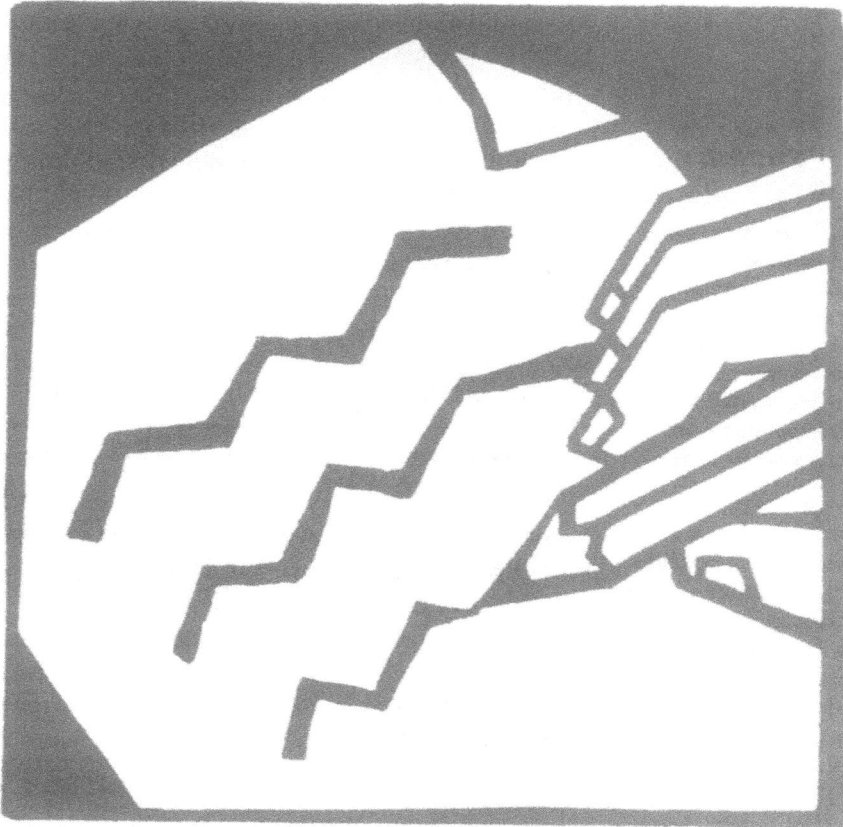

TIP

Do It Now

$ Buy health insurance when you are healthy. Besides the obvious reasons, many policies exclude coverage—either temporarily or permanently—for any health conditions you had before you signed up. For example, many plans don't pay for childbirth in the first nine months a person is a member. During this "waiting period," you'll have to delay care related to these "preexisting conditions" or pay for it yourself.

TIP

Power in Numbers

$ Buy group health insurance if you can, whether through your employer, a union, or an association. The volume of members allows group plans to provide more benefits with lower premiums than individual plans can.

If your only option is a nongroup policy, look for one that is noncancelable or guaranteed renewable as long as you keep paying the monthly premiums. At a minimum, it should be "conditionally renewable," meaning that the insurer can't cancel

■ You're just starting a new job. On your first day at work, the personnel department sends you a thick folder with descriptions of your options for health insurance. Your deadline to select a plan is the end of the week. *How do you pick one?*

■ The company where you work wants to reduce its health insurance bill without cutting your health benefits. Instead of offering several plans, the company will enroll everyone in a single HMO—and it's not the one where you've gotten your health care for years. *How will that affect your health care?*

■ You suspect your daughter may have asthma, and you'd like to consult a specialist. Your health plan has denied your request to see a specialist outside its network of physicians. *What can you do?*

Navigating the seas and shoals of health plans can be difficult and bewildering. Consumers confront a dizzying array of unfamiliar acronyms and options: HMOs, PPOs, managed care, fee-for-service, managed indemnity. . . . The list grows almost daily. It's often hard to know *what* to ask—let alone *whom* to ask—as you try to assemble the best personal health care system for yourself and your family.

This chapter provides some practical suggestions as you take the most common first step in health care: evaluating and selecting insurance. It explains the differences among the major types of health insurance plans and suggests a number of questions to ask yourself and others as you weigh the many options.

First of all, no matter what your situation, *you need health insurance.* Medical bills are one of the major expenses for any family, and the costs are rising. At the very least, protect yourself and your family in case a serious accident or a major illness arises. And remember, you simply can't predict the size of your future medical bills.

Key Insurance Words

Copayments: A fixed dollar amount you pay for health care services. For example, you might have to pay $3 as a copayment at a doctor's office visit.

Deductibles: Amount you must pay before the insurer starts paying the health care bills.

Coinsurance: A percentage you pay for health care services. For example, you might have to pay 20 percent of a hospital bill.

Premiums: What you or your employer pay monthly for insurance coverage.

This Thing Called "Managed Care"

The two magic words in health care these days are *managed care*. A term with many meanings, it generally describes health insurance that attempts to control the rising cost of medical care with one or more of the following methods:

Provider networks. A group of doctors, hospitals, and other health care providers treat plan members, often at reduced rates of payment. Members generally receive the most benefits at the lowest cost if they see a provider in the network.

Utilization management. Medical professionals review proposed hospital admissions, surgery, and other procedures to determine if they are necessary and appropriate.

Case management. In the case of very serious illnesses—AIDS or cancer, for example—the plan works with the member and his or her doctor to coordinate care and arrange for home care, hospice care, or some other alternative treatment that may enhance the person's quality of life and care while also reducing costs.

For information on home care, turn to chapter 16. For information on hospice care, turn to chapter 20.

While managed care is not a new idea, its features are spreading rapidly as employers and other large purchasers of health insurance seek to contain soaring medical costs. Most insured Americans are now enrolled in some type of managed care plan, and soon virtually every plan will include some managed care features.

Consumer Alert: Prior Approval

Some managed care plans require *you* to get approval before going to the hospital, except in an emergency; in others, your doctor obtains the approval for you. Learn the rules of your plan. If you don't follow them, you could be without coverage, even for necessary medical care.

Although you don't need prior approval for emergency hospital care, what does the plan call an emergency? An emergency in the eyes of a

---

your policy unless the plan is eliminating all policies like yours.

Make sure the policy explains clearly when and on what basis the insurer can raise your premiums. Ask the company about its rate increases over the past few years for a person of your age in your community. Don't buy a policy that can increase your rates based only on *your* medical costs.

Check for a policy that:

- Has a "free-look" clause that allows you at least ten days during which you can cancel and get a full refund

- Protects you from large medical costs, *and*

- Has the right coverage for you

State insurance laws determine the kinds of policies and benefits that insurers can sell. Contact your state insurance department to find out about laws that protect you when you buy insurance.

4

concerned parent may not meet the plan's medical standards. To avoid an unpleasant surprise, get a clear, detailed explanation of what your health plan considers an emergency.

Traditional Insurance vs. Managed Care

The alternative to managed care is called *indemnity insurance*. In this form of health insurance, you usually pay your health care provider for each visit, and your insurer reimburses you if your policy covers the particular service you received. However, the provider will often bill the insurer directly, especially for hospital services. Only a few companies now market only pure indemnity plans.

For the consumer, many things distinguish traditional indemnity insurance from managed care—affecting cost, quality, and your well-being. Some of the most common and important differences to you are the following:

Choice of Physician

Traditional plan: You can see any doctor you want, whenever you want.

Managed care: You must use providers in the plan's network, or you have a strong financial incentive to do so. In most plans, you select a primary care provider—often referred to as a "gatekeeper." He or she is almost always a general practitioner, family-practice physician, internist or, for children, a pediatrician. This person handles all routine medical services, as well as authorizing and coordinating your care from other health care providers. The purposes of this primary care provider are to cut down on unnecessary visits to specialists and to make one physician responsible for managing your care. However, critics of this "primary care case management process" believe it has the potential to introduce administrative burdens or delay timely referral to specialists.

For more information on primary care, turn to chapter 5.

How to See a Specialist

Traditional plan: You can consult any specialist at any time, although some specialists may refuse to see you unless your physician sends you to them.

Managed care: Your primary care provider decides when you'll see a specialist and usually sends you to someone affiliated with the plan. Some plans let you see any specialist without a referral, but you may have to pay a larger share of the bill yourself.

For more information on specialists, turn to chapter 13.

How You Are Admitted to a Hospital

Traditional plan: Your doctor decides when you'll enter a hospital and which one.

Managed care: Except in an emergency, your doctor asks the plan to approve your hospitalization beforehand. The plan also approves the hospital to be used.

For more information on hospitals, turn to chapter 6.

What the Plan Covers—and What It Doesn't

Traditional plan: You pay an annual deductible—generally from $200 to $1,000—before insurance kicks in. You also pay some percentage of the bills—most often 20 percent. Your total maximum yearly out-of-pocket payment is generally limited, often to $1,000 or $2,000. In general, the plan doesn't cover prescription drugs or preventive services such as routine physicals, well-child visits, and immunizations.

Managed care: You pay a fixed amount—a copayment—for each office visit to network providers. Copayments vary but generally run $5 to $15. The plan usually includes preventive care and pays the full cost for most other covered services. It may also include prescription drugs. You may be responsible for a deductible before the plan pays anything.

The Paperwork Difference

Indemnity plan: You usually pay your physician and then submit a claim form to the health plan for reimbursement.

Managed care: You usually pay a copayment and submit no forms when receiving care from network providers. The provider handles any paperwork.

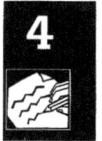

Contraception and Abortion

Two-thirds of indemnity plans routinely pay for abortions, according to the Alan Guttmacher Institute. The remainder either don't cover abortion services at all or restrict coverage, most often by requiring certification of a specific medical reason for the procedure.

About half of indemnity plans don't cover contraception, reflecting their traditional exclusions on preventive care. Only 22 percent routinely cover contraceptive counseling.

HMO coverage for abortions is roughly the same as that in indemnity plans, but contraceptive coverage is considerably superior. About four in ten HMOs cover the most common methods of family planning. Nearly all cover contraceptive counseling.

If these services are important to you, talk to the health benefits personnel where you work. As with most health plan benefits, employers decide whether plans will or won't cover abortions or contraception.

The Varieties of Managed Care

"If you've seen one plan . . . you've seen one plan." In other words, it's risky to generalize about managed care. That said, you'll probably have to select among roughly four types of managed care:

Health Maintenance Organization (HMO). HMOs have a network of health care providers, sometimes located at the plan's own facilities.

Consumers and the Primary Forms of Medical Insurance

Type of Plan	Advantages	Disadvantages	Out-of-Pocket Costs
Traditional indemnity	Choice of any doctor or hospital	Claim forms to file, no quality monitoring, limited preventive care	Varies with plan
Managed indemnity	Choice of any doctor and access to any hospital if the service is approved in advance	More paperwork to get approval for some services, little or no quality monitoring, limited preventive care	Varies with plan
PPO	Choice of any doctor or hospital, preventive care sometimes covered	More paperwork to get approval for some services, may have some quality monitoring, preventive care may be limited	Lower in network, higher outside the network
HMO	No claim forms, may have quality monitoring, preventive care always covered	Only covers affiliated or approved doctors and hospitals	Low
POS	Wider choice of doctor or hospital than traditional HMOs, some quality monitoring if you use HMO providers	Benefits outside the network may be more limited; care may be less coordinated than in a traditional HMO if you get care outside the network	Lower in network, higher outside the network; premiums usually higher than traditional HMO; you may be responsible for charges above HMO fee schedule when using non-network providers

Except in an emergency, HMO members get care from affiliated providers. The plan rarely pays for care from non-HMO providers, unless the member gets approval for such services in advance. HMO members select a primary care provider when they enroll. In general, HMOs cover preventive care, and members don't have to file claims.

Managed indemnity. As with traditional health insurance, a member of a managed indemnity plan can see any medical provider. But typically you get the plan's prior approval for hospitalizations and some outpatient procedures. Such plans don't always cover preventive services, and you may have to file claim forms for some services.

Preferred Provider Organization (PPO). A PPO borrows features from both traditional indemnity and HMO plans. Like an HMO, a PPO contracts with a network of providers. Unlike an HMO, a member may use *any* provider, although financial incentives—usually broader benefits and lower copayments—encourage the use of network providers. Members may have to select a primary care provider and usually need prior approval for all inpatient care and selected outpatient procedures, regardless of whether or not the care is from network providers. Members usually submit claim forms to get reimbursed for services received from non-network providers.

Point of Service plans. Confused by the variety of health plans? Well, a point of service (POS) plan is like a PPO offered by an HMO. A member can go outside the HMO's network by paying higher out-of-pocket costs. In many POS plans, certain services—most commonly preventive care— are covered only if you go to an HMO provider.

Point of service plans are the fastest growing part of the managed care business. They are offered by more than half of HMOs and over 40 percent of employers. More and more employers are using POS products as a way to move reluctant employees into managed care. It's too early to tell if POS plans will be a transitional product or if they are here to stay, but over 9 million people are now enrolled in some type of POS plan.

In general, when you join a managed care plan, particularly an HMO, you sacrifice the freedom to go to any provider and your provider must comply with the policies and standards of practice of the plan. In return, you usually have lower out-of-pocket costs and more comprehensive benefits, and the plan will usually practice more oversight and coordination of the use, quality, and cost of the medical services you receive. It's up to you to weigh the pros and the cons.

HMO Model Types

Besides the different types of health plan, HMOs can also come in different forms, or models. While the distinctions among models are blurring, the major model types are

Staff model HMO: The HMO employs most of the doctors and other medical professionals, and those providers see HMO members in health centers and clinics owned by the HMO

Group model HMO: The HMO contracts with a separate physician group to provide care to members. The HMO pays the groups a negotiated rate, and the groups are not owned by the HMO. A group may contract exclusively with the HMO, or it may also serve other patients.

Independent Practice Association HMO: The HMO contracts with a large number of individual practice physicians who are paid either on a fee-for-service or fee-per-patient basis to take care of HMO members. The physicians in the IPA also see patients who aren't HMO members.

Mixed model HMO: An HMO can include more than one form of HMO within a single plan. For example, a staff model

Other Options for Medical Insurance

Most people get their health plan through their employer or union. However, if you are one of many people who can't do this, you may still have a variety of options.

COBRA. If you are employed, you and your dependents may be able to receive health coverage through your employer even after employment ends, if you or your dependents pay the monthly premiums. Under the federal COBRA law, companies with group health plans and twenty or more workers must allow you and your dependents to continue health insurance if your job ends, you die, you are divorced, or, for your children, their dependent status ends. You and your dependents can remain covered for at least eighteen months and in some circumstances up to thirty-six months.

To get COBRA coverage, you must pay the full cost, which can't exceed 102 percent of the group premium. Your employer must notify you or your family members of your COBRA rights within forty-five days of termination or loss of coverage. You then have sixty days to pay the necessary premium.

Your eligibility for COBRA ends when you become eligible for other group insurance. However, if your new health plan doesn't cover a pre-existing condition, you may continue your COBRA coverage until the new plan's exclusion period ends or your original COBRA eligibility period ends, whichever comes first. If you are receiving health coverage under COBRA, you have the same rights to switch health plans as current workers at your former employer.

The responsibility for administering and enforcing COBRA benefits depends on the type of health plan you have. For insured plans, contact the U.S. Department of the Treasury. If you work for a company with a self-funded plan (see page 50), contact the Pension and Welfare Benefits Administration, U.S. Department of Labor.

Individual (nongroup) coverage. Individuals and their families can often buy coverage on their own directly from insurers. The options tend to be more expensive and offer less coverage than group plans. If you apply for an individual plan, the insurer will usually require you to provide detailed information about your health and your medical history. It might even require you to undergo a medical examination or medical tests. (The process of collecting and evaluating your medical condition is called *underwriting.*) The insurer may use this information to set your premiums and limit your benefits.

In some states, some or all insurers are required to accept any applicant for individual coverage. Many states also restrict the ability of insurers to engage in certain forms of underwriting. *You can find out about individual coverage options in your state by contacting the state insurance department or consulting with an insurance broker. The insurance department can also tell you about any laws that govern underwriting.*

Small group coverage. If you own a small business, you can apply for insurance as a small group. In some states, self-employed individuals are also eligible for such policies.

Most states limit the types of underwriting that health plans can use for small group insurance. For example, many states require health plans to accept any small group that applies and limit restrictions on coverage for preexisting conditions. These small group laws have made it easier—and often less expensive—for small groups to find and keep health coverage. *Contact the insurance department in your state for information about the laws governing health coverage for small groups.*

Many small groups purchase insurance through associations or professional groups. You could contact your local Chamber of Commerce about professional groups offering insurance to chamber members. Or contact a national small business organization, such as the Small Business Service Bureau, National Operations Center, P.O. Box 15014, Worcester, MA 01615-0014; tel. (508) 756-3513 or (800) 222-5678.

A new federal law, the Health Insurance Portability and Accountability Act of 1996 (commonly called the "Kassebaum-Kennedy law" after its two major Senate sponsors), gives significant new rights and protections to health insurance consumers, especially those who get their health insurance as individuals or as members of small groups. In particular, the law limits the ability of health plans to impose limitations on coverage for preexisting medical conditions, even when you change health plans. The law, which went into effect on July 1, 1997, applies to all health plans, including those that are self-funded. The new law is complex, and many states have protections for consumers that are even better than those in the federal law. Consult with your state insurance department to understand the rights you have in your state.

Besides general medical insurance, you may qualify for, or have need of, other types of coverage. Perhaps the most important is Medicare, the federal health insurance program for people sixty-five and older and for certain disabled Americans. It pays for many, though not all, of the health care expenses of millions of Americans.

An additional type of private policy is Medigap insurance, which covers many aspects of health care for elders that Medicare doesn't cover or

HMO might also contract with individual practice doctors.

Shrinking Differences

According to a study commissioned by the HMO industry association, 63 percent of people in fee-for-service plans and 72 percent in PPOs aren't covered for preexisting conditions for several months after they join the plan. HMOs typically have no such exclusions.

However, the coverage differences between HMOs and other types of plans is shrinking. The same study looked at the proportion of employees whose plans covered adult physicals, well-baby care, outpatient mental health, inpatient mental health, and substance abuse. In each case, HMO coverage declined slightly from 1988 to 1993. At the same time, the coverage for enrollees in fee-for-service and PPO plans rose in almost every case, sometimes dramatically.

The major remaining contrasts in coverage are in adult physicals and well-baby care, two services that are key to the prevention orientation of HMOs.

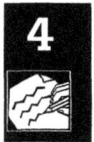

Self-Funded Companies

For many people, their employers pay their health care bills directly instead of through an insurance company or HMO. These plans are called "self-funded" or "self-insured" plans. Some self-funded plans are administered directly by the employer; most are administered by an outside third party, often an insurance company. *You may not even realize that your plan is self-insured.*

Self-funded plans are exempt from state regulation, including insurance laws. Instead, the U.S. Department of Labor regulates self-funded plans.

Self-funded plans don't have to provide state-mandated insurance benefits and may not allow you to convert to a non-group plan when you leave your employment. They *are* required to comply with the federal COBRA law, which gives you rights to continue your group coverage in certain situations.

If you encounter problems with a self-funded plan, first try to work it out with your employer. If that doesn't work, contact the U.S. Department of Labor, Pension and

covers only partially. In addition, insurance companies are marketing a variety of policies, of varying value, for long term care.

For more information on Medicare and Medigap, turn to chapter 11.

Another government program, Medicaid, is a state/federal program for eligible people who cannot afford the cost of health care. It's operated by the states; within federal guidelines, they decide who is eligible and determine the scope of services. Medicaid covers about one-fourth of all children in the United States, and children make up 54 percent of Medicaid recipients.

There are two general ways to qualify for Medicaid. First, you can fall into one of a number of categories, including all those who receive Aid to Families with Dependent Children (AFDC) or Supplemental Security Income (SSI), persons under age eighteen or age sixty-five or over who are eligible for those two programs but choose not to apply, and disabled people who meet certain income and asset requirements. Second, you can become eligible for Medicaid as a "medically needy" individual by spending enough of your income or assets on medical expenses.

Applying for Medicaid is a complicated process, and Medicaid benefits are highly variable from state to state. You can apply for Medicaid at welfare offices or, in some states, at senior citizen centers and other locations. Even if you are turned down, you can file an appeal within sixty days. If you appeal, you should probably seek legal assistance.

Medical Savings Accounts

As the name suggests, a medical savings account (MSA) is like a savings account for medical expenses. Individuals establish an account for medical expenses and also buy health insurance with very high deductibles for protection in the event of a catastrophic illness or accident. You would use the MSA to pay for expenses that are less than the deductible and the insurance for any expenses over the deductible. In most cases, a person can withdraw money from an MSA on a periodic basis.

An MSA is not health insurance. However, in the absence of national health reform, some policymakers advocate them as a way to reduce the number of people without insurance and contain health care costs. In particular, a number of proposals to reform Medicare incorporate MSAs as a key component.

Proponents claim that MSAs encourage consumers to be more conscious of costs and avoid unnecessary care because you pay for medical services out of your own pocket. Opponents of MSAs argue that consumers aren't in the best position to eliminate unnecessary services or contain costs because health care providers make most medical decisions. Critics also believe that MSAs are most attractive to wealthy and healthy individuals, and that widespread use of MSAs would mean higher insurance premiums for people with higher health care needs.

Although some employers now offer MSAs, their use has been limited because contributions to the accounts have not been tax-exempt. However, a new federal law has changed these tax provisions, and the use of MSAs may now increase.

Welfare Administration at (202) 219-8776 or call the office in your state.

Choosing a Health Plan

Many people don't have a choice of plan. For example, their employers may offer only one plan or their health status may limit their options.

If you are fortunate enough to have a choice, however, the process of choosing *and* using a health plan is complicated, and at times very frustrating. Fortunately, a variety of resources can help you. Here are two to get you started:

Your friends and co-workers. Ask people you know about their health plans. What do they think of the coverage and services provided by their plans?

Your health care providers. Ask your present physician and other providers which health plans they recommend and why. If you want to continue seeing a particular provider, find out what plans cover his or her services.

In your search for a good health plan, the information you receive—from your friends and doctors and from the plans' representatives and written materials—will lead you toward a wiser choice. Use the questions in the checklist below to help you in your research. Some questions apply only to certain types of plans; others are important only to certain families. Think about what's most relevant to your own situation and your potential health care needs.

Checklist: Choosing a Health Plan

✓ Can I choose my primary care doctor?
✓ Can I change my doctor if I wish?
✓ Can I get a doctor who understands and is familiar with my culture and my language?
✓ Is my current doctor covered by the plan?
✓ How does the plan pick its doctors?
✓ What do I pay when I see a doctor not covered by the plan?

Promoting Good Health

The best health plans stress health promotion and disease prevention in addition to protecting you when you become seriously ill. Ask about their availability.

In practical terms, this means that they educate their members about ways to stay healthy and cover child immunizations, Pap smears, cholesterol screenings, and other preventive services. Some plans offer low-cost or free classes to help you give up smoking and support groups for cancer patients, their families, or both.

If "wellness" is a major concern for you, look for a plan that not only offers these services—almost all HMOs do—but actively promotes them as well. Do wellness or health promotion take a prominent place in the plan's advertising, member materials, and brochures and posters in waiting rooms? Ask other members if they are encouraged to use such services. Ask the providers about their attitudes toward prevention and about the plan's efforts to keep members healthy.

✓ Does the policy require a deductible and copayment for all services?

✓ Is there a lifetime limit on my out-of-pocket costs?

✓ Is there a lifetime limit on any covered benefits?

✓ Is there a limit on covered days of hospitalization?

✓ Is there an exclusion for "preexisting conditions"? How will this affect me?

✓ Am I likely to need services listed in the "exclusions" section of the benefits description? If so, what will they cost?

✓ Must I get a second opinion to receive specialty care?

✓ What is the procedure to see a specialist?

✓ How quickly can I get urgent care?

✓ How quickly can I get routine care?

✓ How is emergency care provided?

✓ Which hospitals can I use? Are they nearby?

✓ Can I use certain hospitals only for a limited range of conditions or services?

✓ Am I covered for nonemergency care when I travel?

✓ Are all prescription drugs covered? Are my current medications covered?

✓ What are the drug copayments? Do they vary based on the drug?

✓ What health education and wellness programs are provided?

✓ Does the policy cover inpatient and outpatient mental health care?

✓ Does the policy cover dental services? Does the policy cover contact lenses and eyeglasses?

✓ What long term care does the plan cover?

✓ What home care does the plan cover?

✓ What medical equipment does the plan cover?

✓ Are the hours and location of the plan's facilities convenient?

✓ Are lab and other tests conducted in a convenient location?

✓ Is parking or public transportation available?

✓ How long does it take to schedule an initial routine checkup?

✓ Does the staff appear friendly, helpful, compassionate, patient?

✓ What is the procedure for appealing if the plan denies a claim?

✓ How do the plan's members like the plan? Ask the plan if it conducts member satisfaction surveys. If so, ask for a copy of the most recent survey.

✓ Is the plan accredited by the National Committee for Quality Assurance? Does the plan have a quality report card? Ask for a copy.

✓ Does the plan have a member newsletter, health-promotion material, or annual report? Ask for copies to help you judge how well the plan communicates with its members.

✓ If you pick a primary care doctor, how will your care be coordinated by that provider?

✓ What happens if you disagree with the plan's decision not to cover certain services?

Anti-Gag Rules

In some states, anti-gag rules help ensure that physicians and other providers can give you an honest assessment of health plans, without fear of retribution by the plans. Enacted in response to concerns of both physicians and consumers, these laws prohibit a health plan from refusing to contract with, or from terminating the contract of, a provider who discusses the provisions or requirements of the health plan with patients.

Ask your providers if they are constrained in any way from discussing how any health plan may or may not meet your needs. If they do feel constraint, you may want to support the passage of anti-gag legislation in your state.

Cost + Coverage = Your Choice

What you pay and what you get are the obvious issues to consider when selecting a health plan.

Unfortunately, it's often hard to predict your future medical needs. Start by taking your recent health care use as a rough guide. This will allow you to compare the coverage of different health plans and to estimate your total cost under each plan, including your share of the monthly premium or any out-of-pocket costs, such as deductibles and copayments.

It's especially difficult to compare the benefits and costs of different plans because the coverage and copayments vary greatly from plan to plan. If you're lucky, your employer will provide a written comparison of your options. And if you're really fortunate, your employer will require all contracting health plans to charge you the same for exactly the same benefits, making it easier for you to concentrate on finding the highest quality care. Unfortunately, this is far from the norm.

In any case, don't rely only on overviews from health plans *or* your employer, particularly if you have specific medical needs. You can't simply review the plan's marketing material or summary benefit descriptions and make an adequate comparison.

Obtain, read, and analyze the health plan's detailed description of its contract—commonly called the "evidence of coverage," "member contract," or "subscriber certificate." This document will describe, often in deadly detail, the services the plan covers and excludes, as well as other important aspects of the policy. Get your employer's benefits manager or a plan representative to interpret the terms and answer any questions you have.

Keep a record of your questions and the answers, along with the name of the person with whom you talked and the date. Get the answers to any important coverage questions *in writing* on the health plan's stationery.

Although most health plans give you a copy of the member contract only *after* you join, you have a right to see it before making that critical decision. Ask your employer for a copy or get it directly from the health plan. Beware of plans that aren't willing to give you this information.

Cost Comparison

Overall, a 1994 study by the Congressional Budget Office found that managed care, especially the best HMOs, provide equivalent care at a cost about 9 percent less than traditional fee-for-service plans. However, the savings are a mere 4 percent for the average HMO. Even that gap is narrowing, and nearly all fee-for-service plans now include some elements of managed care.

What Else Does the Plan Cover?

Health insurance plans, whatever their general type, can cover a wide variety of services. Among the most important services you might need are preventive care; inpatient hospital services; outpatient surgery; physician hospital visits; office visits, both routine and urgent; hospital emergency care; skilled nursing care; medical tests and X rays; prescription drugs; mental health care; drug and alcohol treatment; home health care; rehabilitation facilities; physical therapy; hospice care; maternity care; experimental surgery or treatments; well-baby care; dental care, both routine and specialized; vision care; hearing aids; and alternative providers (chiropractic, acupuncture, homeopathy, etc.)

The health plan might not provide many of these services directly. More and more health plans contract with specialized firms to provide certain services, most commonly mental health care, dental care, and prescription drugs. In fact, the specialty firm might contract directly with your employer. In other cases, the health plan contracts with the specialty firm and manages the use of covered services.

In other words, the specialty firm, rather than your health plan, could determine what care you'll receive and who will provide it. So you may need to contact the specialty firm, rather than the health plan, to obtain detailed information on the provider network and how to obtain care.

The Typical Employer's Health Plan

In 1992 the health insurance that Americans received through their employers included:

- Mental health in 92 percent of plans
- Substance abuse in 91 percent of plans
- Home health care in 79 percent of plans
- Hospice care in 71 percent of plans
- Skilled and rehabilitative nursing home care in 45 percent of plans
- Well-baby care in 45 percent of plans
- Preventive care in 37 percent of plans

Source: Bureau of National Affairs survey of employer-provided health benefits

4

Domestic Partners

Domestic partners consider themselves a family but either choose not to marry or are legally prevented from doing so because they are lesbian or gay.

A few employers have begun to extend health insurance and other family benefits to domestic partners. Seattle and San Francisco are among the municipalities offering full health insurance benefits to city employees, as do Lotus Development Corp., Ben and Jerry's, New York's Museum of Modern Art, and a growing number of other private employers. Several insurers underwrite domestic-partner policies on a case-by-case basis.

For more information, contact Gay and Lesbian Advocates and Defenders (GLAD), P.O. Box 218, Boston, MA 02112; tel. (617) 426-1350.

Your Choice of Providers

If you're considering a plan with a network of providers, review the list of providers—it's often called the "provider directory." If you join a plan that delivers care in health centers, you'll pick one center, probably near your work or home, and generally pick a primary care physician who practices there. If the plan contracts with doctors practicing in private offices, you'll also probably pick a primary care physician. In any case, check the directory to find out what providers and hospitals you'll use if you need specialty care.

The directory for some health plans covers only primary care. Nevertheless, before you decide to join, you have a right to know about *every* provider who contracts with the plan. Ask for a comprehensive list. And if you want to know if a specific specialist, hospital, or other provider belongs to the plan, call the plan directly and ask.

It's not enough to know that a particular provider belongs to a health plan. You need to find out if you can actually select the provider and what is required to do so.

Does the provider accept new patients from the health plan? A doctor's practice may be full, so he or she won't take on new patients. As strange as it may seem, this could be true even if you now see the doctor through a different health plan. On the other hand, few practices are full under every circumstance. Call the provider to check.

Do you need a referral to see a particular provider? In most managed health plans, your primary care physician must refer you to a specialist. Usually the specialist also contracts with the plan. However, if your primary care physician refers you out of the network, the care is generally covered. Some plans even allow you to go out-of-network without a referral, but you pay a larger share of the specialist's bill.

Can your primary care physician refer you to any network specialist or hospital? While a health plan may contract with a seemingly large number of specialists and hospitals, some plans organize providers into subnetworks—often called "provider units," "referral circles," or "independent practice associations" (IPAs). In these cases, physicians usually refer you only to providers in their subnetwork or provider unit.

It may be important for you to check which specialists you could actually use. For example, if you select a primary care physician in one provider unit, can you continue to use your obstetrician in another unit? Ask your doctor or the plan's member-services department to explain limits on your ability to see specific participating providers.

Similarly, you may want to look into restrictions on your use of network hospitals. A plan may advertise its contract with a particular hospital though it uses that institution only for certain services. Perhaps you want to take advantage of the outstanding maternity services at an affiliated hospital, but the plan sends people there only for cardiac surgery. Again, if this matters to you, check with your doctor or the health plan.

Dissatisfied Docs?

Are many of a plan's affiliated physicians not taking new members as patients? It could mean the doctors are unhappy—and that could have serious consequences for you. Besides the obvious fact that your choice of providers is more limited than you thought, the physicians' attitude could reflect poor quality in the plan as a whole. A rapid turnover of physicians in a health plan could also indicate problems.

How Does the Plan Pay Primary Care Physicians?

Health plans use a wide variety of methods to pay providers, and this could directly affect the type and amount of medical care you receive. Particularly important is how the plan pays your primary care provider.
    You might want to ask the plan:

Are physicians salaried employees? Salary arrangements are less likely to induce physicians to skimp on services or to overtreat you. Doctors who earn a salary will make the same amount of money no matter how much or how little treatment you receive.

Does the health plan still use fee-for-service payment? These plans typically establish fee schedules for paying primary care physicians and specialists for services. Some plans withhold part of the fee for each service—usually 10 to 20 percent—and give it to the physician at the end of the year based on the performance of the individual physician or the plan as a whole. Fee-for-service gives physicians an incentive to provide as much treatment as necessary and potentially an incentive to overtreat you or to favor expensive, high-tech care. On the other hand, some critics believe that fee withholding may result in incentives to undertreat individuals.

Do physicians receive bonuses at the end of the year based on the plan's financial performance? Some plans withhold none of the fee but award physicians a bonus if the cost of referrals and hospitalizations is below the plan's budget targets. Sometimes, the plan links the bonus to member satisfaction and quality.

If it's an HMO, does it pay a primary care physician a fixed monthly payment for each member signed up with the doctor, regardless of how often the member sees the doctor? HMOs may set

TIP

Travel Alert

Does your health insurance cover travel abroad? Under what conditions? Especially if you're planning a long trip, read your policy and consult your insurer and your employer's benefits manager.

If your current policy isn't enough for your needs, consider buying special traveler's insurance. But note that the travel insurance doesn't replace regular health insurance: It probably won't cover you for any care in the United States, even for a problem that arises when you travel.

TIP

Track Record

How long has the HMO been in business? Older HMOs tend to be larger and more stable financially. They also have a track record—for better or worse—with providers and consumers, so it's easier to get information about them.

this "capitation" to cover the expected average cost of treating a member. In some arrangements, the capitation covers only services provided directly by the primary care physician; in other HMOs, the capitation is intended to include the cost of referrals to specialists and other services.

Capitation is a method for insurers to pay for medical services on a per-person or per-member basis rather than a per-service or per-procedure basis (fee-for-service). Under capitation, a health plan pays the participating provider a fixed amount per month for each plan member he or she takes care of, regardless of how much or how little care the member actually receives. The capitation may vary depending on factors such as the age or gender of the member.

According to a 1995 study in the *New England Journal of Medicine,* 84 percent of network or IPA HMOs have some form of "risk sharing" with primary care physicians. Capitation is a primary method of payment in 56 percent of the HMOs, while 28 percent combine fee-for-service payment with a withholding or bonus.

Most HMOs adjust payments to primary care physicians to create performance-based incentives. Half of the group or staff HMOs and 74 percent of network or IPA HMOs adjust payment according to use and cost patterns. More than half of HMOs adjust payments to physicians based on members' satisfaction and the quality of care.

In other words, physician payment arrangements can be very complex, and the effect of different payment methods on quality of care is not yet clear. But this is one factor to consider when evaluating different plans. You may want to ask your current health care providers how satisfied they are with the method and level of payment from particular health plans, and how each plan restricts their ability to refer you to specialists, order lab tests, or otherwise deliver the care that you need.

Consumer Alert: Capitation

While capitation payments eliminate incentives to overtreat, they may create an incentive for undertreatment; your physician could discourage you from visiting the office for minor complaints. Capitation can also discourage referrals to specialists when that referral affects the primary care physician's bonus or withholding.

What If You Leave Your Job or Move Away?

Not all health plans are alike in the coverage they'll provide if you lose your job or move outside the plan's service area. You usually have a legal right to maintain insurance under an employer's plan for between eighteen months and three years, even if you lose your group coverage due to job loss, the death of a spouse, or a divorce. However, you may not be eligible for continued coverage in all circumstances. And if you belong to an HMO or PPO but move outside of the plan's geographic area, you generally can't continue membership. Also, retirees who spend several months a year in seasonal homes may not be eligible for some plans. HMOs generally require you to live in the state a minimum of nine months a year.

Most health plans will give you the option of converting your group policy to an individual or nongroup plan if you lose your group eligibility, even if you move outside the service area. But the benefits are usually lower than in most group plans. HMO policies usually provide better conversion benefits than policies offered by indemnity insurers.

The Quality Question

Traditional indemnity insurers do little or nothing to manage the quality of care their policyholders receive. An advantage of many managed care plans is that they take some responsibility for assuring the quality of service and care rendered to members. In fact, quality management is a hot trend in health care, although many HMOs have engaged in some quality-assurance activities for years.

Unfortunately, it's very difficult to measure quality of care, and few health plans scientifically assess the quality of medical care that members receive. And even the best marks on quality measures don't guarantee that a health plan or its providers will deliver high-quality care to every member every time.

Still, many plans do engage in a variety of activities aimed at improving the quality of your care:

Provider credentialing. Health plans choose providers to join their networks through a process called *credentialing*. Credentialing usually focuses on physicians. Some plans have minimal requirements, such as a state license and hospital admitting privileges. More selective plans require such qualifications as board certification, admitting privileges at particular hospitals, and evidence of cost-effective patterns of practice. A health plan with fewer physicians might have very selective criteria—or physicians may have refused to join the plan for other reasons. Ask a plan what standards it uses to credential providers and how often it updates the information.

Chart reviews and practice guidelines. Many managed care plans review medical records to determine if the care rendered to members meets certain standards. Some common standards include regular immunizations for children, compliance with periodic screening guidelines, appropriate use of consultations, and timely review and interpretation of test results. Ask the plan if it conducts chart reviews, how often, what measures it uses, and how it uses the results to improve the quality of care. You could also ask your physician what she or he thinks of the HMO's quality-improvement activities.

Member satisfaction surveys. Many managed care plans regularly ask members if they are satisfied with the plan as a whole or with specific aspects of care. Often the surveys are extensive enough to provide information on individual primary care physicians, and some plans even use the results to adjust payment to the doctor. Common survey questions include: How easy was it to get an appointment? How long did you have to wait in the doctor's office? How satisfied were you with the care you received? Would you recommend the doctor to others? Many managed care plans also regularly check how many members transfer away from each primary care provider each year and seek the reasons the members switched to other doctors. Ask to see a copy of the latest survey results—but keep in mind that the plan, not an independent researcher, conducts the surveys in most cases.

Outcome measurement. Monitoring "outcomes"—how medical care affects the health and well-being of patients—is ultimately the best way to assess the quality of care that health plan members receive. Although this discipline is in its infancy, some managed care plans are devoting considerable resources to analyzing which types of care work best and improve health—and which don't. For example, healthier members result when plans offer prenatal care, cancer screening, and other preventive and diagnostic programs. Before you pick a health plan, ask for information on its quality-management and improvement efforts.

What percentage of the doctors in a plan are certified by national boards to practice a specialty? If it's below 85 percent, get an explanation from the member-services department. Certification isn't a requirement for physicians, but it suggests a person has successfully completed examinations designed by leaders in his or her field. You may also want to find out if *your* personal doctor is board certified.

Accreditation. Find out if any outside body has accredited the health plan. The two major accreditation agencies are the National Committee for Quality Assurance (NCQA) and the Utilization Review Accreditation Commission (URAC). NCQA, a not-for-profit organization, performs quality-oriented reviews of HMOs and similar types of managed care plans. URAC, also nonprofit, reviews utilization-management firms and the utilization-review departments of insurance companies and certain types of managed care plans. It focuses on managed indemnity plans and PPOs.

In addition, in the late 1970s the federal government set up standards for HMOs. A federally qualified HMO must cover all hospital inpatient services with no limits on costs or days; certain hospital outpatient diagnostic and treatment services, including rehabilitation services; skilled nursing care and home health services; short term detoxification for substance abuse; medical treatment and referral for alcohol and drugs; and preventive care.

This designation is less valuable today as more comprehensive forms of HMO accreditation have emerged. Fewer than half of HMOs are now federally qualified, down from about three-quarters only a few years ago.

Since accreditation programs are fairly new, don't penalize a health plan that is not accredited, but rather award "bonus points" to one that is.

For more information on NCQA, turn to page 63.

To get a list of federally qualified HMOs in your area, contact Department of Health and Human Services, Office of Managed Health Care, 330 Independence Avenue, S.W., Washington, DC 20201; tel. (202) 619-0257.

If Your Provider Leaves the Plan

Despite your most careful research, no one can guarantee that the provider you select will stay with your health plan. Relationships between providers and plans end for a variety of reasons, often with little or no notice to you.

If you are a member of an HMO or other plan that limits your choices, and your provider drops—or is dropped by—the plan, the only way to continue seeing your provider may be to pay the full cost yourself. You could ask the physician you want how satisfied she or he is *before* you join the plan.

If you're in the hospital in the middle of a treatment program when the provider's contract ends, many plans require doctors and hospitals to keep treating you until you're discharged and your care can be transferred safely to another affiliated provider.

TIP

Data Sources

A number of organizations, usually sponsored by coalitions of employers and other large health purchasers, compile, analyze, and publish data on how well health plans do their job. For example, the Pacific Business Group on Health brings together many employers in California, Oregon, and Washington State.

You can find these studies in some libraries or by contacting the organizations directly. Watch the newspaper for articles about these groups, especially when they release studies.

Group Health Cooperative of Puget Sound

The largest HMO in the Northwest, Group Health Cooperative, resembles other health maintenance organizations—except that consumers run it. In fact, with more than 470,000 enrollees, it's the world's largest consumer-run organization. It began in 1947 when a few consumers and physicians joined together to provide what insurance companies and the traditional

Medical Payout Ratios

The *medical payout ratio*—also called the medical loss ratio—tells you what proportion of your premium dollar comes back to you in the form of medical care. While no minimum ratio will ensure that the HMO is providing quality care, this is one factor you can consider as you evaluate health plans.

Consumer advocates suggest that at least 80 to 90 percent of HMO premiums should go to medical care. The national average is about 80 percent, and it's about 93 percent in nonprofit health plans. But in some large national for-profit HMOs the medical payout ratio is as low as 70 percent.

In fact, most managed care plans are very profitable. In the wake of publicity about the relatively low proportion of premiums that many HMOs pay out in medical expenses—and high HMO executive salaries—many states are considering laws that would set a minimum medical payout ratio for HMOs.

Report Cards

Health-plan "report cards" on both quality and cost are emerging across the nation. Many use the Health Plan Employer Data and Information Set, commonly called HEDIS, which looks at quality, access to care, member satisfaction, financial stability, and a number of other factors. By standardizing measures of performance quality, HEDIS will eventually enable consumers and employers to better compare health plans.

However, HEDIS is in its initial stages, and for now, consumers have few sources of data for comparing insurers scientifically. Some plans analyze their own performance and publish the results, but these report cards assess only a narrow range of issues and are not available for every health plan. Still, they are a first step in providing you with better information with which to compare plans. Study a report card if it is available for any plan you are considering.

Among many other measures, a typical report card might include:

Percentage of children immunized. Higher percentages can indicate a plan's commitment to preventive care.

Percentage of women over a certain age who regularly receive mammograms and pap smears. Higher numbers suggest a commitment to early detection and prevention.

Cesarean section rate for deliveries. Lower rates can indicate a commitment to less intrusive childbirth, including vaginal deliveries for women who have had previous cesarean sections.

Member dropout rate. If the rate is high, members may be dissatisfied, although the reasons for disenrollment could also include a job change, a move, or an employer who changes the health plan options.

National Committee for Quality Assurance

The NCQA is one of the organizations leading the growing movement to assess, measure, and report on HMO quality. An independent, nonprofit organization, its board comprises mainly representatives of health plans and employers. It also includes a few consumer and governmental officials, although NCQA doesn't represent consumers.

The two major ways that NCQA measures health plan performance are through accreditation and report cards:

■ In its *accreditation program,* NCQA reviewers assess how well a health plan does in a number of areas, including quality improvement, utilization management, provider credentialing, preventive services, and member rights and responsibilities. Accreditation is voluntary, but more and more purchasers are contracting only with health plans that have been accredited by NCQA. As of March 1996, NCQA had reviewed about half of the country's HMOs. Only about one-third of the HMOs reviewed received full three-year accreditation.

■ To assemble *report cards,* NCQA has developed HEDIS, the Health Plan Data and Information Set, a standard set of 160 performance measures designed to help measure and compare health plan performance in areas such as quality, access, and patient satisfaction.

For information on NCQA, a list of the plans it has reviewed, and the accreditation status of each plan reviewed, call or write NCQA, 2000 L Street, Suite 500, Washington, DC 20036; tel. (202) 955-3535. You can also reach NCQA via the World Wide Web: http://www.ncqa.org.

When It's Time to Complain

Always remember that *you're* the customer: The health plan works for you. You are entitled to get what you pay for and to receive helpful, courteous service. If you have a problem with your health plan, there are a variety of ways to get help.

File a Complaint or Grievance with the Health Plan

Talking with your health plan informally can resolve a great many questions and complaints. Still, keep careful written records of all your con-

medical system didn't: high-quality, comprehensive care at an affordable cost.

An eleven-person board of trustees, elected from the membership, sets the policies. In addition, consumers and trustees serve on a variety of committees, including the Service/Quality Committee that oversees the development of policies, standards, and plans concerning health care and health promotion. On a local level, medical-center councils, composed of elected consumers, the physician chief, the nursing director, and the manager of each center, discuss quality and budget issues.

To find out more, contact Group Health Cooperative, Governance Office, 521 Wall Street, Seattle, WA 98121; tel. (206) 448-5790.

Some HMOs have consumer members on their boards or consumer advisory committees. Find out if your HMO has one and how it selects consumer participants.

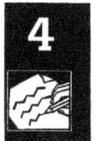

Merger Mania

Health plans, particularly managed care plans, are merging and consolidating at a frantic rate. The plan you join today might become part of another health plan or managed care company tomorrow. Among the possible effects of a merger or takeover on consumers are

Change in covered benefits and/or copayments: When health plans merge, they usually adopt a new, unified benefit package. You could find that your new plan doesn't cover some services in your old plan, or that you have to pay larger copayments for covered services.

Change in provider network: The new plan may not contract with all the physicians or hospitals or other providers in your former plan. While plans generally must give providers notice if the plan wants to end its contract, the notice provisions may be as short as sixty or ninety days.

Conversion of HMO from nonprofit to for-profit status: Many HMOs are converting from nonprofit to for-profit status, often to raise capital through the sale of stock or as part of an acquisition by a for-profit company. Usually,

versations with plan representatives, including the date of your talks, the names and telephone numbers of the people to whom you speak, and a summary of the conversations. Try to talk with the same person each time you call so you can attempt to develop an advocate at the health plan. Be friendly and polite—but persistent. Being assertive often pays off.

If an informal approach doesn't work, many health plans—including most HMOs—have a formal grievance mechanism. Your member contract generally describes how to go about submitting a grievance. You can use this complaint process for any type of problem—for example, if you disagree with a plan's decision to deny your request for certain medical care, if you are dissatisfied with the level of payment made by the plan, or if you have a complaint about the quality of care you received from a plan provider.

Check with your health plan if you are unsure about how to file a complaint or grievance. The plan's rules may require it to respond to any grievance within a given time period.

Talk to Your Employer or Benefits Department

If you belong to the health plan through your employer, you can ask your benefits manager or human-resource department for assistance. Although employers want to limit their health insurance costs, they also usually don't want unhappy employees. Employers can be very powerful allies because they generally represent more than one customer to the health plan. For example, an HMO informed one man that his wife's surgery, scheduled for the next day, wouldn't be covered. He called the president of his company, who contacted the HMO. Just in time, the plan decided it would cover the surgery.

Of course, you will have to decide if you want anyone at your job to have details of your medical problems or those of your family. And if your employer won't, or can't, give you the information you need, go directly to the plan, if you haven't done so already.

Other Options for Complaints

Elicit the support of your health care providers. Ask your doctor and other health care providers to help you document and support your need for services and care. Remember that if the provider is in the provider network, he or she is also an important customer of the health plan.

File a complaint with state regulators. Most health plans are regulated by some state agency, generally the state department of insurance, the department of health, the attorney general's office—or all of these.

While the legal authority and approach of regulators varies from state to state, they may be able to investigate and resolve your complaint. If you have a complaint about the quality of care, you can report it to the appropriate state licensing board. To locate the right regulatory agencies, contact your state insurance department or the National Association of Insurance Commissioners. Every state has insurance counselors to advise older consumers, and many have them for all consumers.

Consult a consumer-advocacy group. The National Insurance Consumer Organization (NICO) has a number of publications, including *The Buyer's Guide to Insurance*. While it doesn't provide direct assistance to consumers, NICO can refer you to your state insurance commissioner for help. NICO, 414 A Street, S.E., Washington, DC 20003. Or contact your state insurance commission directly.

For more information on reaching consumer groups, including a listing of state consumer coalitions, turn to chapter 21.

Go public. Health plans hate negative publicity. If you have tried other approaches, a phone call from an elected official—or even the media in extreme cases—can persuade a health plan to pay for services that it previously denied.

state authorities must approve a conversion, and the charitable assets of the plan must be kept nonprofit and used for the plan's original charitable purposes.

For more information on how mergers might affect you, contact a consumer-advocacy group, such as those listed in chapter 21.

4

The Ten Largest HMO Companies (1994)

Name	Members	Percentage (%) of national enrollment
Kaiser Foundation Health Plans	6,599,043	12.9
CIGNA HealthCare	3,309,335	6.5
United HealthCare	2,751,137	5.4
Prudential HealthCare	2,076,734	4.1
U.S. Healthcare	1,768,094	3.5
FHP, Inc.	1,718,854	3.4
Humana, Inc.	1,589,760	3.1
PacifiCare Health Systems	1,417,018	2.8
Health Systems International	1,339,253	2.6
Aetna Health Plans	1,103,585	2.2

Note: Some HMO companies operate more than one HMO under different names.
Source: Patterns in HMO Enrollment, Group Health Association of America, June 1995

Estimating Your Family's Annual Health Care Costs

Fill out a worksheet like this for each plan you consider. To collect the necessary information, consult the plan or your employer's benefits manager. Use your experience to date as a rough guide to your future health care needs. And consider new needs you may have, such as a planned pregnancy.

Type of Care	Name of Provider	Your Cost Per Use	Uses Per Year	Your Annual Cost
Primary care provider				
OB/GYN				
Prescriptions				
Mental health care				
Substance abuse care				
Hospitalization				
Chronic or home care				
Emergency care				
Other				
		Your annual out-of-pocket costs		
		PLUS Your deductible		
		PLUS Your annual premium contribution		
		Estimated Total Annual Health Care Costs		

Resources
Organizations

National Association of Insurance Commissioners
120 W. 12th Street
Kansas City, MO 64105
(816) 842-3600
The association can direct you to your state's insurance commission.

National Committee for Quality Assurance
2000 L Street, N.W., #500
Washington, DC 20036
(202) 955-3500
Contact NCQA for a copy of its pamphlet, "Choosing Quality: Finding the Health Plan That's Right for You." For a list of health plans accredited by NCQA, call (202) 955-3515 or via the Web:http://www.ncqa.org

U.S. Department of Health and Human Services
Health Care Financing Administration Medicare Information Hotline (800) 888-1770 (recorded message); (800) 888-1988 (to request written material or ask questions)

Publications

Castle Connolly Pocket Guide: How to Find the Best Doctors, Hospitals, and HMOs for You and Your Family (Castle Connolly Medical Ltd., 1995), $9.95.

"Checkup on Health Insurance Choices." Free from Agency for Health Care Policy and Research, P.O. Box 8542, Silver Spring, MD 20907; tel. (800) 358-9295.

Choosing the Right Health Plan, by Henry Berman and Louisa Rose (Consumer Reports Books, 1989), $14.95.

"Consumer's Guide to Health Insurance." Sixteen-page pamphlet available free from Health Insurance Association of America, P.O. Box 41455, Washington, DC 20018; tel. (202) 824-1600.

Consumers' Guide to Health Plans (Center for the Study of Services, 1994), $12. Order from the Center for the Study of Services, 733 15th Street, N.W., Washington, DC 20005; tel. (202) 347-9612.

Fighting Back Health Insurance Denials, by Robert Peterson, with David Tenenbaum, $3.50 plus shipping. Order from Center for Public Representation, 121 South Pinckney Street, Madison, WI 53703; tel. (608) 251-4008.

Health Care Financing: A Guide for Families, by Julie Becket, $5.50 plus $2.50 shipping and handling. Order from National Maternal and Child Health Resource Center, Law Building, University of Iowa, Iowa City, IA 52242; tel. (319) 335-9073.

Health Insurance Made Easy . . . Finally: How to Understand Your Health Insurance So You Start Saving Money and Stop Wasting Your Time, by Sharon L. Stark, $14.95 plus $2 postage and handling. Order from Stark Publishing, P.O. Box 8693, Shawnee Mission, KS 66208.

The HMO Health Care Companion: A Consumer's Guide to Managed Care Networks, by Alan G. Raymond (HarperCollins, 1994), $10.

4

5 Primary Care

Harriet Tolpin

Harriet Tolpin, Ph.D., is Dean of the Graduate School for Health Studies and professor of economics at Simmons College. She is also clinical professor in the department of community health at Tufts University School of Medicine. As a health economist, her interests are the financing, organization, and delivery of health care services.

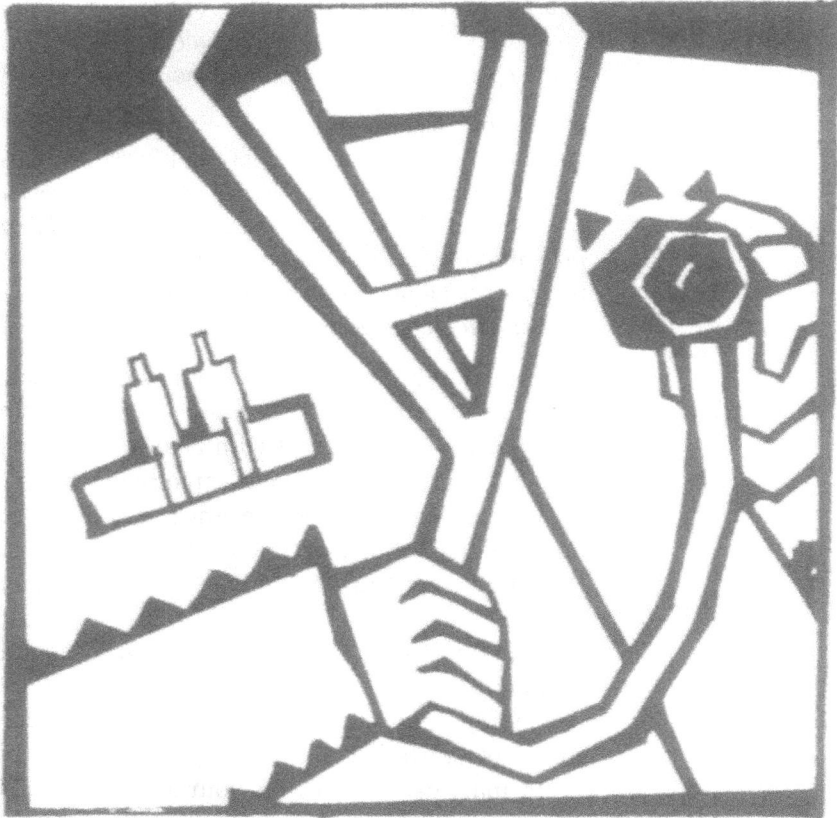

Everyone needs primary care.

■ You and your eight-year-old daughter, Elizabeth, visit your family physician for your annual exams. A discussion of Elizabeth's school problems raises the possibility of attention deficit disorder. *The doctor refers her to a pediatrician who specializes in child development for further evaluation.* In your own exam, the doctor says your weight and blood pressure are a little higher than the year before, and your family has a history of heart attacks. *You and the physician discuss ways to lower your risk. Rather than take medication, you settle on a plan of more exercise and a better diet.*

■ Your father has had mild Alzheimer's disease for several years. Recently, he entered a hospital for treatment of a blood clot in his leg. A routine chest X ray showed that he probably has lung cancer, although it's most likely curable with surgery. He hasn't prepared a living will, and the hospital environment has made him more confused than ever. Do you put him through the ordeal of surgery? *His internist convenes the family and lays out alternatives, including risks and benefits. Jointly, you decide not to operate but to provide more home care after this hospitalization.*

■ At your sister's annual gynecological visit to her nurse practitioner, she complains that she's sleeping poorly and having trouble concentrating. *Your sister and the nurse practitioner review a number of possible causes, leading to a tentative diagnosis of mild depression. They review the pros and cons of different types of treatment. Although the NP favors counseling, your sister opts for medication for the time being. The NP will monitor the medication but suggests a visit to a counselor as well.*

Each of these examples of your family's health needs falls within the province of primary care. Primary care is the appropriate place for you to make your *first* contact with health care providers. It also constitutes your regular source of care on an ongoing basis.

Primary care aims to prevent premature death and disability *and* to enhance your ability to function well and maintain a high quality of life. It focuses on you first as a whole person, and then on specific diseases or illnesses. It works to keep you healthy—by promoting good health and preventing disease as well as by diagnosing and treating illnesses and accidents that do arise. And it's your primary care provider who should collaborate with you to coordinate and manage all your health care— from specialists, social service agencies, and others.

Primary care also lowers your health care bills by detecting an illness early and initiating treatment before the problem becomes more serious and costly to manage. For example, a nurse practitioner's familiarity with you could alert her or him to heart disease that may run in your family or to stress in your life that might affect your health. Familiarity can also lessen the need for tests at each visit and for each condition.

Familiarity Breeds Respect

It's important to get regular checkups, whether you are sick or well, to detect problems early. Just as important, these checkups establish a "baseline" of what healthy means for *you*. When caregivers know you in a healthy state, they're likely to take out-of-the-ordinary complaints more seriously. They gain a better basis for assessing your health and feel safer about recommending treatments.

When you are healthy, providers can focus on you rather than your symptoms. They have time to get to know you, answer your questions, and counsel you about good health.

Primary Care Is . . .

- *Comprehensive:* It focuses on you as a whole person.

- *Coordinated:* It holds together your personal health care system.

- *Continuous:* You need it from birth to death.

- *Accountable:* Your primary care provider works for you. If you have problems with the health care system, a good primary care provider is your first resort—as well as your strong advocate—in obtaining the services you need.

What a Good Primary Care Provider Does

Primary care is your appropriate first point of contact with the health care system. As your care coordinator and care manager, a primary care provider makes sure you receive timely and suitable care from all the various agencies and people in the health care system.

Primary care:

- Promotes and maintains your good health
- Prevents disease and disability
- Detects and treats common health problems
- Educates and counsels patients and families, *and*

■ Refers you to other providers and community agencies when appropriate

This comprehensive approach means that primary care providers deliver any or all of a wide range of specific services at each visit. These include:

■ Physical exams and health histories
■ Health screenings and immunizations
■ Assessments and evaluations of acute illnesses, such as colds and infections
■ Advice on managing common, acute, and chronic conditions, such as flu, ear infections, high blood pressure, and diabetes
■ Prescriptions and instructions for common and acute conditions
■ Prenatal care, family planning, managing normal pregnancies, and delivery
■ Identification of conditions that require more specialized care and referral to the appropriate professionals
■ Counseling on health-related lifestyle factors, such as physical activity, fitness, nutrition, smoking, substance abuse, family planning, and violent or abusive relationships.

One, Two, Three

Primary care refers to first-level or generalist care that you get outside a hospital.

Secondary care, often provided in hospitals and facilities for long term care, makes more use of caregivers with specialized training.

Tertiary care is highly specialized care for severe health problems, such as that given in intensive-care, coronary-care, and trauma units.

Priorities

Until recently, primary care ranked low among the hierarchy of doctor specialties in the United States, but today primary care physicians are in demand. This is partly due to the rise of managed care, which stresses the role of primary care providers.

In California and Minnesota, where managed care is especially prevalent, about half of all doctors "specialize" in primary care. Experts say this is roughly the proper proportion for average communities. Unfortunately, only about one-third of U.S. doctors work in primary care.

Patient-Centered Care

A good primary care provider will ask you questions and share with you responsibility for your health and decisions about it. Primary care fosters a strong partnership between the provider and the patient.
For more information on patient-centered care, turn to chapter 6.

Life Work: Promoting Health and Preventing Disease

Primary care is critical to you, whatever your age, because it emphasizes screening for diseases, immunizations to prevent them, and advice on lifestyles that keep you healthy. Indeed, *Healthy People 2000*, a major federal report, sets out specific national goals for promoting health and preventing disease for people of every age. Many of these goals relate to your access to—and use of—primary care:

Infants. Primary care for pregnant women improves their own health and that of newborns. Comprehensive prenatal care reduces the occurrence of infant deaths and low-birthweight babies. It can also lessen the incidence of infant illnesses that result from the mother's health habits, such as smoking, substance abuse, and poor nutrition.

Children. Primary care helps children stay healthy with immunizations, early detection of developmental problems, timely treatment of infections and respiratory illnesses, and the management of asthma and other chronic conditions. Primary care providers also educate children about the dangers of tobacco and alcohol and the importance of exercise and good eating habits. And through ongoing relationships with children and their parents, primary care providers are in a good position to identify possible child abuse and other threats to children's health and well being.

Adolescents and young adults. Primary care is an important vehicle for improving attitudes and health practices that form in adolescence and continue into adulthood. In particular, education and counseling can address smoking, alcohol and drug use, high-risk sexual behaviors, and depression. Also, the relationship primary care providers develop with their patients as children enables them to work together better during the years of adolescence and early adulthood. This may reduce the risk of suicide, the second leading cause of death among young white men between ages fifteen and twenty-four.
For more information on primary care for children, turn to chapter 8.

Adults. The ongoing relationship between primary care providers and adults offers opportunities to reinforce healthy behavior. For example, cancer, heart disease, stroke, injury, and chronic lung disease are the major causes of death in the United States. Many cases of all these illnesses are preventable or curable. Regular screening of women could reduce deaths from breast cancer by 30 percent; cervical cancer can be cured if detected early by Pap smears. Smoking causes more than 85 percent of all deaths from lung cancer, the most common cancer in the United States for both men and women. Smoking raises the risk of chronic lung disease, heart disease, and stroke as well. The risks of heart disease and stroke also relate to diet and exercise. A primary care provider can encourage people to receive appropriate screenings and to stop high-risk behaviors.

For more information on primary care for adult women, turn to chapter 9; for adult men, turn to chapter 10.

Older adults. People over age sixty-five need primary care to maintain their health and prevent the early onset of life-threatening diseases and conditions. For older adults, primary care includes screening for cancers, immunizations against pneumonia and influenza, control of high blood pressure, counseling to promote healthy behaviors, and management of such chronic conditions as arthritis, osteoporosis, and incontinence. Primary care providers also monitor medications and work with patients to offset depression by recognizing early warning signs.

Elders are especially likely to benefit from the familiarity and coordination of care that primary care providers offer. As people age, they are more likely to have multiple complex problems that require coordination.

For more information on primary care for elders, turn to chapter 11.

Preventable Illness

Two important components of primary care are screening to detect diseases early and patient education and counseling. These proven health strategies can help you avoid disease and reduce your health care costs.

Drug and alcohol abuse, smoking, failure to use seat belts, and unsafe sex are among the behaviors that together account for more than one-fourth of the dollars Americans spend on health care.

Some of the many preventable medical expenses relate to:

■ Heart disease, affecting 7 million people. Bypass surgery costs $30,000.

- The complications of alcoholism; 18.5 million Americans abuse alcohol. A liver transplant costs $250,000.
- Low-birthweight infants; 260,000 are born every year in the United States. The cost is at least $10,000 for intensive care for one infant.

Who Provides Primary Care?

You'll receive primary care from a generalist—a practitioner who can pay attention to all of your body's systems, as well as to factors in your environment that could influence your health. Most often, this person will work in your community, in a location you can reach easily.

At least three types of providers may be trained to provide primary care:

- Physicians
- Physician assistants
- Nurse practitioners

Primary Care Teams

Consider getting primary care from an interdisciplinary team comprising primary care physicians, physician assistants, and nurse practitioners. Additional team members can reflect your individual situation; for example, if you're an older person, the team might include a nutritionist and a social worker.

The team approach enhances your opportunities to receive integrated medical, nursing, and social services. You can find and request teams in many of the settings that provide primary care services—community health centers, some HMOs, and private practices.

Physicians

About 280,000 physicians in the United States deliver primary care, including family physicians and general internists for all adults. Obstetricians/gynecologists often function as primary care providers for women, while pediatricians can fill that role for children. In addition, some physicians have begun to specialize in women's health or geriatrics. These fields have a primary care orientation.

In addition, several types of nontraditional providers do offer primary care. These include naturopaths and chiropractors.

For more information on alternative primary care, turn to chapter 19.

The Limits of Primary Care

While primary care is essential, a generalist's capabilities do have limits:

- It may be difficult for a generalist to know when a particular condition is unusual. Primary care providers may recognize a problem more slowly than would a specialist, in part because a provider who knows you well may be more likely to accept a broader range of conditions as healthy.

- Primary care providers may be familiar with the "whole" you, but they may also be less competent than specialists at treating a particular part of you.

- As the health care system currently operates, no individual or system can coordinate all the needs of a person or family with multiple, complex problems. Inevitably, some concerns fall through the cracks.

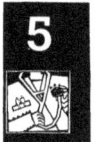

5

Family practitioners receive the broadest training in primary care. They bring to mind the general practitioner you may have grown up with, but their training is far more extensive. Many general practitioners receive no specialist training, whereas family practitioners take extra preparation after medical school in a half dozen fields. As a result, they see the medical, social, and psychological factors affecting health, and they look at both individuals and families as a whole. They can manage the entire range of primary care services, including immunizations, physical exams, medication, and routine pregnancies.

Family practitioners have several advantages as primary care providers. They can care for everyone in your family and recognize problems that arise from interactions in the family. They receive training in psychiatry and the psychological and social aspects of illness. And they can deliver care over the years, working with you from infancy to adulthood through old age.

Family practitioners also have disadvantages as primary care providers. While they must know something about everything, no one can have comprehensive knowledge of every health problem. Any given family practitioner will be more comfortable with certain conditions than with others—although weaknesses and strengths relate more to a person's knowledge, experience, and skill than to the field of family medicine.

Internists can be either generalists or subspecialists. General internists correspond more closely to the definition of primary care providers than do subspecialists, but internists who further specialize in such fields as cardiology (the heart) and oncology (cancer) often serve as primary care providers for their patients.

In their favor as primary care providers, internists have more training than family practitioners in certain types of problems, such as heart disease. They are also more likely to provide total management for adults during a hospitalization.

There are also a few disadvantages of internists as primary care providers. They tend to order more tests than family practitioners. And an internist may not be as comfortable as other primary care providers with the full gamut of health concerns and the factors that contribute to them.

Osteopathic physicians (D.O.'s) provide comprehensive medical care, including preventive medicine, diagnosis, surgery, hospital referrals, prescriptions, and other medications. About 37,000 D.O.'s practice in the

United States, with over 64 percent delivering primary care, compared with 26 percent of M.D.'s. All fifty states license osteopathic physicians to perform surgery and prescribe medications, and hospitals grant privileges to both M.D.'s and D.O.'s.

Osteopathic medicine rests on the theory that the entire body must be considered when treating disease. It focuses on preventive care, emphasizes the interrelationship of structure and function, and has an appreciation of the body's ability to heal itself. In diagnosis and treatment, osteopathic physicians pay particular attention to the patient as a person—a holistic approach. In addition, they are specially trained in osteopathic manipulative treatment—using their hands to diagnose, treat, and prevent illness.

Allopathic Medicine vs. Osteopathic Medicine

While osteopathic physicians (D.O.'s) are sometimes considered to offer "alternative health care" because of their holistic orientation, they share much the same scientific foundation as allopathic physicians (M.D.'s). For example, D.O.'s apply the same standard methods of diagnosis and treatment as M.D.'s, and specialize in the same fields as allopathic physicians. In fact, these specialists are often board certified by the American Osteopathic Association as well as the American Medical Association.

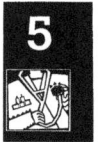

5

Specialists as Primary Care Providers

Certain specialists perform some of the functions of primary care providers—for example, coordinating and managing care during a major illness. However, it's still important to have a regular primary care provider if at all possible—that is, a person who comes to know you well over the years.

Physician Assistants

Physician assistants provide diagnostic and therapeutic medical services. Most PAs have three or more years of college-level education, with additional specialized schooling and on-the-job training. A physician always directs or supervises a PA.

Physician assistants take health histories, perform comprehensive physical exams and minor surgery, order and complete routine diagnostic tests, develop diagnostic and management plans, treat common illnesses, counsel patients on staying healthy, and facilitate referrals to local health care and social service agencies. In some states, they can prescribe certain medications. They also may specialize and receive certification in specific fields, such as women's health.

Advanced Practice Nurses

Advanced practice nurses can provide primary and preventive care services. And like physician assistants, they usually do so at a lower cost than doctors. Currently, more than 100,000 nurses provide primary care in the United States.

Nurse practitioners. NPs, the major nonphysician providers of primary care, provide a full range of primary care services. They can assess your general physical condition, diagnose and treat common illnesses and injuries, educate you in ways to promote health and prevent disease, and coordinate your care. NPs train as generalists but some specialize in caring for particular groups: newborns, children, women, adults, employees, families, or elders. Many studies have documented the cost-effectiveness of nurse practitioners, the high quality of care they provide, and the satisfaction of their patients.

Of the 25,000 to 30,000 nurse practitioners in the United States, most practice in community settings—neighborhood health centers, worksites, and family-planning clinics, for example. They provide care independently or in collaboration with physicians.

Individual states have the authority to determine whether or not NPs may practice independently. At least thirty-six states require NPs to be nationally certified by the American Nurses Association or a specialty nursing organization. In at least thirty-five states, NPs prescribe medications.

Certified nurse-midwives. CNMs provide primary care for pregnant women. With specialized education beyond nursing school, they offer prenatal and gynecological care, deliver babies in homes, hospitals, and birthing centers, and care for a mother in the months after she gives birth. CNMs refer complicated cases to physicians, consult with physicians, or work jointly with them. They also counsel women on family planning and provide postnatal care for normal newborns and infants born without major health problems.

CNMs often collaborate with physicians. Individual states determine the regulations for scope of practice.

Finding Primary Care

Primary care services are generally offered through:

- Private practices
- Outpatient clinics
- HMOs
- Neighborhood health centers, *and*
- Community sites such as workplaces and schools

One for All?

It's often more efficient to use one primary care provider for everyone in your family. Among other things, the provider will learn about family interactions that affect the health of each member.

On the other hand, some people prefer separate providers. For example, a child could feel less inclined to confide in a doctor who might share too much information with his or her parents—and vice versa.

Private Practices

Traditionally, primary care takes place in an office in your community. A physician may practice alone or in conjunction with a nurse practitioner or physician assistant. More often, physicians work in group practices, with several physicians and other health professionals who offer primary care. Sometimes several specialists are part of the practice, and some primary care providers are on the staff of health plans or other health care organizations.

Group practices may offer you several pluses:

- More of your needs will be met at a single location, especially if it includes several specialists.
- Information is more easily shared—and tests less often repeated—than when referrals occur among isolated practitioners.
- Care tends to be better coordinated.

On the other hand, large group practices can be hectic and more people have access to your medical record, which may threaten confidentiality. With a small practice, you're more likely to have privacy and see the same doctor each visit. Moreover, modern communications and other technology can bring many benefits of group practices into the offices of private practitioners even in isolated areas.

Consumer Alert: Outpatient Clinics, Ambulatory Care Centers, and Primary Care

Hospital outpatient clinics typically provide specialty care that doesn't require an overnight stay in the hospital. Usually, the clinics are located in the hospital.

As a source of primary care, however, hospital outpatient clinics offer few advantages to the consumer:

- They focus on disease and treatment rather than on promoting wellness.
- A clinic focuses on a particular set of conditions, not on the whole person.
- Most facilities follow up on inpatient hospital stays rather than deliver primary care.

Ambulatory care centers, sometimes referred to as "doc-in-the-box medicine," are convenient for routine problems, such as cuts, sprains, and respiratory infections. Usually created and owned by physicians or hospitals, they provide walk-in service and offer evening and weekend hours.

Do not substitute ambulatory care centers for a primary care provider. These centers don't take responsibility for either ongoing care or coordinating a variety of health care needs. Rather, they handle routine conditions *if* your primary care provider isn't immediately available—for example, when you're away on vacation.

Consumer Alert: Primary Care and Emergency Rooms

Consumers without a regular source of primary care—both people with health insurance and those without it—often go to a hospital emergency department for basic care. This is inappropriate, costly, and generally unsatisfying. Perhaps most significantly for you, the staff lacks a primary care provider's invaluable knowledge of you, your medical history, and your medical records.

Even worse, many people, especially those without health insurance, call the fire department for emergency medical care!

Community Health Centers

Community health centers play a major role in primary care, especially but not exclusively for the poor and the uninsured. Also known as neighborhood health centers, public health clinics, and community health clinics, these organizations have strong local roots and serve communities with accessible and affordable health care.

An interdisciplinary team often provides care at community health centers—to the benefit of patients. Moreover, many centers offer excellent services that address language, culture, finances, transportation, and other barriers that make it hard for some people to get good health care. Most centers are affiliated with nearby hospitals.

To an even greater extent than other primary care providers, health centers emphasize public health, seeking to improve the health status of their communities as a whole. As integral members of the communities in which they are located, health centers maintain ties with other neighborhood organizations, such as schools, churches, and social service agencies. These organizations and the health centers often collaborate in projects to educate people about particular health problems and high-risk behaviors such as domestic violence and substance abuse.

Managed Care and Primary Care

"Staff model" HMOs typically have facilities that resemble large multi-specialty group practices or community health centers. Because such facilities also often handle minor surgeries and such diagnostic services as laboratory tests and X rays, they offer "one stop" health care for members. Also, they tend to have nurse practitioners on staff who collaborate with physicians.

HMOs are built on a foundation of primary care—it's the "health maintenance" part of their name. However, there is a growing concern that pressures to control costs in HMOs and other managed care organizations limit the time primary care providers can spend with patients, reducing the opportunity for education and counseling. Moreover, primary care providers in some HMOs make less money if they refer patients to a specialist. This potentially puts the doctor's financial self-interest and the patient's health into conflict. As an educated consumer in an HMO, consider this potential conflict and make sure you receive the attention you deserve.

Most doctors in solo and group private practices participate in one or more managed care networks, and the number of physicians is rising rapidly. Such organizations rely heavily on primary care providers to manage and coordinate their patients' care.

For more information on managed care, turn to chapter 4.

TIP

Care for Everyone

Community health centers are open to everyone, regardless of income or insurance. They attract patients of diverse ages, incomes, and backgrounds, and most consumers find that they excel at delivering high-quality, affordable care for the entire family.

5

TIP
Personal Preferences

Your choice of a primary care provider is personal. Weigh *your* preferences in such matters as a provider's age, gender, or personality.

Be realistic, however. Basically, most consumers want a primary care provider to be highly ethical and skilled, with superior training, availability, and compassion.

At Work and School

In recent years, many employers have developed employee health services that provide some primary care services, including screening, counseling, and education about lifestyle behavior. And some large companies have developed primary health care centers that provide basic care close to the worksite and offer a wide range of services, including physical therapy, pharmacy, radiology, and some laboratory services.

Another new initiative is the introduction of health clinics into schools to improve primary health care for adolescents. Most often, the clinics are in middle and high schools.

Choosing Your Primary Care Provider

Choosing a primary care provider is one of the most important decisions a consumer makes. The person you select will be responsible for managing all your health care—day to day and year to year. Trust and rapport, in addition to professional training and technical competence, are leading qualities for you to consider.

It's important to select a primary care provider who will accept you as a partner in your care. You'll feel more in control and participate more fully in health care decisions that affect you and your family. This can make diagnosing problems easier, lead to the most appropriate care, improve your response to treatment, and speed your recovery.

In choosing your primary care provider, look for a person who communicates well with you. Good communication with your primary care provider is critical to the patient-provider partnership. You want a primary care provider who is open to your questions, asks your opinion about your symptoms, gives you advice on staying healthy, discusses the potential side effects of prescribed medications, and encourages you to talk about whatever concerns you may have.

Getting Started

In most cases, step one in selecting a primary care provider is to examine your health insurance, consulting your employer's benefits manager if you get insurance through your job. Does it restrict your choice in any way? For example, does your plan pay for the services of nurse practitioners and certified nurse midwives? HMOs, other health insurers, and public programs such as Medicare and Medicaid determine which providers are eligible for reimbursement and for what specific services.

If you belong to a managed care plan, you'll probably choose a primary care provider from a list of affiliated practitioners or clinics. The member-services department will give you information on the plan's primary care providers to help you decide. This information often includes a provider's training and availability. However, it might not cover many other facts you really want to know—for example, the provider's skill, knowledge, and "track record." In any case, state your preferences, if any, on matters like age, gender, and training—and be willing to exercise your option to change providers.

Some health insurance plans require you to get a primary care physician to authorize specialist services. Such plans may place few limits on your choice of provider—and give you little information to help with your choice.

For more information on insurance, turn to chapter 4.

No matter how you pay for primary care, consider many factors in choosing a primary care provider. Talk to your friends, look in the library for medical directories and other reference materials, and call each provider's office. Ask your relatives and friends about their primary care providers. Gather information from other consumers who use—or have used—particular primary care providers.

For guidance on finding candidates for your primary care providers, turn to the sidebar on page 84.

At this stage, you may already have a list of several possible providers. Which ones accept new patients? For those that do, find out more. If one person stands out, proceed to get answers to all the questions that are important to you:

■ Does he or she deliver *primary care?* For adults? For children? For both? Does he or she treat the whole family (if that's what you want)?

■ Does he or she focus on areas of particular relevance to your health concerns and those of your family, such as women's health, adolescent health, or elder care?

■ What is his or her training?

■ Is this a group or an individual practice? How likely is it that you'll see the provider you want in a group or team practice? Can you decide whom to see? Can you benefit from a team perspective?

■ With which hospitals is the provider affiliated?

■ What is the provider's reputation with other physicians? With patients?

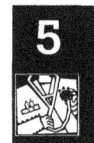

Finding Candidates

Despite the shortage of people trained in primary care, in most communities you can choose from a number of health professionals. Don't feel compelled to accept the first one you contact.

To compile a roster of potential primary care providers:

■ Ask friends, colleagues, and any medical personnel you know whom they use.

■ Contact local hospitals, medical schools, and nursing programs. They'll identify providers on their staffs or in affiliated group practices.

■ Contact a referral service, whether a local nonprofit agency, a hospi-

■ Does the office provide other services that may be important to you, such as interpreters, relationships with social service agencies, hours that fit your schedule, and arrangements for watching your children while you are with the doctor or nurse?

■ Is the practice easily accessible? Is it open evenings or weekends? Does the provider make house calls if you can't get to the office? Can you readily get advice on the telephone, both before scheduling an appointment and for follow-up advice? What diagnostic facilities are available on site, such as laboratory and X-ray facilities?

Credential Check

Although quality is central to your choice of a primary care provider, judging it is extremely difficult. Two indirect—and imperfect—indicators are education and experience. Did a person train specifically as a primary care provider? Also, check for evidence that she or he tries to stay current through continuing professional education: board certification and recertification suggests this (although they may actually indicate knowledge rather than skill in applying it). About two-thirds of physicians are board certified these days, compared to 46 percent twenty years ago. Credentialing organizations also certify increasing numbers of advanced practice nurses.

Check for the dates of graduation and certification. Some consumers prefer a recent date, implying up-to-date training; others look for more years of experience.

For information on education and credentials, a variety of sources may prove useful, including medical and nursing directories and state licensing boards.

Also, find out whether a provider teaches in a medical school or nursing program. Teaching indicates that a provider's colleagues consider a person knowledgeable in a particular field.

The Try-Out

When you narrow your list of potential providers to one name, make an appointment. Use this visit to decide if you feel that you can establish a comfortable relationship of trust and mutual respect with this individual. Remember, you are looking not only for someone to provide medical care but for a partner and a strong advocate in the health care system. (Some people who can afford it try out two or three providers. The point is to find a person you *want* to work with, rather than one who will merely suffice.)

A visit helps you judge the atmosphere of the office, even if you don't arrange for a regular appointment or full physical examination. Does the office appear well organized and efficient? Is the staff friendly on the phone and in person? Do interactions among the staff and between staff and patients seem smooth? If the answers are yes, you have a better chance of receiving quality care. Your health will benefit from good record keeping, shorter waiting times, and enough time with caregivers.

Find out who handles routine calls and matters: Is it a doctor, a nurse practitioner, or someone else? It's important that whoever handles such calls has access to the information necessary to respond appropriately. It's also important that you have direct access to the person ultimately responsible for your care in nonroutine and emergency situations.

If you do schedule a regular appointment, *ask a potential primary care provider:*

- What is your approach to health maintenance?
- What do you routinely check for?
- How often will I need regular checkups?
- What tests do you routinely perform and why?
- Can a friend or family member be in the exam or consulting room with me?
- Who covers for you if you are unavailable? What is his or her training or specialty?

In addition, use the checklist below to help you make a decision before, during, and after your visit. Remember, look for a person who can provide high-quality health care and be your partner and advocate in the health care system.

tal-based service, or a for-profit agency. Referral services may be listed in the Yellow Pages under the headings for "Hospitals" and "Physicians and Surgeons Referral and Information Bureaus."

■ Consult publications such as the *American Medical Directory, Directory of Osteopathic Physicians,* and the *Official ABMS Directory of Board Certified Medical Specialists.* These are available in many libraries.

■ Consult your state or local medical and nursing societies for names of certified primary care providers in your community.

■ Consult a local consumer's guide, if one is available.

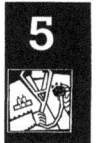

5

Checklist: Choosing a Primary Care Provider

✓ Does the primary care provider take enough time to learn about you and your family, or does she or he act rushed and impatient?

✓ Does the initial health assessment include questions about your lifestyle and your health habits?

✓ Does the provider's philosophy toward medical care include a strong commitment to prevention?

✓ Does the primary care provider encourage you to ask questions, and are your questions answered satisfactorily?

TIP

In an Emergency

Can you reach your primary care provider in an emergency? Make sure you'll have an effective system for covering emergencies *twenty-four hours a day.*

Registering a Complaint

The best place to lodge an initial complaint about care or bills is with the primary care provider. Everyone makes mistakes and deserves a chance to learn from and correct them. If you make the complaint in writing, keep a copy. If you pursue a problem further with the provider, send a certified letter and request a reply within ten days. If it's a billing dispute, include a copy of the bill, keeping the original in your files.

Address more serious, recurrent, or unresolved grievances to the insurance company, HMO administration, or the state medical board. Use legal action only as a last resort or in the most serious cases of negligence or harm.

For more information on registering a complaint about a health care provider, turn to chapter 3.

✓ Does the primary care provider share information with you that is relevant to your current and future health?
✓ Does he or she explain the reasons for all tests and treatments?
✓ Does the provider seem to prefer to teach or to give orders?
✓ Does he or she present you with options and welcome your efforts to participate in all decisions about your health care?
✓ Does the provider offer you a copy of your medical record?
✓ Does the office appear well organized and efficient?
✓ Do interactions among the staff and between staff and patients seem smooth?

Forging the Partnership

Your real responsibility as a health care consumer doesn't end once you choose a primary care provider. Developing and maintaining a strong working relationship with the person you select is critical to your good health.

For primary care to be effective, this relationship must be one of trust, cooperation, and support. Primary care is a joint enterprise. You need to feel comfortable talking frankly and openly with your primary care provider, and vice versa. It's up to you to disclose all relevant information, including your chief complaints, symptoms, worries, current medications, family circumstances, and any history of alcohol or drug abuse. And it's your responsibility to ask questions, follow advice, and notify the primary care provider if problems arise. The provider's responsibilities include presenting you with your full range of options and inviting you to express your values and preferences concerning them. These are ethical and legal obligations.

Before every appointment:

■ Plan your visit.
■ Determine the most important issues you want the appointment to address.
■ Be familiar with your own and your family's medical history.
■ Assemble any written records of your health care since your last appointment.
■ Write down questions as you think of them.

At the appointment:

■ Be as specific as possible.
■ Ask for explanations of diagnoses and treatments.
■ Ask for written summaries of X rays and other tests.

- Volunteer facts you think may have been missed.
- Ask for drugs to be prescribed by generic name.

Consider bringing a friend or relative with you to all appointments, not just the initial visit. He or she can help you ask questions and take notes about instructions the primary care provider gives you.

Money Matters

Health maintenance, or preventive care, can help you feel better and enjoy your life. It is also efficient and economical. It costs far less to prevent most health conditions or to treat illnesses early than to deal with them when they become more serious. Prevention and early action reduce the expenses associated with tests, medications, hospital stays, and sometimes even surgery and other expensive procedures that may accompany acute illnesses.

Primary Care and Insurance

Even for healthy consumers who aren't at high risk for particular diseases and illnesses, coverage for physical exams, health assessments, and screenings varies from plan to plan, as does coverage for wellness programs and other health-maintenance activities. When you are considering a new primary care provider, check:

- Will the provider deal with your insurance carrier?
- How do the provider's fees compare with what your insurance will pay?

Generally, insurance plans and HMOs cover those primary care services that relate to diagnosing and treating common acute and chronic conditions. The typical benefit package also includes immunizations. Follow-up visits for the ongoing management of common and chronic conditions are also typically covered. You'll usually make a small copayment for these services.

Generally, HMOs offer more comprehensive primary care benefits than do other insurers. HMOs encourage wellness and health maintenance through a variety of mechanisms that may include patient education, wellness programs, nutrition counseling, and vaccinations and other screening tests. Participation in these activities may require a small payment from you.

TIP

Print or Type

Ask your doctor to follow the recommendation of the American Medical Association to print or type prescriptions. Poor handwriting on prescriptions leads to more illnesses, longer hospital stays, and even death.

5

TIP

Ask in Advance

- What is the cost for an initial office visit, consultation, or exam?

- What is the cost for a routine office visit?

If You Lack Insurance . . .

For people who must pay out of pocket for their health care, primary care often seems a luxury rather than a necessity. People with no regular source of care typically enter the health care system through an emergency room when a health problem becomes acute or life-threatening. They also often forgo necessary services related to managing chronic conditions.

There are options. In particular, you can find quality providers that charge less for services, such as community health centers. Moreover, most health centers charge sliding-scale fees based on income, making them affordable for people without insurance.

In addition, you can seek help from special programs that pay for health care services for those

All HMOs and many insurance plans, especially those with managed care features, now require a primary care provider, generally a physician, to authorize the services of a specialist. Primary care providers thus act as "gatekeepers" who give approval for a patient to move into other parts of the health care system. This makes the relationship between you and your primary care provider even more central to all of your care.

For more information on specialists, turn to chapter 13.

Pioneers

The inclusion of health promotion and disease prevention in benefit packages is a relatively recent phenomenon. It rests on the idea that preventing illness costs the insurer less than treating it, and insurers structure their benefits accordingly.

The Smart Consumer

You can take a number of steps to save money, especially if your health insurance doesn't cover primary care. Even if it does, you can often save on your portion of the bill.

Ask about the fees for certain procedures in the office of a provider you are considering. The American Medical Association recommends that doctors post fees prominently, but if the information isn't visible, don't hesitate to ask. You might get fee information over the phone, but you may have to go to the office.

Here are a few other steps you can take:

■ Schedule a preliminary visit just to meet the provider. Such a visit might be free, but even if there is a charge, it's probably worth the investment in your future health.

■ Shop around. Prices vary from city to city as well as within any community. The national average for a complete physical is $103, while in New York City it's $265.

■ Don't shop around endlessly. You could organize your search by interviewing three recommended providers in a relatively short time period. Keep a list of attributes you consider the most important and use them to compare the providers.

■ Don't use a specialist for primary care. It's expensive, and most specialists aren't trained in this area.

■ If you can, contact your primary care provider before going to an emergency room.

Typical Physician Charges for a Complete Physical

Boston	$148
New York	$265
Washington	$147
Phoenix	$111
National average	$103

Source: Medirisk

Resources
Organizations

American Academy of Family Physicians
8880 Ward Parkway
Kansas City, MO 64114
(816) 333-9700
Call or write for referrals to family physicians and a publications catalogue.

American Academy of Nurse Practitioners
P.O. Box 40013
Washington, DC 20016
(202) 966-6414
Call or write for publications on what nurse practitioners do, the quality of care they provide, and why they are cost-effective. Also contact the AANP for referrals to local NPs.

American Academy of Physician Assistants
950 N. Washington Street
Alexandria, VA 22314
(703) 836-2272
Call or write for publications and for referrals to local PAs.

American Medical Association
Physician Data Services

525 N. State Street
Chicago, IL 60610
Write for a profile of any member of the AMA. The profile will include the person's medical education, specialty, board certifications, location of internship and residency, AMA membership, and any successful malpractice lawsuits. Send a written request with the doctor's name, address, specialty, and other pertinent information. Include a self-addressed envelope.

American Osteopathic Association
142 E. Ontario St.
Chicago, IL 60611
(800) 621-1773
Contact the AOA for information about osteopathic medicine. For referrals to osteopathic physicians, call ext. 7401.

Medical Data Source
5959 W. Century Boulevard, #1000
Los Angeles, CA 90045
(310) 641-3111
(800) 776-4MDS
Call for an annual membership and to receive comprehensive, easy-to-use information on medical conditions, prescription drugs, and physician backgrounds, and for referrals to local health facilities, such as nursing homes, rehabilitation centers, and support groups. Subscription rates vary depending on the level of service you choose—usually not more than $48 per year.

Mediguard/Medirisk, Inc.
Two Piedmont Center
3565 Piedmont Road
Atlanta, GA 30305
(404) 364-6700
Medirisk, Inc., supplies physician fees and other health care information to subscribing payers, providers, manufacturers, and self-insured employers.

National Association of Community Health Centers

unable to pay themselves. A call to legal-services offices or to the state department of health, public health, human services, or public welfare can help you find out about such programs.

TIP
Use Ma Bell

If you can, get advice over the phone from your doctor or nurse instead of scheduling a visit. Ask a potential provider if he or she gives help by phone and what the charge is, if any.

5

1330 New Hampshire Avenue, N.W.
Washington, DC 20036
(202) 659-8008
Call or write for information on and referrals to community health centers.

National Clearinghouse for Primary
    Care Information
8201 Greensboro Drive
McLean, VA 22102
(703) 821-8955
The clearinghouse provides a wide variety of publications on primary care, mostly for administrators and practitioners, although a few publications on AIDS and on medicines for elders are geared to consumers. Call or write for a list of publications.

Prologue/Consumer Health Services
(800) DOCTORS
Call for free physician referrals in Chicago, Dallas/Ft. Worth, Denver, Houston, Kansas City, Miami/Ft. Lauderdale, Philadelphia, Pittsburgh, and Washington, D.C. This service matches patients and doctors on over 500 variables, such as gender, specialty, location, hospital affiliation, and age. Doctors pay to be included, with about 30 percent of doctors listed.

Publications

American Medical Directory (American Medical Association, 1988). Available in many libraries.

Examining Your Doctor: A Patient's Guide to Avoiding Harmful Medical Care, by Dr. Timothy B. McCall (Birch Lane Press, 1995), $22.50. Available in bookstores, by calling (800) 447-BOOK, or through *Consumer Reports* magazine.

Healthy People 2000 (U.S. Department of Health and Human Services), $25.75 plus $4 for shipping and handling. Order from National Health Information Center, P.O. Box 1133, Washington, DC 20012-1133; tel. (301) 565-4167.

"How Is Your Doctor Treating You," in *Consumer Reports,* February 1995.

How to Choose a Doctor, edited by Michael Rooney, $4 plus $3 for shipping and handling. Order from People's Medical Society, 462 Walnut Street, Allentown, PA 18102; tel. (800) 624-8773.

How to Talk to Your Doctor: The Questions to Ask, by Janet Maurer (Simon & Schuster, 1986), available in many libraries.

Smart Patient, Good Medicine: Working with Your Doctor to Get the Best Medical Care, by Richard L. Sribnick and Wayne B. Sribnick (Walker and Co., 1994), $8.95.

6 Hospitals

Joseph Restuccia, Alan Labonte, and Jeffrey Gelb

Joseph Restuccia, D.P.H., is professor of health care and operations management at Boston University School of Management. He also holds faculty appointments at the university's medicine and public health schools. His work focuses on issues pertinent to health care quality and productivity.

Alan Labonte has twenty years of experience in hospital management. He is currently a doctoral candidate and research associate at Boston University School of Management.

Jeffrey Gelb, M.D., is a physician with clinical training in general and orthopedic surgery. He is medical director for Total Learning Concepts, Inc., developing multimedia educational materials on medicine and managed care.

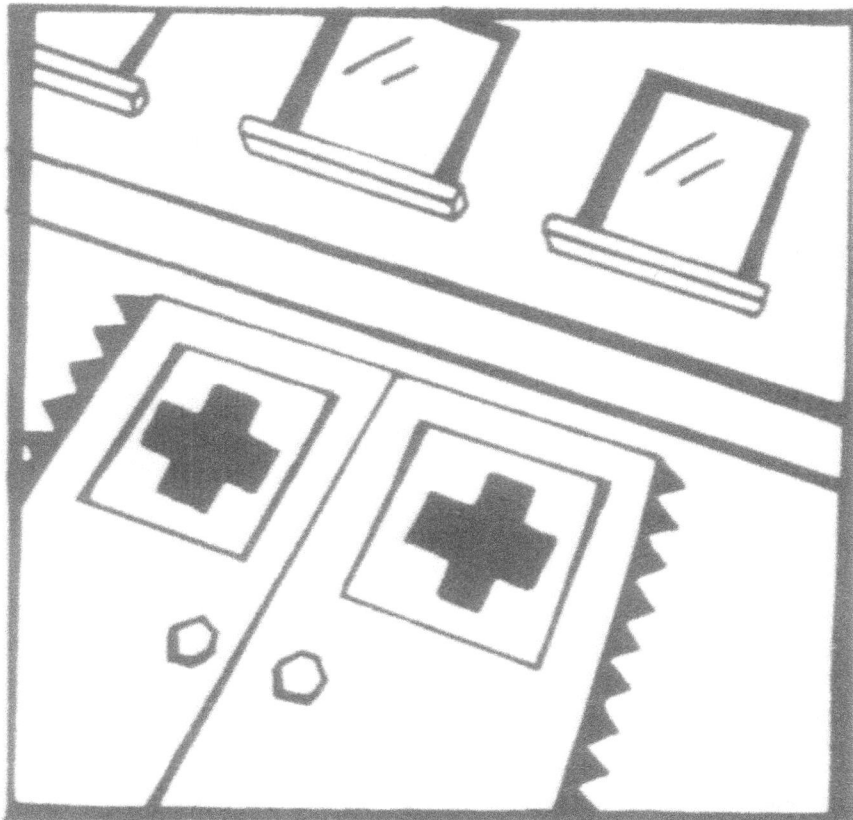

TIP

Take Charge

Don't let medical person-
nel treat you like a child.
They may have more
medical training, but you
are in charge of your
own care. It's your body.

Who Does What

You have a right
to know about
the doctors and other
caregivers working with
them, including their
training. Every hospital
employee wears a tag
showing his or her name
and title. If a person isn't
wearing a tag, ask why
not and make a note of
his or her name. And if
you don't know a doctor
who comes to your
room, be prepared to
refuse care from him or
her. Otherwise, you might
be charged for the visit.

The doctors at nonteach-
ing hospitals are mainly
attending physicians who
also practice outside the
hospital. Each physician is
fully responsible for the
patients he or she admits,
with other physicians acting as consultants. Non-
teaching hospitals also
have a small number of
hospital-based physicians
on their staff, mainly to
provide emergency care,
radiology, anesthesiology,
and pathology services.
They also may help man-
age the hospital.

Western hospitals date from medieval times when monks provided hospitality and care for weary and sick travelers. In fact, the word hospital derives from the Latin word for guest. How different those welcoming images are from the high-tech, fast-paced, and seemingly impersonal institutions of today.

Fortunately, some of the anxiety about hospitals can fade if you know how they are organized. With careful planning and knowledge, you can be a valuable—and valued—partner with your hospital and the team of caregivers you encounter there.

As with many of your health care choices, the time to learn about hospitals is when you are well and in a position to make a careful, informed, and objective decision. Try to get a sense now of your family's potential need for hospital care, taking into account current illnesses or conditions, your family's medical history, your insurance coverage—and your personal preferences.

The Hospital: A Capsule View

Most hospitals handle patients in two basic ways:

- *Inpatients* stay in the hospital overnight.
- *Outpatients* visit the hospital for a specific treatment, procedure, or test but don't stay overnight.

The Varieties of Hospitals

Most hospitals fit into one of two main categories: general medical-surgical and specialty. There are several varieties of the latter, including psychiatric, rehabilitation, and chronic disease hospitals. Within all the categories, hospitals can be teaching or nonteaching, for-profit or nonprofit, small community-based facilities or large tertiary care centers serving whole metropolitan areas.

The vast majority of the community and specialty hospitals in the United States can provide the care you need when you are sick or injured. Many hospitals also encourage medical research, educate doctors and other health care professionals, and promote public health through such programs as prenatal education. Some hospitals emphasize one goal, but most address a combination of goals.

Dear Diary

Write down all the hospital care you receive *as you receive it*. A friend or family member can help with this. Record the dates you are in the hospital and the dates and nature of the services you receive, including tests, prescriptions, doctor visits, and so on.

Teaching and Nonteaching Hospitals

A *teaching hospital* is affiliated with a medical school and has a teaching program for medical students, interns, and residents. Some teaching hospitals have schools of nursing and train other health-related professions as well.

Many teaching hospitals are also *community hospitals*. A community hospital primarily serves its local area with general medical and surgical services. About 5,300 hospitals in the United States are community hospitals.

For severe problems, *tertiary care hospitals*—usually major teaching hospitals—provide highly specialized services, such as that given in intensive-care, coronary-care, and trauma units. Community hospitals that aren't equipped to handle such cases often refer acute-care patients to tertiary hospitals.

From the consumer's point of view, the principal strength of a teaching hospital lies in its ability to provide round-the-clock physician services and highly sophisticated technology and medical techniques. Interns and residents—the "house staff"—manage day-to-day care under the guidance and supervision of fully trained in-house "attending physicians" who are members of the hospital and medical-school faculty.

Despite the temptation, don't automatically select a prestigious teaching hospital as your family's primary hospital. You and your physician may very well prefer a smaller hospital that is close to your home. The quality at smaller community hospitals often compares to that at large teaching institutions, particularly for routine illnesses or surgeries. And the accessibility of a local hospital for family and friends is also important: The support of loved ones can be integral to healing.

Specialty and General Hospitals

About a thousand hospitals *specialize*—that is, they treat a specific category of patient or patients with a specific type of disease or condition. You can find hospitals dedicated to a number of special purposes or constituencies, such as cancer, psychiatry, rehabilitation, orthopedics, elders, and children. If someone in your family has a chronic condition that warrants ongoing, specialized medical support and access to the latest treatment, talk to your current providers about establishing a relationship with a hospital specializing in that condition.

In a teaching hospital, you'll receive care from attending physicians plus first-year residents (interns), advanced residents, physicians gaining advanced training in a specialty or subspecialty (fellows), and full-time teaching faculty who may also be attending physicians.

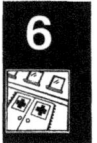

6

Contracting Resources

The number of community hospitals is declining due to attrition, takeovers, mergers, and, most significant, the fact that far fewer procedures now require an overnight stay.

The proportion of specialty hospitals in the United States is declining as well. Hospitals are finding that they need to offer wider services to survive in today's competitive health care marketplace.

With fewer hospitals to choose among, it becomes more important to be an informed consumer. In 1994, 735 hospitals were involved in mergers and acquisitions.

Has your local hospital merged with another one in town or with a chain? Or is the hospital contemplating some type of joint venture in the future? You may want to investigate the following questions to determine how you and your community might benefit or lose:

■ Would my local hospital remain open?

■ Would the merger change a nonprofit hospital into a for-profit one? Would this affect the services it offers? Would this

However, specialty hospitals may be far from your home and lack the facilities and staff necessary to treat unrelated medical complications. Even if you use a specialty hospital for one problem, think about your family's general medical care. Select a primary care physician and a hospital that will work together to address your family's needs.

For-Profit and Nonprofit Hospitals

A hospital can be owned by a city, a county, a state, the federal government, a church, investors, or a nonprofit corporation.

For-profit hospitals are owned by corporations or, less often, by individuals, such as doctors who practice at the hospital. Hospital corporations usually own a chain of institutions located in several states, and they often own nursing homes or other types of health care facilities as well. The largest companies now own hundreds of hospitals and other health care facilities.

Nonprofit hospitals are owned by private nonprofit corporations, as well as by cities, states, the federal government, and church groups. Sometimes, the nonprofit "owners" hire for-profit companies to manage the hospital.

Some studies suggest that for-profit hospitals make much of their money by *cream-skimming*—targeting patients who are fully insured and have less serious illnesses. Other studies point to a lower quality of care in for-profits as a result of lower employee-to-bed ratios than nonprofit hospitals. In response, for-profit hospitals maintain that their profits and lower staffing ratios derive from efficiency.

In fact, most studies have found for-profit and nonprofit hospitals to be similar in efficiency and quality. Both types receive most of their revenue from insurance companies. And except for hospitals owned by local governments, neither nonprofits nor for-profits provide much "free care." Thus, check the facts about *each* hospital individually, seeking the best providers and the best care, whether it's at a nonprofit or a for-profit institution.

Hospitals for Veterans and Their Families

Millions of Americans have access to the 174 hospitals and clinics run by the federal Department of Veterans Affairs. Tailored to veterans, the hospitals are typically affiliated with medical schools and staffed by the school's faculty, residents, interns, and students.

Advantages of VA hospitals include free care or reduced rates for veterans, programs for abuse of alcohol or drugs, and access to specialty care. Among the downsides are the bureaucracy, the increased likelihood of receiving care from physicians in training, and the possibility of having to travel far for specialty care.

For more information about VA facilities and your eligibility to use them, contact the Department of Veterans Affairs, Washington, DC 20420.

Veteran's Resource

The Department of Veterans Affairs has an excellent guide called *Federal Benefits for Veterans and Dependents.* This 96-page handbook describes federal benefits such as medical care, education, and disability compensation. It explains the eligibility requirements for different benefits and provides addresses and phone numbers for all VA offices, medical centers, and other facilities.

To order a copy, send $3.25 to the Superintendent of Documents, Government Printing Office, Washington, DC 20402-9325; tel. (202) 512-1800. Refer to stock number 051-000-00-198-2.

Outpatient Care

If you imagine a hospital in your future, you probably picture an overnight stay. However, this isn't all—or even most—of what many hospitals provide today. Outpatient care is a major part of the services provided by hospitals: Americans made 383 million outpatient visits to community hospitals in 1994, up from 212 million in 1984. In contrast, Americans spent 207 million days in community hospitals in 1994, down from 257 million a decade earlier. About 88 percent of community hospitals provide some form of outpatient care.

The Emergency Room

The most common outpatient service in a hospital is the emergency room. The staff there treat and manage patients who suddenly become seriously ill or injured. Emergencies include severe and uncontrollable bleeding, severe burns from heat or chemicals, bullet or stab wounds, unconsciousness, a drug overdose, a temperature over 103°F, eye injuries, and more.

Hospital emergency rooms are required by law to care for everyone who comes in for help. The emergency-room staff makes a judgment call

affect the amount of free care it provides?

■ Would any departments close, such as the emergency room or outpatient clinics?

■ Would the merger create additional local services?

■ Would the merger affect ethical health care decisions at my local hospital, such as those concerning abortions?

■ Would the merger affect my insurance coverage?

■ Would the new owners be concerned about my community?

For more information, contact the Center for Community Health Action, c/o Families USA/Boston, 30 Winter Street, Boston, MA 02108.

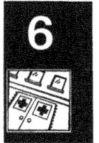

6

TIP

Bring a Friend

Bring someone to the emergency room with you to help monitor your care, explain your problem, support you emotionally, and advocate for you with hospital staff.

Nonemergency Alternatives

For routine care, *after-hours* and *urgent-care* health care centers are less expensive and more convenient than emergency rooms for immediate—but nonemergency—medical problems. With 80 million patient visits in 1994, urgent-care centers are a growing alternative to emergency rooms for treating nonemergency cases, and insurers encourage people to use them for this purpose.

Similarly, the popularity of outpatient surgery has stimulated the growth of independent, for-profit *ambulatory treatment centers*. If you're considering a center that isn't hospital-sponsored, find out how it handles an emergency. Remember, a medical complication can arise at any time. Is a hospital emergency department nearby? Does the center have an agreement with the hospital to take patients from the center when necessary?

Ask in advance about the credentials of the physicians, nurses, and other staff who will be responsible for your care. Make sure the facility is licensed by the proper state agency and subject to regular professional standards surveys.

about how quickly you need to receive care. If needed, the staff can draw on all the hospital's resources, twenty-four hours a day.

Don't wait until you need urgent care to find out about the emergency resources available at your local hospital. Determine where the closest emergency room is—not every hospital has one. And know how to call an ambulance: Does your community have a 911 telephone emergency-response system? Or would you call the police department, the fire department, or a private ambulance company? If an ambulance isn't needed or is unavailable, do you know the quickest route to the emergency room?

When you reach the hospital, the chances are quite high that the emergency-department physician won't have much information about your medical history. To get the most effective care in the least amount of time, be prepared to provide accurate information about:

- Your current medical problems
- Your medical history, especially previous hospitalizations and surgery
- Current medications (with the name and dose of each one, along with how often you take it), *and*
- Allergies

Don't rely on a hospital emergency room for regular medical care. This is expensive and time consuming. You and your family need and deserve a personal physician to manage your overall medical care on an ongoing basis. A personal physician is better able to provide quality care for nonemergency illnesses because he or she knows you as a patient.

If you're unsure about the seriousness of your condition, try to reach your primary care provider first. He or she may help coordinate your care by providing emergency personnel with critical medical information. Your insurance may require you to do this anyway in some circumstances.

If you have a choice among several emergency departments, you may want to inquire about their comparative capabilities.

One strong indicator of quality is volume. The more visits a department handles, the more capable it's likely to be.

Another important factor is staff training. Better hospitals use only doctors who are board certified in emergency medicine, surgery, or other specialties geared to the emergencies commonly seen—for example, pediatricians in a children's hospital. Others rely on residents or other physicians with little training in treating emergencies.

Testing and Treatment: Hospital Clinics

Throughout your lifetime, health care providers will refer you and your family to a hospital for outpatient care for specific procedures or treatments. For example, before entering the hospital for an overnight stay, you'll probably get some routine diagnostic tests as an outpatient, particularly if your condition isn't urgent. Usually, this is done to record certain information about your blood and heart activity, reducing the length of the inpatient stay—and reducing your total cost.

Because inpatient hospital stays are expensive and some patients prefer not to stay overnight anyway, the trend is toward performing surgery and other treatment on an outpatient basis. Thus, most people get eye and knee surgery in an outpatient day surgical unit. Moreover, compared to an overnight stay, outpatient care exposes a patient to less risk of acquiring an infection from the germs that are inevitably present in hospitals. Other advantages of outpatient care—ones that contribute to a faster recovery—include less anxiety and less disruption of your family life.

If you do receive outpatient surgery, it's important that you determine exactly what kind of care you'll need afterward. Make sure that someone can provide it—a family member, a friend, or a nurse or home-health aide arranged through a hospital clinic.

Searching for Quality

Hospitals are big business. About 30 million people spend a night in a hospital each year. And Americans make over 300 million visits to hospitals for outpatient services annually.

Hospitals employ a number of methods to maintain and improve the quality of care they deliver to these millions of customers. For example, most hospitals have written policies intended to help prevent the spread of infection. In addition, committees examine every unexpected death and accident, as well as cases that may have been handled improperly. And hospitals must document the reason for all unusual occurrences in delivering care.

Unfortunately, it's beyond the ability of most health care consumers to assess the quality-control procedures of a given hospital. Your doctor can give you some advice, and nurses are often a good source of information. Also, ask the hospital quality-assurance department to explain its efforts to ensure that you receive the best care possible. The hospital's

However, none of these centers are equipped to handle life-threatening situations, and they don't replace a regular relationship with a primary care provider. Always arrange to forward copies of the medical records for service to your regular provider. And check with your insurer for coverage.

TIP

Ambulance Service

In many situations, you'll want to call an ambulance for transportation to the emergency room. For example, you may need urgent care when no one is available to drive you to the hospital. Also, some ambulance services are staffed by trained emergency medical technicians (EMTs) who can provide some medical assistance immediately. And if you need emergency care, EMTs can get to you much faster than you can get to the hospital.

6

The Outpatient Experience

Follow this hypothetical experience of Steve Tripton as he receives high-quality medical care without the trouble and expense of spending a night in the hospital:

Tripton twisted his knee while skiing. When his knee pain didn't improve with medication and physical therapy, his family physician referred him to Dr. Joel Caputo, an orthopedic surgeon. Dr. Caputo diagnosed torn cartilage inside the knee and recommended surgery to remove the torn portion. Tripton agreed.

On the day of the surgery, Tripton arrived at County General Hospital and was checked in by Jane Crawford, a nurse. She asked Tripton questions about his last meal, his medical history, and drug allergies. An anesthesiologist, Dr. Raphael Muñoz, came in and reviewed the medical history, asked about any previous difficulties with anesthesia, and examined Tripton. A few minutes later, Dr. Caputo arrived.

Dr. Muñoz and Nurse Crawford wheeled Tripton into the operating room and gave him medication to fall asleep. The next thing Tripton

accreditation and indirect signals such as services and staffing can also play a role in your evaluation.

Accreditation and Quality

Everyone wants high-quality care. But how can you know how good your local hospital is, or any hospital that your health care providers recommend? It isn't easy. The simplest potential indicator—cost—provides no reliable signal on quality.

That said, *accreditation* indicates that a hospital meets at least minimum standards of quality—and perhaps much more. The Joint Commission on Accreditation of Healthcare Organizations (JCAHO), an independent, nonprofit organization, assesses the quality of most hospitals every three years. This process is voluntary, and about 80 percent of U.S. hospitals participate.

You are entitled to know a hospital's level of accreditation. The overwhelming number of hospitals receive simple accreditation, which does little to differentiate them from one another. A few hospitals receive accreditation with commendation, conditional accreditation, or no accreditation. Conditionally accredited facilities have six months to correct deficiencies cited by the JCAHO.

The JCAHO recently began to make detailed data on hospitals available to the public. Reports cover a wide range of areas, including nursing care, infection control, patient rights, and safety.

Besides accreditation, *board certifications* can be used as a sign of quality. Medical and surgical specialty societies certify physicians to practice a particular specialty if they receive extra training and pass advanced tests in the field. Although certification measures knowledge more than skill, a high proportion of board-certified physicians on a hospital's medical staff suggests a higher level of expertise on hand. About two-thirds of U.S. physicians are certified.

Make sure the hospital you use is accredited. Among other things, that means it has programs, staff, or procedures related to:

Handling patient complaints. The hospital has a patient advocate or representative on staff or at least a clearly stated process for handling complaints.

Infection control. The hospital has an infection-control practitioner on staff and a clear system for conducting such activities.

End-of-life decisions. An ethics committee or consultant is available to help patients, providers, and families deal with these difficult questions.

JCAHO Check

You are entitled to know the JCAHO accreditation for any hospital, when the commission last surveyed a facility, and when the next survey will occur. The hospital's director of quality assurance or quality management or another manager should be able to give you the information. If no one at the hospital will tell you, call the Joint Commission on Accreditation of Healthcare Organizations Service Center at (708) 916-5800.

Call that same number if you wish to order the detailed JCAHO report on a hospital. The cost is $30 per report.

Services, Staffing, and Quality

Several indirect measures can indicate that a hospital delivers quality care. Among these indicators are the types of nurses on staff and the kinds of services offered.

Nurses. Generally, nurses are the only medical personnel available to you immediately around the clock. And they're the ones most likely to be familiar with all aspects of your care.

Registered nurses (RNs) have more medical education and training than licensed practical nurses (LPNs). Registered nurses can tailor and implement the plan of care prepared by your doctor.

The national average for hospitals is four registered nurses to every licensed practical nurse. A higher proportion of registered nurses indicates that a hospital has a higher level of nursing expertise. Unfortunately, you'll have trouble getting statistics on nursing staffs. Ask the hospital or your state's affiliate of the American Nurses Association, or consult the American Hospital Association.

It's also important to learn about a hospital's nursing practice in general. For example, what are the overall staffing levels? Generally, one nurse can care for three to six patients. If a hospital has a higher average ratio of patients per nurse, seek an explanation. If the ratio is lower, the hospital's overall philosophy *may* be based on a commitment to patient-centered care (see pages 101–102). In addition, the higher the proportion of nurses who are *permanent* employees, rather than "registry" nurses, the better the nursing care.

remembers is waking up with his leg bandaged. He spent a few hours in the recovery room, where a physical therapist came to demonstrate the use of crutches and exercises to perform at home. Dr. Caputo scheduled a follow-up appointment with Tripton and gave him a prescription for pain medicine and written instructions, including a number to call in case of an emergency.

A friend took Tripton home a few minutes later. The next day, Tripton received a checkup call from Nurse Crawford to make sure that he was doing okay.

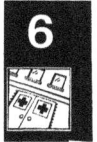

6

Hospitals Can Make You Sick

By their very nature, hospitals are dangerous. They are occupied by sick people, many of whom have serious and unknown infectious illnesses. They are also filled with dangerous machinery. And health care personnel, even the best ones, practice a necessarily imperfect and imprecise science.

It should come as no surprise that about one in twenty U.S. patients get sick *from* their stay in a hospital. *Iatrogenic* illnesses (caused by physicians or other care providers) result from infections that are carried by doctors, nurses, and others; complications of surgery and other procedures; and a wide variety of other sources, including, ironically, many of the technologies that save lives.

Hospital-acquired illnesses are a major concern for both patients and caregivers, but they don't always indicate low-quality care. About one-third to one-half of hospital-acquired infections are preventable or result from carelessness.

People with illnesses affecting their immune system—such as patients undergoing cancer treat-

Perhaps the clearest indicator of nursing-care quality is organizational structure. Two methods of organization are common in nursing. With functional nursing, nurses are assigned particular tasks, such as medication, dressing changes, or clinical examinations. With primary nursing, the hospital assigns a nurse to be the main caregiver for each patient. In general, the latter model results in better patient care.

Discharge planning services. In addition to medical services, quality hospitals have a comprehensive set of discharge planning services, as well as handrails, walkers, and other equipment or appliances needed to assist in daily life. Discharge planning is especially helpful to people who continue to need care after leaving the hospital—an increasing proportion of patients with today's shorter hospital stays.

Case management. Some hospitals assign nurse case managers to patients not only to help with discharge planning but to play a central role in coordinating overall care. This method of coordinating patient care is compatible with either primary or functional nursing and can improve the quality of care.

If you or someone in your family requires home-health care, rehabilitative care, long term nursing care, or hospice care, for example, trained discharge planners or case managers can help you find and select these services. Preferably, planners are full-time hospital employees—typically nurses or licensed clinical social workers—whose job is to assess patient needs and work with patients and their families, physicians, and insurance companies.

Find out ahead of time who does case management or discharge planning for inpatients. A good hospital will start a case manager when you enter the facility. This makes it easier to prepare for any possible access problems or a lack of caregiver support.

For more information on home care, turn to chapter 16.

Consumer Alert: Nursing Cutbacks

Is a hospital replacing registered nurses with licensed practical nurses, and LPNs with unlicensed aides? If so, find out why. Are cost concerns driving the change in staffing, and will this affect your care? For example, the remaining RNs or LPNs could be overwhelmed with higher workloads.

Consult your physician, the hospital, or a nursing association or union. Ask the hospital how it's maintaining the quality of care as it employs a higher proportion of less-trained personnel.

Practice Makes Perfect

An effective way to compare the ability of hospitals to treat you is to determine how often each hospital encounters cases like yours. In general, look for hospitals—and specialists—that often perform the procedure in question. How many patients with your condition has a hospital treated? What is its success rate with the procedure?

Ask your doctor or the hospital for data on the relevant experience of both the facility and the people who would handle your surgery or other care. Your doctor will help you interpret it.

Patient-Centered Care: A Quality Perspective

More and more hospitals are instituting a *patient-centered* approach to quality, and patients are the beneficiaries. The elements of, and level of commitment to, this idea vary from hospital to hospital. According to the Picker/Commonwealth Program for Patient-Centered Care, look for a hospital that:

Respects your values, preferences, and expressed needs. Do caregivers consider your short-term and long-term goals? Do you decide what role you will play in decision making? Do caregivers ask what you need, want, and expect?

Coordinates care and integrates services within the hospital. Is your care from various providers effectively coordinated? Do you get consistent information from all providers?

Encourages communication between patient and providers. Make sure you receive accurate, timely, and appropriate information. Expect caregivers to educate you about the long-term implications of disease and illness. Ask for the information you want about your health, diagnostic tests, and treatment options. Do you and your family know what you need to know to manage your care?

Enhances your physical comfort. The hospital staff should alleviate your pain as much as possible and provide the help you need with such regular activities as bathing and eating. Are limits on your ability to function adequately addressed?

Provides for your emotional support and alleviates fears and anxieties. Do caregivers consider your concerns about your illness and its

ment and those who routinely take several medications—have a particularly high risk of acquiring an infection in a hospital. These are known as *nosocomial* infections. If you feel you may be at high risk, ask the hospital if it has a program of surveillance, prevention, and control of such illnesses. Is an infection-control practitioner on staff? If not, what does the hospital do to control infection? And don't hesitate to ask doctors, nurses, and other caregivers if they have washed their hands before examining or treating you.

6

TIP
Ask a Nurse

Nurses are the true coordinators of your medical care. Find out which nurse is assigned to you. She or he is central to your care in the hospital.

Death Rates and Quality

The federal government compiles mortality data—death rates—for hospitals. Unfortunately, these statistics are hard to interpret, particularly given the overwhelming number of variables involved. A high rate could indicate a quality problem but may also indicate an excellent hospital that accepts the most troubling cases or focuses on a very sick or elderly population.

Although *adjusted rates* can correct somewhat for the fact that some hospitals treat patients who are more frail or desperately ill, death-rate statistics mainly serve to help hospitals monitor their own quality. The federal government stopped publicizing the data in 1993.

Nevertheless, *U.S. News & World Report* uses mortality rates as one criterion in compiling its annual list of America's best hospitals. And the rates for 5,500 hospitals are available to the public in the *Consumer's Guide to Hospitals*, which advises readers to use the mortality rates only as a starting point, not as a definitive mark of hospital quality.

effect on your ability to care for yourself or your family? Do they consider the principal stresses in your life? Do they consider your concerns about paying medical bills or about lost income due to illness? Do you have access to appropriate support networks to help with these worries?

Involves your family and friends. The hospital staff should involve family and friends in planning and providing care. Do family and friends have the support they need to perform this function?

Provides for a smooth transition from one location for receiving care to another. When you leave the hospital, you and your family must understand the medications to take, treatment regimens to follow, activities to pursue or avoid, and the danger signals that may arise. The hospital should make sure you receive written plans for continuing care and treatment.

The Best Hospital

There is no such thing as the "best hospital" for everyone, but in general, better hospitals will have:

- Coordinated care among administrators, physicians, and support staff
- Communication among staff from different departments
- Family-centered, patient-centered care, *and*
- Comprehensive discharge planning on such matters as diet, side effects, medication, danger signals, and follow-up care.

Making a Choice

You may have some choice about a hospital, although your options are often limited by the type of care you need, where your doctor has admitting privileges, where you live, and your health plan. No matter which hospital you use, the more you know about *any* hospital, the better off you'll be and the more likely you are to be a competent partner in your care.

You want to find two aspects of good hospital care: the right *medical care* and a *caring atmosphere*. Both are critical to the outcome of your hospital visit.

Of course, the quality of the care is the most important component in your choice of a hospital; it's a universal concern. But other factors depend on your personal preferences and needs. Do you prefer a less expensive hospital? One closer to home? A smaller one? One with a national reputation?

Check the Services: High-Quality Care

Every hospital offers a distinct mix of services. For example, 93 percent of the hospitals in the United States have emergency departments, but only 17 percent have open-heart facilities. At 19 percent of hospitals, you can receive radiation therapy; 11 percent offer organ transplants. An impressive 85 percent have physical-therapy facilities, but for occupational therapy, the figure is 52 percent. Although only 17 percent have facilities for hospice care, 73 percent have high-tech CT scanners.

If you need, expect to need, or simply prefer to have on hand a particular type of service, talk with your primary care provider or the admitting physician to make sure the hospital you select can provide what you are seeking. For example, if you want to give birth in a more homelike environment, seek hospitals with an "alternative birthing center" or similar facility.

Inquire about a hospital's ability to meet your particular needs, such as care for cancer, heart disease, or kidney disease: Does it have the right services and specialties? What is its experience with conditions you or your family have now or anticipate in the future? What is its success rate with specific medical procedures? Think about your family's medical history and its current health.

In addition, ask whether a hospital has:

- Staff trained and designated to prepare and manage your plan of care
- Staff trained and designated to prepare and manage your discharge plan
- Preadmission testing services so you can obtain as much care as an outpatient as possible
- Referral networks if you need to transfer to a more specialized facility
- JCAHO accreditation
- Social workers available to help you access social, clinical, physical, and financial services, *and*
- Education programs for patients and members of the community

To order the *Consumer's Guide to Hospitals,* contact the Center for the Study of Services, 733 15th Street, N.W., #820, Washington, DC 20005; tel. (800) 475-7283. The cost is $12.

TIP

Firsthand Look

Take the time to visit hospitals you are considering to get information about the medical staff and to find out about the availability of services that may be important to you, such as chaplain services or women's health services. A visit will also give you a good sense of the hospital's atmosphere.

Call the hospital and ask for the public relations or administrative office. Ask who to talk with. Arrange a time to visit.

6

TIP

Consumer Alert: Required Reading

The patient handbook can answer many of your questions about a hospital. If the hospital doesn't give you a copy when you enter, ask to see it. At the same time, ask for a copy of the Patient Bill of Rights and get full information on your rights and responsibilities.

Consumer Alert: Quality Check

Does the hospital you are considering admit Medicare patients? If not, check with the state health department: The hospital may have been suspended for some reason.

Check the Services: The Caring Hospital

Your recovery depends on environmental factors as well as medical ones. Is your hospital a *caring* institution?

A caring atmosphere is almost as difficult to identify as highly skilled care. Among other factors to consider, a hospital should offer emotional support to your friends and family if you are seriously ill.

Obviously, the staff is key: Are nurses, doctors, and other staff members courteous, polite, and friendly toward patients and visitors? Do they answer questions, or are they rushed and distracted when you try to talk with them?

It's hard to know about these matters before you enter the hospital, but if you experience problems while using the hospital, talk to your admitting physician or your primary care nurse. And you should be able to determine ahead of time whether a hospital:

- Provides accommodations for parents to spend the night with their children and helps make arrangements for other out-of-town visitors
- Accommodates special diet requests
- Allows visitors to bring food to patients if a doctor approves
- Sets liberal hours for when you can receive visitors and make phone calls
- Has hospice services available
- Allows patients to sit outside their rooms
- Provides full information on patient's rights
- Keeps waiting rooms and patients' rooms clean

Getting Recommendations

The phone book isn't a good place to start your search for a hospital. How you *do* start your search depends on the stage you have reached in your efforts to construct a personal health care system for yourself and your family.

If you already have a primary care provider, begin by discussing hospital options with him or her. Most primary care providers are affiliated with one or more hospitals. Ask how each facility excels or lags in general—and what that means for someone like you. In addition, your primary care provider, whether a physician or someone else, can give you good advice on other hospitals, why you'd use them, and how you would be admitted should the need arise.

If you belong to a managed care plan, also talk to its member-services department. Just as primary care providers are affiliated with a limited number of hospitals, many health plans will send you to certain hospitals for certain conditions. The plan should be able to provide you with information about the available options

For more information on managed care and your choice of hospitals, turn to chapter 3.

On the other hand, your search for information on hospitals could be one aspect of your efforts to select both a primary care provider and a health plan. In this case:

■ Ask your employer's or union's benefits department to recommend good hospitals and to provide information about them.

■ Consult any nurses you know. Hospital nurses have direct experience with such basic factors as the coordination of each patient's care, the caring atmosphere, and staff satisfaction. One telling question to ask a nurse—or any other health care provider—is whether she or he would send a family member to a particular hospital.

■ Talk to friends, family, and colleagues about their experiences. Use the questions throughout this chapter to guide your conversation and look for the elements of hospital care most important to you and most relevant to your health care needs.

TIP
Special Needs Referrals

If you have a special need, the appropriate organization can refer you to both local facilities and, for the most complex cases, nationally recognized facilities. For example, cancer patients may wish to contact the American Cancer Society.

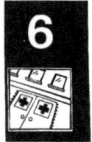

Building a Health Care Partnership

No one is as interested in the health of you and your family as you are. It's your responsibility to be informed, maintain records of your medical history, evaluate and select hospitals, and question your physician, nurse, and others about medical advice. Your doctor and the hospital's staff are professionals who want to do a good job. For them to do so, you have to play an active role in the treatment process by offering your opinions and asking questions.

When a doctor recommends a hospitalization, whether for an inpatient stay or an outpatient visit, make sure you need to go to a hospital.

If it's for a surgery, you'll often need a second opinion from another doctor. In fact, your insurer may require a second opinion to provide coverage.

Ask your physician:

- What is the diagnosis? What are the chances it might be wrong?

- Why does your condition require hospitalization? Can it be treated adequately without a hospital visit?

- What does the recommended treatment entail?

- What is recovery like? What can you expect? How long will it take?

- What level of equipment sophistication does it require?

- What happens if you postpone the hospital visit?

- If it's for surgery, are there nonsurgical alternatives? What are the pros and cons of other ways to treat the condition?

- Can you get the surgery or other service as an outpatient?

- Why does the physician recommend *this* hospital? Is it because of the complexity of the treatment, the special equipment or personnel available, the convenience of the location?

- What are the risks or possible complications of the procedure? What is the chance that complications will occur?

- What are the benefits? What is the chance of achieving them?

Look Who's Talking

If you have concerns about your medical care, *talk to your physician, your nurse, and other caregivers about them.* A major factor in the success or failure of medical care is your compliance with recommended treatments. If you aren't clear about—or disagree with—these recommendations, you can't comply well with the treatment and you lessen your chances of getting better. Don't be afraid to ask questions because you feel ignorant or don't want to waste a doctor's time. After all, you hire the doctor and the hospital, not the other way around.

Your Role in the Partnership

Shared knowledge enhances the physician-patient relationship and improves the efficiency and effectiveness of medical care. To get the most out of your hospital visit, carefully evaluate why you are going. Review your symptoms and questions in advance, and make a list of questions or comments. This way, you won't forget to mention anything, and your physician is better able to focus the discussion, eliminate unnecessary tests, and provide you with better treatment.

Discuss any medical problems you have had in the past—the more specific the better. For example, it's better to tell caregivers you have a history of high blood pressure and had a small heart attack five years ago than to say you have heart problems. Still, give whatever information you have, even if you don't know details.

List your current drugs, including the exact name, the amount of medication in each pill, and the number of pills you take daily. Limited information—such as, "I take a green pill for my stomach once or twice a day"—is rarely sufficient. It's better to say, "I take Zantac for a peptic ulcer, 150 milligrams, twice a day." Know what allergies or reactions to medications you have had, specifying the name of the medication and the nature of your reaction—a rash, nausea, difficulty breathing, and so forth.

Record any previous operations, including the reasons for the surgery, what was done, any complications, the name of your surgeon, the hospital, and the date. At any time, you can get a copy of the actual report on an operation by sending a written request to the hospital. This report can be very valuable to a new physician or hospital.

In the hospital, keep a careful record of your medical care. Keep track of any tests you receive, including X rays, lab tests, EKGs, and so on. Make sure to request a copy of the test results; at times it's worthwhile to have actual copies of the X-ray films in your possession after you are discharged.

Before leaving the hospital after either an inpatient or outpatient visit, make sure you understand your physician's treatment plan:

- What medications do you need?
- When and how should you take them?
- Should you change or stop your previous medications?
- What dietary and other restrictions should you observe?
- What additional procedures or tests will you need?
- What preparation will you need to perform for those procedures?

TIP
Medication Alert

Find out as soon as possible which medicines are prescribed for you, why they were chosen, and when you should take them. That way, you can monitor your care, raise a warning flag in case of an error, keep records, and check the bills.

Don't immediately swallow pills that a nurse brings you. First, confirm the name, dose, and purpose. Also, be sure to reemphasize the other medications you are already taking and ask about possible interactions with your new prescriptions.

For more information on medications, turn to chapter 7.

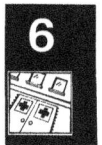

6

Checklist: If You Are Hospitalized . . .

If you receive either inpatient or outpatient care from a hospital:

✓ Inform your caregivers of drug interactions, allergies. Make sure they document this in your medical record.

TIP
Patient Advocates

Hospitals often have patient advocates on staff to help you understand and deal with the hospital bureaucracy. They can help you understand how the hospital works and address minor problems you encounter during your hospital stay.

Hospitality Houses

Friends and families are integral to health care. However, many patients must use hospitals far from home. For example, a person needing major surgery or complicated radiation treatments may travel to a specialty hospital far away for several weeks or more.

To provide affordable lodging for patients' families and friends, *hospital hospitality houses* are located near many hospitals. For the most part, these are nonprofit organizations that offer a variety of services— overnight lodging, kitchen and laundry facilities, transportation, and children's playrooms. They offer a warm and supportive alternative to the isolation and expense of hotel rooms. The charge for an overnight stay

✓ As an inpatient, make sure the information on your wristband is correct.

✓ Be sure any caregiver you use calls you by name before beginning treatment.

✓ Ask questions about any treatment, procedure, medication, or anything else that you are not clear about. If you can't do so, ask a family member or friend to do so for you.

Your Hospital Record

Parallel to your own written notes, the hospital will maintain an official record of the care you receive. Many states guarantee your access to this medical record, although you may have to pay a fee to get a copy. And you may have to fight the hospital bureaucracy.

Patient medical records provide a considerable amount of detailed information about your stay in the hospital. Generally, they are in chronological order, beginning with a *medical history and physical* and ending with a *discharge summary* that records your condition and status the day you leave the hospital. The middle part of the record contains the *orders* your physician gives to the hospital staff, notes on your day-to-day *progress*, the daily record of your *nursing care* and nurses' observation notes, your *test results*, and finally, an *operative summary* if you have a surgical procedure.

Read the nurses' notes first. They are usually neat and easy to read and provide a highly detailed story of your hospital stay.

You may be hospitalized at the same facility several times over the years, and all of these encounters should be included in your total medical record. For this reason, specify the dates of the encounters you want to review when requesting access to your record. To speed up access, include your Social Security number and date of birth.

If you move to another area, request a copy of your complete hospital medical record, as well as your family's physician records. Carry them with you to your new home. These are invaluable resources in your family's continuing medical care.

When Problems Arise

As a patient, you have a number of rights, many of which are supported by law. Others may come with your health plan. Others simply make sense.

As a hospital patient, you have the right to confidentiality and privacy. And no one can deny you care on the basis of race, sex, or religion.

You have the right to all the information you need to make decisions about your care. If you are an adult, only you can accept or refuse a treatment.

You have the right to refuse to be examined by anyone, from an intern to the head of staff, and for any reason. You might want to ask how often a particular doctor has performed a given procedure, even if it's very basic. If an intern or resident has never done a procedure before, you can refuse to be treated by that person or insist on close supervision.

Learn your rights. The hospital should provide you with a statement describing them. Ask for the statement if the hospital can't offer it to you. Talk to your physician and insurer at once if the hospital doesn't make the statement available.

For more information on patient rights, including the hospital bill of rights, turn to chapter 3.

If you feel you've received poor care or unfair treatment in a hospital, first talk with the staff concerned. Next check with the nurse you see most often or the head of your nursing unit. And consult your attending physician. If you can't resolve a complaint through the attending physician, bring your problem to the attention of hospital authorities: Try talking with the patient advocate, the director of quality, the chief of service, or the chief of staff. You may also need to find a personal advocate, whether it's a friend, a family member, or your primary care provider.

As a last resort, you may decide to talk with your doctor about a transfer to another unit or another hospital. And you always have the right to leave the hospital on your own at any time, even if it's against medical advice.

tends to be low, and in many cases free.

For more information and referrals to facilities in a particular location, call the National Association of Hospital Hospitality Houses at (800) 542-9730.

Families of seriously ill children can ask a hospital social worker if there's a Ronald McDonald house in the area, or look in the local phone book.

Registering a Complaint

If you aren't satisfied with an institution's response to your concerns, you can register a complaint with a number of organizations either while you are in the hospital or afterward. State your case as clearly as possible. Document it with information from your own record and the hospital's official record, if you have a copy. If you don't have a copy, get one.

To lodge a complaint about hospital care, you can contact:

- The Joint Commission on Accreditation of Healthcare Organizations, 1 Renaissance Boulevard, Oakbrook, IL 60181; tel. (708) 916-5800
- The American Hospital Association, 840 N. Lake Shore Drive, Chicago, IL 60611; tel. (312) 280-8209
- The state licensing agency for health care facilities—usually this is in the department of health or the department of public health

Understanding the Language

If you or someone in your family doesn't speak English fluently, you'll need a competent language translator the moment you enter the hospital, preferably at no cost. If possible, consult the hospital before admission about any language services you may need. More and more often, hospitals are training and enlisting translators for the languages they encounter regularly.

In the past, hospitals and patients used anyone available as a translator: a relative or a friend, another patient, a person employed in another capacity at the hospital. All of these choices are inadequate. For one thing, rarely will any of these people understand medical terminology in one, let alone two, languages. Also, you want a translator available twenty-four hours a day. After all, who will translate for a patient who wakes up in pain at 3 o'clock in the morning?

Most important, few relatives, friends, or even hospital employees have training in a critical part of health care: respecting each patient's right to privacy and information. For example, a parent

■ The state Peer Review Organization. For the phone number in your state, call the Medicare hotline and ask for assistance: (800) 638-6833.

Consumer Alert: Early Discharge

Speak up if physicians or hospitals want to discharge you, but you don't think you're ready for discharge. Talk to the staff. They are responsible for your well-being.

Ask for home services, such as a visiting nurse, if you think they're needed. Ask how soon and how often home services will be provided. With more and more early discharges, home-health agencies increasingly lack the staff to provide enough services and to do so in a timely manner.

If you are a Medicare patient, you have the right to appeal the hospital's decision. During the appeal, which usually takes a day or two, you can remain in the hospital.

The appeal steps are explained in the materials you receive when you enter the hospital. If you don't receive these, ask for them.

Tell your doctor you want to appeal, and then contact the organization in your state responsible for overseeing the quality of Medicare services. Call (800) 638-6833 to find out who to contact in your state.

Money Matters

While insurance may pay most of your hospital bill, you're often responsible for up to 20 percent of the bottom line. Thus, you have a strong incentive to keep that cost as low as possible while getting the best care. Fortunately, the prices a hospital charges for a particular service generally don't relate to the quality of care it delivers.

Before you are treated at the hospital, the admitting department will ask you for information about your health insurance and require someone to guarantee payment. However, if you have no insurance and can't pay for your hospital care, you may be entitled to free care:

■ Each state has a Medicaid program that covers basic medical services for low-income people.

■ Most states also have other programs to provide free care to people who can't pay their bills. Ask the hospital about possible arrangements for free care. Speak with the hospital's social-services office or the admissions office

Free Care

Most nonprofit hospitals were built with federal "Hill-Burton" funds. As a condition of receiving these funds, they must provide a limited amount of care to people who can't pay. For referrals to facilities that provide free or below-cost care for low-income people, call (800) 638-0742 or, in Maryland, (800) 492-0359.

Price Questions

One of the best ways to avoid a future misunderstanding about billing or payment is to educate yourself, before admission, on the intricacies of your family's health insurance. As you seek cost-effective health care, your insurer will play a major role, mostly on the side of saving itself money. Your interest differs: You want to get the best care possible—and you want the insurer to foot most or all of the bill.

As in many other situations, a little preplanning can save lots of effort, pain, and confusion later. Take the time to investigate the following:

■ Does the hospital that you'll use have a contract with your insurer? For example, HMOs typically pay the full amount of insurance only if you use participating or network hospitals.

■ What copayments and deductibles are your responsibility?

■ How long a stay is approved?

■ If your insurance doesn't cover a private room, how much would an upgrade cost you?

■ What does your insurance cover—and not cover?

■ What happens if the hospital charges more for your projected care than your insurance considers reasonable?

For more information on hospitals and insurance, turn to chapter 4.

Be aware that doctors' fees for hospital services are typically billed separately. Beforehand, ask your family physician what bills you'll receive from his or her office and what other physicians will provide medical services during your hospital stay. Then check with your employer or health insurer to determine if you are responsible for paying a portion of these bills. And once you get the bills, make sure you received all the services listed.

may hesitate to speak frankly if his or her child is the translator. Or an adult translator may censor the conversation between a child and a physician. The patient needs to know the doctor heard everything she or he says, and vice versa.

For emergencies, many hospitals subscribe to the AT&T Language Line; it provides translators for 140 languages, twenty-four hours a day. While they don't replace in-person interpreters, the Language Line and other services like it are excellent supplements.

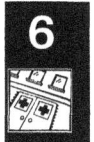

6

When you enter a hospital, a variety of factors affect the cost. Among the questions you can ask your physician in advance are

■ What are the room-and-board charges? What is the price for a semi-private room? For a bed in intensive care? What do these charges include, and what is billed separately?

■ What is the usual charge for my anticipated procedures?

■ Does the hospital have a payment counselor to help me arrange such things as installment payments?

Price Pointers

Ask a hospital for a written list of services and fees. Even though these rarely match the actual fees patients or insurers pay, the listed prices can help you decide among options, compare rates at hospitals, and check if your insurer will cover what you require.

At least thirty states monitor hospital charges. Check with the state health department to find out what agency is responsible. If there is such an agency, it can provide you with much of the cost information you seek. Otherwise, your best bet is to call the business office of the hospital.

The Hospital Bill

After you are treated, request a *detailed* bill that itemizes all the services you received. Simply reading it is a major challenge. Hospital bills are filled with obscure codes, seemingly meaningless abbreviations, and unending jargon. Just as annoying, it's impossible to predict what a given hospital will bill you for—a toothbrush, ambulance fees, phone calls, and so forth.

Moreover, besides the hospital bill, patients often receive bills directly from their own physicians—and from physicians they don't even know. These fees are usually legitimate, such as bills from the person who reads your X rays. But you'll want to check.

On top of that, hospital bills contain a surprising number of errors. You'll have to wade through the details carefully, separating the legitimate charges from possible errors. For example, some services may appear twice under different names. If you find a mistake—such as a service you didn't receive—ask the billing department for an explanation and, if indicated, an adjustment. Many employers reward employees if they find a hospital billing error and secure an adjustment.

You do have several potential aides, allies, and teachers in this educational experience:

- Many states *require* hospitals to provide you with an itemized bill.
- Your physician and other health care providers can help you decipher the language and check that you received all the care that is in the bill.
- Your insurer shares your concern that the bill is accurate.
- The staff of the billing office may try to clearly explain your bill. If so, ask particularly about all charges labeled "miscellaneous."

When you receive the bill, review the dates of your stay to determine if they are correct. And don't be charged for a private room if you used a semiprivate room.

In addition, consult your memory, the hospital's medical record, and your own written records of your hospital care to test the bill's accuracy. And get your doctor's advice as soon as possible. Examine the bill carefully to spot:

- Tests and room supplies you didn't receive
- Canceled tests
- Treatments and special services you didn't receive
- Double billing for a single service
- Telephone charges you didn't make, *and*
- Charges for a higher class of service than you received

If you were given a few days worth of a medication while in the hospital, the bill should only reflect that amount of the drug, not a full month's worth. In other words, does the bill cover only the medications you actually took? If the bill includes take-home prescriptions, make sure you got the medicine to take home.

If the billing department doesn't answer your questions to your satisfaction, you can contact the hospital's administration. You can also contact the state agency that licenses hospitals.

No Free Lunch

Don't accept supplies you don't need—you may be billed for them. Bring items such as a comb, a toothbrush, razors, shampoo, and a robe and slippers from home, or have a friend bring them.

Similarly, make sure you aren't billed for *buying* a toothbrush, thermometer, or any other item the hospital didn't let you take home.

TIP

Negotiate a Payment Schedule

If you can't afford to pay your hospital bill all at once and are not eligible for free care, talk to the billing department about a payment schedule. Most hospitals are happy to arrange monthly payments that you can afford.

6

Resources
Organizations

American Hospital Association
840 North Lake Shore Drive
Chicago, IL 60611
(312) 280-8209
The annual *AHA Guide to the Health Care Field* is available in libraries. It contains data on accreditation, approval for special facilities, medical-school affiliations, size, and major services. Call or write for an excellent consumer guide to hospitals and other publications.

American Nurses Association
600 Maryland Avenue, S.W., #100W
Washington, DC 20024-2571
(800) 274-4ANA
Contact the ANA to receive a free copy of the brochure "Every Patient Needs a Nurse," explaining what consumers should expect from a nurse.

Hill-Burton Hospital Free Care
(800) 638-0742
Call for information on health facilities that participate in the Hill-Burton Free Care Program.

Joint Commission on Accreditation of
    Healthcare Organizations
1 Renaissance Boulevard
Oakbrook Terrace, IL 60181

To find out if a hospital is accredited, call the commission's service center at (708) 916-5800. You can also ask for the hospital's accreditation history and the date of its most recent survey and the next one scheduled. For $30 each, you can order detailed data on a hospital. Reports cover a wide range of areas, including nursing care, infection control, patient rights, and safety.

Shriner's Hospital Referral Line
(800) 237-5055
Call for free referrals to Shriner's Hospitals for children under age eighteen with orthopedic problems or burns.

Publications

Consumer's Guide to Hospitals (Center for the Study of Services, 1994), $12. Order from the Center for the Study of Services, 733 15th Street, N.W., #820, Washington, DC 20005; tel. (800) 475-7283. (Updated periodically, so request latest edition.)

Take This Book to the Hospital with You, by Charles B. Inlander and Ed Weiner (Rodale Press/People's Medical Society, 1993), $14.95 ($12.95 to members of People's Medical Society).

7 Medications

Joe Graedon and Teresa Graedon

Joe and Teresa Graedon have been writing about health for over twenty years. Their People's Pharmacy books, syndicated health column, and weekly radio talk show reach millions of health-conscious people across the United States, Canada, and other countries. Their newest books are *The People's Guide to Deadly Drug Interactions* (St. Martin's Press, 1995) and *The People's Pharmacy: Completely New and Revised* (St. Martin's Press, 1996). Joe Graedon, M.S., is a pharmacologist; Teresa Graedon, Ph.D., is a medical anthropologist.

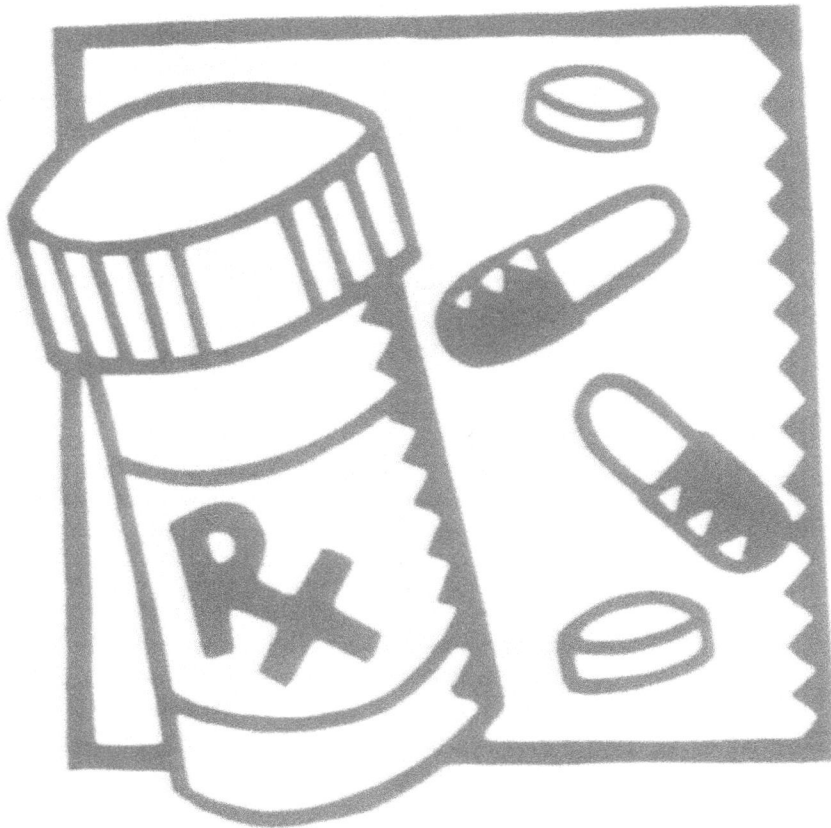

Consumers are swallowing more pills than ever before, and paying unprecedented prices. In 1995 Americans shelled out almost $58 billion for prescription drugs in pharmacies, up from $11 billion in 1976. This does not include the additional billions spent for medications they took in hospitals. By the year 2000, it is projected we'll spend $20 billion for over-the-counter products—up from $2.6 billion two decades ago. Clearly, we are spending an extraordinary amount of money on pills, but are we getting our money's worth?

More than ever, consumers need accurate and reliable information on the medicines they take most often. Fortunately, there is some good news:

■ People are taking more responsibility for learning about their medications. Fewer consumers are willing to swallow pills passively without any knowledge of what the drugs are supposed to do. They want to be informed about why and how to take medicine, what the potential side effects may be, and what other medications they need to avoid.

■ Generic prescribing—by the scientific name instead of the brand name—is on the upswing and growing faster each year. Many health professionals and health plans have accepted the fact that most generic drugs are good drugs and can represent significant savings for consumers.

• When you receive a prescription, you should get important information on how the drug works and what its dangers might be. This can come in the form of the official package insert for M.D.'s and pharmacists, or a pharmacy insert prepared by the chain or independent pharmacist. Inserts don't substitute for good communication between you and your health care providers, but they do help you to be an informed partner in your treatment program.

This chapter doesn't replace a trip to the clinic. Rather, it explains in everyday English how to find out just what those pills really do.

Consumer Alert: When a Claim Isn't a Claim

The U.S. Food and Drug Administration rules on the safety and effectiveness of anything that claims to be a medicine, except for herbals and homeopathic remedies. According to the law, the FDA's jurisdiction over drugs includes "articles intended for use in the diagnosis, cure, mitigation, treatment, or prevention of disease in man or other animals, and articles (*other than food*) intended to affect the structure or any function of the body of man or other articles."

The emphasis on the words *other than food* is added. A drug is supposed to have therapeutic benefit, and it undergoes years of studies to establish that it's both safe and effective. The FDA has no power to insist on proof of the safety and effectiveness of food, only that the food is clean.

Manufacturers of herbal, homeopathic, and other nontraditional remedies are using this "other than food" loophole to get around the regulations. That's why you will often see instructions such as "Take one serving" instead of "Take one pill" on the label of some herbal products.

Working with Health Care Providers

Instead of acting as a passive receptacle for the pills and potions prescribed for you and your family, you can be an active health consumer and a partner with your doctors, the pharmacist, nurse practitioners, and other health care providers, learning about the significant consequences of medications and evaluating the benefits as well as the risks. You can also monitor your response to the drug therapy and remain vigilant for side effects.

Golden Rules

■ *Don't take anything for granted.* Drugs can accumulate gradually and cause serious side effects even after you have taken them a long time. Let your doctor know if a troublesome or unexpected symptom arises. If you've taken a drug for many years, ask your doctor to reevaluate your therapy from time to time.

■ *Double-check with the pharmacist about precautions, interactions, side effects, and how to take your medicine.* The pharmacist can also tell you how to store the drug. If you're having trouble taking a medicine—for example, you can't pry a childproof cap off or the pill tastes so foul you gag on it—your pharmacist may be able to suggest a solution.

■ *Contact your doctor's office promptly if you don't understand any instructions or you notice a new symptom shortly after starting the medication.* If it's an emergency, say so when someone answers the phone.

Understanding Your Medicine

Before initiating any drug therapy, here are some key rules of thumb for what you need to learn.

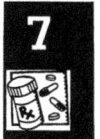

TIP

Easy Access

Ask the pharmacist for a bottle you can open. If you get a bottle with an easy-open cap, keep it out of reach of children. And if you can't read the fine print on the label, ask for a label or separate sheet with the information in large type.

TIP

Memory Aids

Do you need help remembering to take your medicine? It's not smart to skip doses of a drug that should be taken regularly. Your pharmacist can recommend a pillbox organizer, a record-keeping chart, or a bottle with a built-in timer to help you remember.

Such systems should include the schedules for taking each medication and special instructions for their proper use. Keep these records right where you take your medicines, check off each dose as you take it, and make a note if you miss a dose.

Know why this drug is being prescribed. All too often people focus exclusively on the side effects of a medication. It's equally important to understand the anticipated benefits so that you can weigh the benefits against the risks.

Know the name of your drug. Find out its *exact* brand name *and* its generic name. Many drugs look and sound a lot alike. While most pharmacists double- and triple-check their work, accidents do happen. If a heart medicine like digoxin were confused with a close cousin called digitoxin, a disastrous overdose could put you in the emergency room. Make sure your doctor tells you the name of the drug carefully and slowly, and then you pronounce it back until you get it right. You can also ask to have the name of the drug (and its generic components) typed out or printed neatly on a separate piece of paper. If any bad reaction occurs, you can immediately identify the medicine instead of trying to describe a little white tablet or a black-and-green capsule.

Learn how to take the drug. Many people take their medicine incorrectly, if they take it at all. Some studies have shown that one-quarter to one-half of all patients either don't get the prescription filled or fail to take the drug after buying it. Of those who take their medications, more than half may make serious errors by doing so at the wrong time.

To avoid these mistakes, ask your doctor for simple, easy-to-understand guidance, make sure you understand exactly how to take your medicine, and follow the instructions. And make sure the instructions are specific: "Before meals" is ambiguous, but it's easy to understand the meaning of "A half hour before meals."

Check the dose. Even if the pharmacist neatly spells out your instructions for taking the medicine, check the dose. You are the final quality-control inspector. After the doctor writes the prescription and the pharmacist fills it, you are the last person who can realize that something is wrong.

Using sources like those listed in this chapter, find out a reasonable range of doses for the drug. If the amount prescribed for you differs significantly, call the pharmacist. If the pharmacist appears to have filled the prescription incorrectly, call the doctor to make certain it's the right dose.

Find out the drug's side effects. Every drug has the potential to cause some side effects in some people. Your health care providers have the legal and ethical responsibility to inform you about the most common and the most dangerous adverse reactions associated with any medication. Ask about any tests that could detect early signs of these side effects—such as an occasional blood check or urine analysis. If you experience a side effect, even a minor one, contact your physician.

Learn about drug interactions. A great many drugs are totally incompatible with other medicines. In particular, problems can occur when more than one person prescribes drugs for you. Always take a list of every remedy you take—including nonprescription medications like laxatives, antacids, or cold pills—when you visit each health care provider. Ask for a list of any foods or beverages that might not mix well with your medication.

For more information about drug interactions, turn to page 124.

Get it on paper. Visiting a medical office is a traumatic experience for most people. A lot of anxiety is associated with sickness, and often the doctor-patient relationship itself can be stressful. You may not be in any frame of mind to understand or remember what the doctor or nurse tells you. So ask them to write down all important instructions and warnings. Another option would be to take a small tape recorder or dictating machine that will allow you to record the conversation for later playback.

For a checklist of these and other questions to ask about your medications, turn to page 123.

The Types of Medications

Once upon a time the distinction between over-the-counter (OTC) remedies and prescription drugs was clear. OTC products were thought of as mild medications, with few if any serious side effects, that might help relieve simple symptoms. Prescriptions were considered "strong" medicine. You had to go to medical school to understand the intricacies of such powerful medication.

Of course all that has changed. So many prescription drugs have been cleared for OTC sale that it's harder to draw a clear distinction these days. People can buy products such as Actron, Advil, Aleve, Pepcid AC, Tagamet HB, Motrin IB, Orudis KT, and Zantac 75 "off the shelf."

There are also varieties within the two categories. For example, both prescription and OTC products may come in generic or brand names. Also included among OTC remedies are vitamins, food supplements, and

---

TIP

Expiration Dates

The expiration date on a label is valuable information. Although nothing magical happens on the last day a drug is supposed to be "good," this date is in a sense the end of the manufacturer's promise that a pill will deliver a certain amount of medication to the bloodstream. Beyond that, it might work—and it might not. It might deliver a full dose, or half. Or it might deliver some useless—or even harmful—by-product of the chemical breakdown of the drug. It's not a risk worth taking.

7

The Pharmacist

Shopping for a pharmacist will save you money—and keep you healthier. The pharmacist is a highly trained health professional who can provide you with crucial information about your medicine and help you avoid serious mistakes.

You want a pharmacist who will:

■ Keep accurate and up-to-date records of your use of medications, their side effects, and their interactions.

■ Answer all your questions well and give you written information to take home.

■ Talk to you without other people hearing you.

■ Be available by phone in an emergency, *and*

■ Accept payment from any insurance you have for medications.

herbal remedies and other alternative medicines. But no matter what the drug, follow the rules laid out in this chapter; in general, they apply to *all* medications.

For more information on alternative medicine, turn to chapter 19.

Prescription Drugs

A prescription is basically a simple thing. It's the order from a doctor—or, in many states, a nurse practitioner—to a pharmacist to provide you with a certain quantity of a particular drug and to label the package with certain instructions.

Are prescription drugs safe just because the doctor or nurse practitioner prescribed them? The truth is, with over thirty thousand prescription medicines on the market, doctors often don't have the time to keep track of all the reported difficulties with the many drugs they prescribe. Too often their information comes not from medical journals but from drug company salespeople whose presentations usually emphasize the benefits of their products. Doctors are supposed to read detailed information about each drug before prescribing it, but sometimes they don't. In other words, you share the responsibility for your own welfare.

Physicians most often consult the *Physician's Desk Reference,* or *PDR,* published annually by Medical Economics, Inc. You can purchase this book yourself, or it's available in many libraries. Other sources to consult include:

■ *The People's Pharmacy: Completely New and Revised* (St. Martin's Press). Yes, we admit it, we're biased. We think our latest *People's Pharmacy* edition will provide you with valuable information about your medicine. We also offer *The People's Guide to Deadly Drug Interactions* (St. Martin's Press). This book will help you protect yourself from dangerous drug combinations.

■ Another excellent resource is *PDR Family Guide to Prescription Drugs.* It's easier to understand than the doctors' bible (the *PDR*) and is more affordable.

■ An inexpensive and handy drug guide is *The Pill Book* (Bantam Books). Updated every couple of years, it's quite comprehensive.

Skipped Medication

Generally speaking, if the directions read "Take two tablets twice a day," take them at evenly spaced intervals. Keep in mind the goal of drug therapy is to get a more or less constant supply of a medication into your bloodstream.

If you skip your morning pill and instead double up at noon, several possible things could happen. Your body might simply shed the excess drug. Or you might have no medication in your bloodstream for a while. These may be relatively benign outcomes.

The dangers are greater with medications that have a powerful effect on the heart, kidneys, or your hormones. In some cases, the distance between "just enough" and "too much" is small, so doubling up can mean double trouble.

What to do if you miss a dose depends on the drug. In some cases, do nothing; just keep taking the medicine as if nothing had happened. In the case of low-dose birth control pills, however, you'd better use some other form of contraception for the rest of the month. There is no hard rule: When in doubt, check with both the physician and the pharmacist.

Over-the-Counter Medications

Self-treatment is a growing phenomenon, but you can't take good care of yourself unless you're fully informed about the medicines you can get without a prescription. These are called over-the-counter (OTC) or off-the-shelf remedies.

Unfortunately, you can't assume that *all* the nonprescription products you'll find on the pharmacy or health food shelves will be safe *or* effective. Remember, the FDA has little or no jurisdiction over herbal products, "natural" treatments, or food supplements. Consequently, there are lots of things that may or may not live up to the ads.

Is everything you buy over the counter either ineffective or dangerous? The answer is an emphatic *no*. In fact, only a handful of drugs and chemicals in the stores could be considered ineffective or hazardous.

But before you start building up your own little black bag of nonprescription medicine, develop a resource library so you *can* become a knowledgeable consumer. You don't have to buy lots of expensive medical books; your local library should be well stocked with the books and magazines. Besides *The People's Pharmacy: Completely New and Revised,* an excellent source is *The Handbook of Nonprescription Drugs.* Compiled by the American Pharmaceutical Association, this book not only lists the ingredients in most products, but it also gives an overview of the various families of medicines, such as asthma products, laxatives, menstrual products, and antacids. Check your library or call (800) 878-0729 to order a copy ($124).

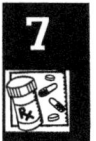

Storing Your Medications

Do *not* store drugs in the medicine cabinet. To see why, look at the mirror after your next shower. All you'll see is steam. Nothing damages drugs faster than heat and humidity.

Where *should* you store drugs? Almost anyplace else is fine, as long as it's away from sunlight and heat. Perhaps a kitchen closet that's out of children's reach, or a high shelf in a bedroom.

Temperature can be a tricky issue. "Store in a cool dry place" may be a harder task than you think. If you order drugs by mail and they are delivered by the postal service or even a commercial carrier, the pills may sit in a hot delivery truck for hours. Temperatures may rise to well over 100°F. Even if you pick up your medicine at the pharmacist and leave it in the car while you do other errands, the heat and humidity could cause rapid deterioration. Childproof caps are not airtight, and humidity can cause problems for many medicines. The bottom line: Treat medications as if they were precious gems. Handle them carefully; at the price they cost, they may well be worth more than gold.

Consumer Alert: OTC—Not Wimpy Drugs

It's easy to walk into a pharmacy, supermarket, or convenience store and buy something for your sniffle. All you have to worry about is driving or operating heavy machinery, right? If you don't need a prescription, it's not really a drug, right? Wrong on both counts. OTC drugs have real benefits and risks.

Remember that the *combination* of prescription and over-the-counter (OTC) medications could be responsible for drug-induced symptoms. Tell your doctor about *all* drugs you take, even those as seemingly innocuous as cough remedies. Only then can she or he determine whether a drug interaction is at the root of an illness that shows up after you've started the medication.

Herbal Remedies

Americans spend over a billion dollars each year on natural remedies, buying them not only at health food stores but also from supermarkets and pharmacies and by mail order. Sales are growing 15 percent a year, with no end in sight.

Herbal treatments often have histories that go back thousands of years, and plants are the source of many of today's successful prescription medicines. Nevertheless, few medical schools teach about these therapies. And pharmacy schools, which once took pride in "pharmacognosy" classes on medicinal plants, now mostly shun the topic. As a result, the health professionals most Americans turn to about drugs—physicians and pharmacists—are often unprepared to answer questions or make recommendations about these natural remedies.

The difficulty of knowing exactly what's in an herbal preparation makes consumers vulnerable to fraud and unexpected hazards. The U.S. Food and Drug Administration has almost no legal authority to require that herbal products are effective or safe. You can't trust that a product actually contains the ingredient on the label, and you have no way of knowing how much is in a dose.

Given this lack of protection, the most important ingredient in any herbal remedy is a strong dose of common sense. This is essential at every step of the way, including the decision to treat yourself. Serious conditions deserve medical attention, so start with a clear diagnosis from a health professional. If the disorder may be treated with herbs, by all means do so, but tell *all* your health care providers about *all* your medications. And check with the expert if the symptoms don't go away in a reasonable amount of time.

If you are taking any other medications regularly, check carefully to see whether the herb may interact with your prescription or OTC drugs. Certainly, if any negative symptoms arise, discontinue the herb and consult a health professional.

Remember that herbs can have side effects just like any drug, and certain herbs are potentially dangerous. Growing in the ground doesn't make a plant safe, as you are reminded every so often when someone inadvertently consumes poisonous mushrooms.

To be on the safe side, check with your pharmacist about proper storage. Always keep the medicine in the bottle it came in. And if the label falls off, tape it back on or replace it immediately.

Avoiding Drug Dangers

The majority of medications can't cure anything. Rather, most drugs temporarily relieve symptoms. And there's almost always a price for such relief: The U.S. Food and Drug Administration estimates that anywhere from 3 percent to 11 percent of Americans are hospitalized each year because of adverse drug reactions. That translates to somewhere between 1 million and 3 million Americans hospitalized due to bad side effects. Today's potent drugs carry even greater risks, raising the ante for consumers.

Even with the best testing, no drug can be guaranteed safe for everyone. Every drug has some side effects.

Checklist: How to Avoid Medication Miseries

7

Good communication is crucial for taking medicine safely. Get answers to these questions from your doctor, nurse, or pharmacist.

✓ *What is the name of my medicine?* Know the generic as well as the brand name.
✓ *What is this drug supposed to do?* Will it cure my basic problem or just relieve my symptoms? Do I take it to prevent a problem or only "as needed"?
✓ *Are there other ways to treat my problem?* Sometimes nondrug approaches keep a medical condition under control or supplement a medicine. An old-fashioned drug may be less convenient but considerably easier on your wallet.
✓ *What is the prescribed dose of my medicine?* Is it tailored to me and my body? For example, lower doses of certain medications reduce the risk of bad reactions for older people.
✓ *How should I take this medicine?* Should I take it with a meal or on an empty stomach? Should I swallow the pill with water, juice, or milk? Should I avoid coffee?
✓ *How long should I take this medicine?* Sometimes drugs intended for a temporary problem end up being taken for years because nobody tells the patient when to stop.

Herbal Resources

If your health care professional doesn't know about the safety and effectiveness of herbal preparations, how can you take these drugs wisely? It's hard to tell if the clerk at the health food store is quite knowledgeable or totally ignorant.

An excellent source of information is the American Botanical Council (ABC). It offers a variety of publications, including the journal *HerbalGram* and a number of books. Contact the ABC at P.O. Box 201660, Austin, TX 78720-1660; tel. (800) 373-7105.

For further information, you can consult these resources:

- *The Healing Herbs*, by Michael Castleman (Rodale Press, 1991), $27.95

- *Nature's Cures*, by Michael Castleman (Rodale Press, 1996), $27.95

- *Herbs of Choice*, by Varro E. Tyler (Pharmaceutical Products Press, 1994), $12.95

- *The Honest Herbal*, by Varro E. Tyler (Pharmaceutical Products Press, 1993), $15.95

- *Handbook of Medicinal Herbs*, by James A.

✓ *How should I discontinue this medicine?* Stopping a medicine can sometimes be more complicated than starting. Withdrawal reactions, especially with some new antidepressants, can be awful. Find out the best way to phase out your pills.

✓ *What are the most common side effects?* What might I experience? Are these reactions likely to diminish with time?

✓ *What are the most serious side effects?* Are any reactions so dangerous that I should call my doctor immediately if they occur? What are the warning signs?

✓ *Will I need lab tests to detect reactions?* What tests will I need and how often?

✓ *How will this medication interact with other drugs I'm taking?* Tell your doctor about all of them, including over-the-counter and herbal remedies.

✓ *How should I store my medicine?* Your pharmacist can advise you on the best place to keep your drugs.

Interactions between Drugs

Many of the unexpected side effects from medicines come from combining more than one drug at a time. Indeed, improper combinations could be fatal.

Drug interactions are complicated and confusing, and the complexities can be mind-boggling. With so many combinations and permutations, it practically takes a computer to sort out the matter:

One drug may cancel the benefits of another. For example, some antibiotics may reduce the effectiveness of birth control pills and lead to an unwanted pregnancy.

One drug may amplify the side effects of a second drug. For example, antihistamines may magnify the lack of coordination and drowsiness that sedatives often cause, or the combination of an over-the-counter cold pill and a prescription drug for nerves could be lethal if you try to drive your car.

The combination of two or more drugs could create a totally unexpected reaction. If a woman takes a medicine for a vaginal infection (metronidazole) and also has a few drinks, the unpleasant reactions might include a headache, flushing, nausea, and vomiting.

Drug incompatibilities present a tremendous challenge to health care providers. For one thing, there is just too much information to memorize. Another problem is that doctors rarely know all the nonprescription drugs their patients are taking. Laxatives, painkillers, and cold remedies are just a few of the over-the-counter medications that can have a profound effect on prescription drugs. A dangerous interaction could occur if the doctor doesn't know you take these nonprescription products. And most people don't even think to mention that they take a vitamin-and-mineral complex or an herbal remedy, yet this kind of incomplete communication is almost guaranteed to cause problems.

Drug-to-drug reactivity is an especially acute problem when you get prescriptions from two or more people. The cardiologist who puts you on medicine for angina and high blood pressure may be unaware that the rheumatologist has prescribed another medication for arthritis. The combination could well decrease the ability of the medicine to lower blood pressure effectively.

Duke (CRC Press, 1985), $316

■ *The Review of Natural Products.* Subscription is $65 per year. Order from Facts and Comparisons, 111 West Port Plaza, #300, St. Louis, MO 63146-3098.

Drugs That Affect Sexuality

Many factors can affect sexual desire. Romance, psychology, stress, hormones—and drugs—can all stimulate or depress passion.

Changes in libido can be subtle and hard to measure, but the scarcity of literature on drugs affecting sexuality means that you must rely on your own judgment. If a medication seems to be having a negative effect, you and your doctor should consider whether another medicine might be less likely to interfere with sexuality. Trial and error could be the best process, since the doctor may not be able to confirm the reaction by looking it up in a standard reference.

Drug and Food Interactions

Almost by accident, scientists have discovered that certain drugs and foods do not mix well. In some cases, people didn't get better when they took their medicine with meals or particular beverages. In other instances, a food produced an unexpected and alarming reaction.

Food can affect your medicine in three basic ways:

1. Food can reduce the absorption of a pill you swallow, so you get less of the drug into your bloodstream.

2. In a few instances, food may enhance absorption.

3. Some medicines irritate the digestive tract, causing stomach pain, heartburn, indigestion, nausea, vomiting, or diarrhea. Often these medications pose less of a problem if you take them either during a meal or just after eating.

In many instances, food may not affect the medication at all. However, there's no data about food interactions for many drugs, making it very difficult for physicians and pharmacists to give you sound scientific recommendations. And with over thirty thousand prescription medicines on the market, it's impossible to list food-drug interactions here. Check with your physician and pharmacist. They may have to contact the manufacturer for information, so allow some time for a response. You can also consult some of the resources listed at the end of this chapter

Drug and Nutrient Interactions

As nutritional supplements gain in popularity, the significance of their interactions with medications also increases. Postmenopausal women are taking calcium and vitamin D to ward off osteoporosis; many men are taking vitamin E to help prevent heart attacks. Any number of health-conscious people take vitamins or minerals for a variety of reasons: to help ensure a healthy pregnancy, to strengthen the immune system, to reduce the risk of cancer.

Although more studies are needed to confirm the significance of such health benefits, doctors and patients can't assume that drug-nutrient interactions are esoteric or unusual. All of the possible ways food can affect drugs also apply to nutrients.

Psychological Side Effects

Hallucinations, anxiety, depression, suicidal thoughts, insomnia, nightmares, paranoia, memory loss, and delirium aren't always signs of mental illness. In some cases, psychological and emotional changes *may* be unanticipated reactions from common medicines. If these symptoms aren't recognized as drug side effects, they might be treated with other medications. It can turn into a vicious cycle.

Clearly, not all psychiatric symptoms are brought on by medicine. Sometimes depression, anxiety, or hallucinations happen because of severe stress or biochemical changes in the brain. But all psychological symptoms deserve careful evaluation by a health professional capable of determining if a medication is contributing to the problem.

This is especially true for seniors, who are more susceptible to drug side effects and are usually less likely to complain about them. All too often an older person will accept a symptom as another sign of the aging process, when in fact the cause could be a prescription drug, an over-the-counter medication, or a combination of both.

If you notice psychological or emotional changes while taking any drug, notify your physician at once. Family members must also be vigilant for personality changes that may be brought on by medicine. Drug-induced mental problems are far too often overlooked or ignored.

If you suspect a medication you are taking is producing psychological symptoms, first of all, *don't stop taking that medication* and *do contact your physician.*

The next step is a little tricky, however. Quite possibly, you will need to find a professional—perhaps a psychiatrist—who understands neuropharmacology in order to get you back on the road to good health, mentally and physically. Your family physician may be fully aware of the physical side effects that are common for the drug in question but less knowledgeable about how that drug affects the central nervous system. Or your physician may not be aware of other drugs you are taking, including over-the-counter medications.

Consumer Alert: Withdrawal Dangers

Some psychological symptoms associated with medications don't start until a person stops taking the drug. Stopping an anti-anxiety drug suddenly may cause disorientation, fear, insomnia, anxiety, and agitation. Seizures have occurred in people with no history of epilepsy.

How do you get off such medicines without suffering from withdrawal symptoms?

The first thing—and this can't be stressed enough—is that cutting back requires medical supervision. Consult a health care professional. *This is under no circumstances a self-help project.*

Children and Medication

Children are not just little adults, either mentally or physically. They don't always react to medications the same way adults do.

Physicians writing in the *British Medical Journal* have reported cases of children who suffered terrifying hallucinations—most of which involved insects or spiders—after taking a cold medicine that contained both an antihistamine and a decongestant.

One wonders how many times irritability, dizziness, and nightmares are blamed on the illness rather than the treatment. After all, if a parent takes an over-the-counter remedy safely, why can't a child? In fact, antihistamines, common in allergy and cold remedies, can cause drowsiness in adults, but they can act as a stimulant for children. A child who gets a multisymptom medication for a cough could be wired for hours.

Money Matters

Prescription medicines used to be a health care bargain. The average prescription would cost less than $10, and most people felt they were getting their money's worth. Now, it's not unusual for pharmaceutical manufacturers to raise prices every few months.

Who pays for those drugs? For the most part, you.

Drug Plans

More and more people have some coverage for prescription drugs in their health insurance plans. Also, most health plans that cover your hospital care cover at least the prescriptions you receive during your inpatient stay in the hospital (but not always those you take for follow-up care after leaving the hospital).

Insurance coverage for medications can save you a lot of money, if you understand and follow the health plan's rules. For example, you may have to buy your prescriptions by mail or from a restricted list of pharmacies.

If your health insurance covers prescriptions, find out:

■ What medications does it cover? Does it cover drugs for chronic conditions only? Does it cover experimental drugs? Any nonprescription drugs?

■ What rules must you follow for the insurance to pay for your medications?

■ What is your out-of-pocket cost? Does this vary depending on whether you use a generic or a brand-name drug? Does it vary depending on where you buy the prescription?

Lower-Cost Prescriptions

An easy way to save money is to ask the doctor what drug he or she is prescribing and whether it's available in generic form. With rare exceptions, generic drugs are every bit the equal of their brand-name twins. The FDA holds every manufacturer—brand-name and generic alike—to high standards designed to assure consumers that the final product is what it's supposed to be in terms of dose, potency, cleanliness, and other critical factors. In fact, Brand Name A and Generic B may be *identical* because they're the same pill, made by the same manufacturer, in the same factory, at virtually the same time.

If your insurance covers prescriptions, check the rules. It may be that you *have* to use the generic form if it's available and your doctor hasn't specified otherwise.

If a drug isn't available in generic form, ask if any acceptable alternative medicine might be available generically. Many conditions can be treated by a variety of medications, and a doctor who knows you are on a tight budget may choose an older medicine that costs less than the very latest development.

"Dispense As Written"

When a physician writes "Dispense as written" or "Do not substitute," the pharmacist must give you exactly the drug called for, which usually means a specific brand name. This can cost you money.

Why would the doctor do that? He or she may have absolute, scientific knowledge that one company's preparation of a drug causes the drug to act differently than one produced by another company. Or the doctor may think that's true but lacks scientific proof of such a conclusion.

Ask your doctor to explain why the prescription says "Do not substitute."

Mail-Order Pharmacies

Consider shopping by mail. This won't work if you need a one-time prescription for an immediate illness, but it can save big bucks for medications you know you'll need for a chronic problem that requires ongoing medication. Your insurance might even specify a mail-order supplier for long-term medications.

The notion of ordering medication by mail may seem a bit strange. In reality it's a simple, easy process. You put your prescription form in an envelope, along with a check for the number of pills. Back comes the prescription, delivered to your mailbox.

On the other hand, you may have good reason to pay more at the local pharmacy. In addition to immediate service, you can get personal attention, including information on the drug: how to take it, any possible adverse effects, interactions with other drugs, and so on. And keep checking on prices: Your local drugstore may charge the same price as a mail-order source for some medicines. And don't buy more than you need just to get a mail-order discount: Wasted medicines are costly, too.

There is another advantage to buying locally. The medicine will not sit in a hot delivery truck all day or in your mailbox. Temperature extremes (too hot *or* too cold) can be devastating to some of today's complex chemical compounds.

7

TIP

Take Your Medicine

$ The most important step in getting the best value at the pharmacy is to take your medicine properly. Make sure you get clear instructions on when and how to take it and follow them.

Claims That Are Hardly Ever True

- "Breakthrough"—Medicine, alas, usually works its way forward by inches.

- "Miracle"—A few unexpected recoveries may be difficult to explain, but these are also almost impossible to predict.

- "A Doctor's Formula" or "A doctor's discovery" or doctor's anything

- "It worked for me!" or "It saved my life" or any other kind of testimonial

- "New from Europe" or someplace other than nearby

- "Contains Foo-Goo" or some other strange, vaguely nauseating ingredient

- "The doctors don't want you to know this"—If there's a conspiracy, it's one of conservatism. It

Mail-Order Sources

A number of superdiscount pharmacies operate mail-order services. The American Association of Retired Persons (AARP) runs one of the largest and best known. For information, contact the AARP Pharmacy Service, 500 Montgomery Street, Alexandria, VA 22314; tel. (800) 456-2277.

Here are some other mail-order pharmacies:

- Action Mail Order, P.O. Box 787, Waterville, ME 04903-0787; tel. (800) 452-1976
- American Preferred Plan, P.O. Box 9019, Farmingdale, NY 11735; tel. (800) 227-1195
- Systems Pharmacy, 6109 Willowmere Drive, Des Moines, IA 50321; tel. (515) 287-6872
- Medi-Mail, P.O. Box 98520, Las Vegas, NV 89193-8520; tel. (800) 331-1458 or (800) 922-3444

More Money-Saving Options

Generic drugs and mail-order pharmacies are the most obvious ways to save money on medications, but they aren't the only ones. Here are a few more:

Consider nondrug alternatives. The best way to reduce your drug bill is to eliminate the drugs. Sometimes a nondrug approach can be successful—for example, exercise and diet to lower cholesterol or weight loss and relaxation practice to control blood pressure. This requires good communication with health care professionals, who will guide you and evaluate your progress. A nondrug regimen may require more effort on your part, but it can be just as effective as medication, less expensive, *and* result in fewer side effects. Of course, no one should ever stop medication without medical supervision!

Ask about nonprescription options. In the past few years, many medicines once available only by prescription have been approved for over-the-counter sale. Ibuprofen, originally sold as Motrin, was once the best-selling arthritis prescription. Now you can buy it as Motrin IB, Advil, Nuprin, Medipren, and, at substantial savings, generic ibuprofen. There are also amazing savings on stomach medicines like cimetidine (Tagamet HB), ranitidine (Zantac 75) and famotidine (Pepcid AC).

Ask the doctor for a free sample plus a prescription for enough medication to last a moderately long time. When you start a new medication, ask for enough samples to find out if you can tolerate the medicine. You can't check the drug in the store to make sure it fits, as you might a pair of shoes. And prescription drugs aren't returnable.

If no samples are available, ask the pharmacist for enough medicine to last several days (unless your health plan charges a fixed copayment per prescription, in which case you want the largest supply each time). It costs more per pill to buy a small amount, but if the medicine gives you a horrible rash, you won't have wasted as much money overall.

Once you know a medicine agrees with you, save by buying in quantity. Prices often show discounts at quantities of fifty and a hundred, so if the prescription can reasonably be written for those amounts, ask the doctor to do it. *But make sure the expiration date is on the label.* Don't get so much medicine that it expires before you can use it.

Of course, your immediate cash outlay may be a factor. If a drug is expensive, you might not want to pay a lot at one time to save a relatively small amount per pill.

Comparison shop. Call several local pharmacies to check out the price of your new prescription before you go get it. Even if a pharmacy has a "lowest price" policy, you'll still have to do some shopping by phone to find out that lowest price.

Comparison shopping is especially important with a long-term prescription for a drug you take daily, such as drugs for heart problems, high blood pressure, arthritis, and other chronic problems.

Treat your prescription right. To get the most for your drug dollar, take care of your medicine. Improper storage could shorten its effective life, waste money, and endanger your health.

Free Medicine!

A number of pharmaceutical manufacturers provide free prescriptions. To qualify, you can't have insurance that covers drugs, and you must be low-income. Ask your doctor to help you access the program, or call the pharmaceutical industry's Patient Assistance Hot Line at (800) 762-4636 for eligibility information and a directory of programs.

Connecticut, Illinois, Maine, Maryland, New Jersey, New York, Pennsylvania, and Rhode Island have state-funded programs that provide assistance for older people who are financially strapped. Minnesota has made provisions for both children and older people. If you are fortunate enough to live in one of these states, check with social services agencies

may sometimes slow down the appearance of a new drug, but it is, by and large, to doctors' credit and your advantage. It's unethical for a doctor to prescribe a regimen that won't help a patient. It is also unethical to experiment with an unproved therapy unless the patient has no other hope and agrees, with full knowledge of the potential risks, to be part of a study.

■ *"FDA approved"*—If something is flashing the FDA at you as an implied endorsement, ignore what's being sold.

■ *"Cures everything"* or at least lots of things. Fewer than a handful of drugs work against more than either a limited number of diseases or a limited number of bacteria. If it sounds too good to be true, most likely it is.

■ *"It cures an incurable disease"*—If you never go for a "cure" for any of seven conditions, you could avoid almost all of the fraud come-ons. The Big Seven are *weight loss, arthritis, cancer, impotence, baldness, wrinkles,* and *aging.*

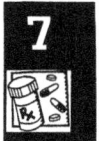

or special programs like PACE (Pharmaceutical Assistance Contract for the Elderly) in Pennsylvania and PAAD (Pharmaceutical Assistance to the Aged and Disabled) in New Jersey.

WORSHEET
Drug Safety Questionnaire

Copy this questionnaire and take it to your doctor or pharmacist. Ask him or her to fill it in or to help you do so. You will take your medicine more safely if you know the answers.

Purpose of medicine: _____

Name of medicine: _____

Brand: _____

Generic:_____

Dose: _____

When to take: _____ A.M.   _____ P.M.

Take medicine:_____ with food _____ an hour before or two hours after meals

Foods to avoid, if any: _____

Special precautions, if any:_____

Contraindications or situations when this drug might be inappropriate, if any:

_____

Interacting medicines to avoid, if any: _____

Common side effects: _____

Serious symptoms: _____

I should notify my doctor immediately at phone number: (office): _____

(home): _____

Date to discontinue (if any): _____

_____

Resources
Organizations

Health Research Group
2000 P Street, N.W.
Washington, DC 20036
(202) 588-1000
Call or write to order *Worst Pills, Best Pills II,* edited by Sidney M. Wolfe, or to subscribe to the monthly newsletter *Worst Pills, Best Pills News* ($10 per year).

Medical Economics
P.O. Box 162
Montvale, NJ 07645-1742
(800) 232-7379
Call or write for a list of publications for health care professionals and consumers, including *The PDR Family Guide to Prescription Drugs,* 1995 ($25.95) and *The PDR Family Guide to Women's Health and Prescription Drugs,* 1994 ($24.95).

The People's Pharmacy
P.O. Box 52027
Durham, NC 27717-2027
(800) 732-2334
Call or write to order materials or to receive a literature list. Books available are *The People's Guide to Deadly Drug Interactions* ($26.95), *Graedon's Best Medicine* ($15.95), *The Aspirin Handbook* ($4.99), *The People's Pharmacy: Completely New and Revised* (St. Martin's Press, 1996) ($16.95), *The Pill Book* ($6.99). Also available are brochures ($2 each) on such topics as gastrointestinal drugs, drug-food interactions, and drugs and older people. Audio tapes ($10 each) are available on such topics as sex after forty, anxiety and its treatment, and dealing with grief and bereavement.

U.S. Food and Drug Administration
Consumer Information Line: (301) 443-3170
Call to get information on a specific drug.

U.S. Pharmacopoeia Practitioner's Reporting Network
(800) 638-6725
(301) 881-0256 in Maryland
Call to report problems with medical devices.

Publications

American Drug Index, by Norman F. Billups and Shirley M. Billups (Facts and Comparison, 1995), $45. Updated annually, health professionals use these monographs for identifying, explaining, and correlating pharmaceuticals.

The American Medical Association Guide to Prescription and Over-the-Counter Drugs, edited by Charles B. Clayman (Random House, 1990), $39.95.

Complete Drug Reference (Consumer Reports Books, 1996), $39.95. A guide to over-the-counter and prescription drugs.

Complete Guide to Prescription and Non-Prescription Drugs, by H. Winter Griffith (Body Press/Perigee), $15.95. Updated annually.

The Consumer's Medical Desk Reference: Information Your Doctor Can't or Won't Tell You—Everything You Need to Know for the Best in Health Care, by Charles B. Inlander and the Staff of the People's Medical Society (Hyperion, 1995), $24.95.

7

"Herbal Roulette," in *Consumer Reports,* November 1995. To order a reprint ($3), call (800) 234-1645.

The Pill Book: The Illustrated Guide to the Most Prescribed Drugs in the United States (Bantam Books, 1996), $24.95.

Prescription Drug Handbook, by AARP Pharmacy Service (Harper, 1992), $17.95.

"To Your Good Health: Advice for Older Adults About Medicines for Self-Care." For a copy of this free pamphlet, contact the Nonprescription Drug Manufacturers Association, Publications Department, 1150 Connecticut Avenue, N.W., Washington, DC 20036; tel. (202) 429-9260.

Part Three

Focusing on You

8 Parents as Health Care Consumers

Nora Wells

Nora Wells is the parent of sons ages twenty-five, twenty-one, and fifteen, one of whom has cerebral palsy. She has been active in parent advocacy activities for the past twenty years at both the state and national levels. She is a national coordinator for Family Voices, a grassroots network of families of children with special health needs. She is coauthor of *Paying the Bills: Tips for Families on Financing Health Care for Children with Special Needs.*

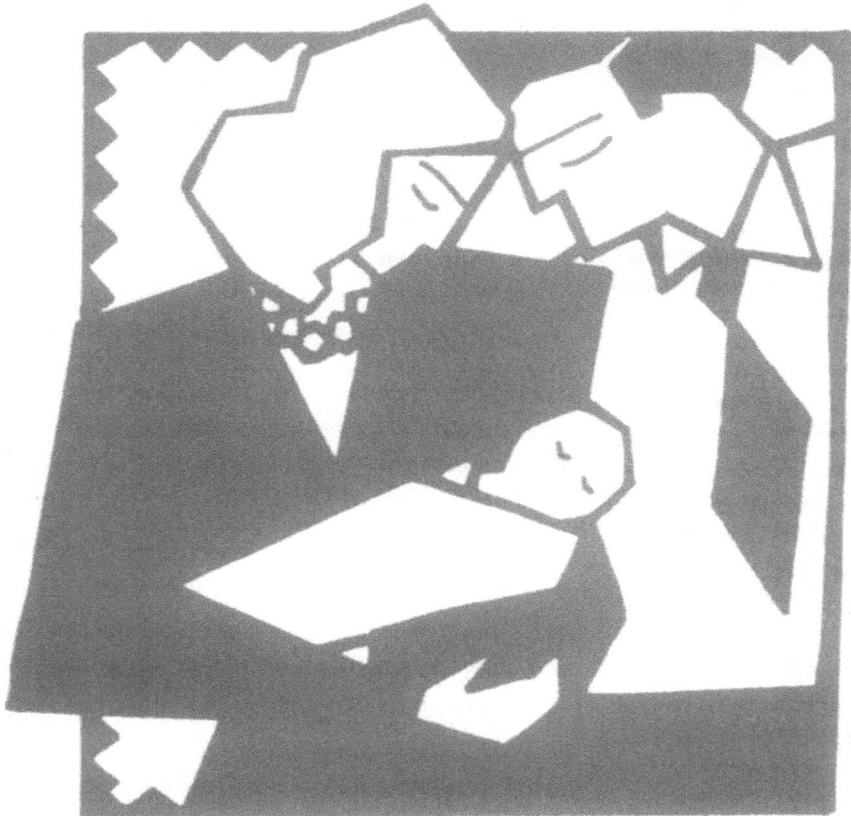

TIP

Guidelines for Parents

For a free copy of the pamphlet "You and Your Pediatrician: Guidelines for Parents," send a stamped, self-addressed envelope to the American Academy of Pediatrics, 141 NW Point Boulevard, Elk Grove Village, IL 60007.

Special Questions

If your child has special health care needs and you are seeking a physician or other health care professional, ask specific questions of potential providers about their experience with your child's condition. For example, if your child has asthma, you might want to know how a provider handles this special need. How will you and the provider cooperate to handle emergencies? Ask a provider:

- Do other children in your practice have similar special needs?

- What specialists and agencies do you work with on a regular basis?

- How do you communicate with these other providers?

As a parent, you make many major decisions in the life of your child. Few choices you make matter more than those surrounding health care. From the mother's pregnancy into the child's infancy and through the teen years, you decide when to seek medical care, and you choose the people who are best qualified to provide it.

As you take these steps, you also serve as a role model for your daughters and sons. With your help—and that of their health care providers—your children will prepare to take over their own care and decision-making responsibilities as they reach adolescence.

Primary Care for Children

The first important decision you must make is the choice of a primary care provider for your child. This is the all-important person who will:

- Provide "well child" care—that is, the preventive measures you, your child, and health care professionals take to keep your child healthy.
- Maintain basic medical records on your child.
- Treat your child when he or she is sick.
- Refer your child to specialists when needed.
- Give you medical and developmental advice on caring for your child, *and*
- Work with you to monitor your child's growth and development.

Providers of Primary Care for Children

Every child needs a primary care provider from the day he or she is born. Parents can get this basic, ongoing care for their children from many kinds of providers. Depending on where you live, certain types may be more plentiful than others:

- *Pediatricians* are medical doctors who specialize in the care of children.

- *Family practitioners* are medical doctors with special training to care for all members of a family, including children.

- *Nurse practitioners* are nurses who are trained to perform a number of well-child and other routine procedures. Many are also the primary care providers for children and families.

Public Health Departments

In many places, county and city health departments operate clinics and special programs for youth, including providing some primary care services. Among other services, these offices may provide child health and pediatric care, as well as adolescent services, immunizations, family planning services, pregnancy tests, pregnancy counseling and referrals, maternity services, and childbirth education classes.

To locate your local health departments, look in the blue pages of your phone book.

Choosing a Provider for Primary Care

Often, a key factor in the choice of a child's primary care provider is the family's medical payment plan. Sometimes you can choose any provider, but many plans limit your options. Traditional insurance, if it covers primary care, usually allows you to choose any board-certified physician. However, more and more families now participate in managed care plans, such as HMOs. Managed care plans almost always include primary care, but you usually must choose your providers from the plan's network. Sometimes you have many choices of providers; sometimes you're limited to the physicians at a center near your home. In either case, it's up to you whether everyone in your family will share the same primary care provider, or whether you will each see a different person.

Tap into a variety of resources to find the primary care provider who suits your needs. Word of mouth is one excellent source: Talk to your family and friends. Whom do their children see? What do your friends like—or dislike—about these providers? Ask your own doctor for recommendations. Seek referrals from local agencies, such as day care centers, preschools, schools, and early-intervention programs.

School-Based Adolescent Care

More and more adolescents can now get health services through their schools. The schools help health care providers reach this group, which is often medically underserved.

School-based centers make use of multidisciplinary teams—nurse practitioners, physicians, social workers, nurses, and health educators—to provide comprehensive care to adolescents, including on-site appointments, referrals, and follow-up.

- With which hospitals are you affiliated?

Note that you may want to consider similar issues when you select a health plan.

8

For more information, contact your local Department of Public Health's School Health Department.

TIP

Before Birth

Select a primary care provider for your child before an emergency arises—ideally, before or during your pregnancy. If you move to a new area, make identifying a primary care provider for your child a high priority.

After you have chosen a provider, don't throw away the other recommendations. You may need a second opinion or a new provider in the future.

The Factors to Consider

When picking a provider for your child, think about what matters to you. No one provider is perfect in every way. Only you can evaluate the importance of each factor.

Think about personality and style. Do you like the way the provider interacts with children and parents? Do you think his or her style fits the needs of you and your child? Does the provider support the right of families to be with their child for procedures and treatments? Does he or she believe in sharing all information with patients?

Keep in mind a number of other points as well:

■ Do you find it easy to communicate with the provider and to ask questions? *Just as important, does your child?*

■ Is location important? Can you get to the office or health center quickly if your child has an emergency? Is there a beeper number you can call? An answering service? How quickly does the doctor respond when a parent calls about a sick child? Is there a phone number you can call for routine questions? When can you call?

■ How do you get an appointment if your child is sick? Is this a group practice, with providers covering one another's patients when they aren't available themselves?

■ Are the office hours convenient for your child's regular appointments? If you work days or your child is school-age, can you readily arrange evening or weekend appointments?

■ Will your insurance cover the provider's services?

For more information on choosing a primary care provider and questions to ask, turn to chapter 5.

Primary Dental Care for Children

Just as several types of professionals handle medical care for your children, a variety of choices are available when it comes to their routine dental care as well:

■ *Pediatric dentists* specialize in the care of children.
■ *General dentists* treat both children and adults.

■ *Orthodontists* specialize in straightening teeth for both children and adults.

For more information on dental care, turn to chapter 17.

Your Role in the Partnership

Once you identify a health care provider for your son or daughter, build a partnership in which you each clearly identify your needs. From the point of view of a quality provider, you're an essential source of information about your child's development. Your perspective on your child is unique.

Before you call or visit your child's provider, write down your questions and concerns so that you remember them at your visit. *All of your questions and opinions are legitimate and important.*

Some of your questions may not be easy to answer—many medical questions have no certain answers. This makes it extremely important that you share all your concerns and questions openly with providers and listen carefully to their replies. *If you don't understand a reply, don't hesitate to ask again—and again.* Because many medical situations are emotionally charged, it can help if you try to articulate your concerns and worries and ask questions when you need more information. If you think of an additional question when you return home from an appointment, never hesitate to call the provider's office and ask.

You can also learn a great deal, and gain a great deal of support, from other adults. Talk with other parents and your children's teachers, day care providers, and baby-sitters about your health concerns for your child. These people can be important sources of information about your child. Likewise, advocacy and mutual-help organizations provide information, support, and other forms of assistance to parents of children with a variety of specific health conditions.

For more information on mutual-aid groups, turn to chapter 22.

The most important aspect of your relationship with your child's medical providers is the quality of trust and communication you establish. At the most basic level, medical treatments probably won't succeed if you and your child can't follow the instructions carefully. And providers can't give reasonable care to your child if you don't openly report your concerns. Your child's providers will rely on you to follow the treatment plan and to report any changes you see in your child during treatment. If the plan isn't working or causes you or your child concern, check back with your provider. The plan may need to be adjusted.

Families need to completely understand:

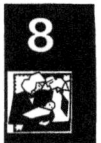

TIP

Two Appointments

Sometimes you have so many questions about your child's health that you can't cover them all during a single exam or treatment. If need be, schedule a separate time to discuss your questions with your child's providers, whether in person or on the phone.

- Prescribed treatments
- The reasons for the treatments
- The expected results
- What might happen during treatment, *and*
- What to do if the treatment doesn't go as planned

Make sure you understand what might happen if you refuse the treatment. What are your options? Particularly if you are considering a complicated procedure such as surgery, ask for materials to read and for the names of other families whose children have had the procedure.

Whenever your child receives care, give providers feedback. Discuss those aspects of care you particularly liked as well as those that worried or displeased you. Providers usually listen carefully to this kind of input and find it very helpful. It could also significantly improve the care your child receives in the future.

Time to Change Providers?

If you are genuinely unhappy with your child's care, be willing to change providers. However, remember that continuity is important for good health care, as is the relationship that you and a particular health care provider build over the years.

In other words, try to select your providers carefully from the first, and always communicate with them fully. Invest the time and effort required to build a strong relationship.

Keep Records

Build and maintain a complete record of every contact with your child's health care providers, both in person and over the phone, and write down what providers report and recommend. Include in this record a log of all immunizations, medications, and other treatments prescribed for your son or daughter. For immunizations, note the type of shot, the date, the location, and the provider. For medications, write down the dosages and the times when the child takes each medicine. Keep note of any special considerations:

- Could a drug interact dangerously with any foods or other medications?
- What possible side effects should you look for?
- What should you do in case of a reaction to the medication?

These records will improve the health of your children in several ways. First, even if you think you'll remember instructions after a visit, it's easy to forget critical details a few days later—or even a few hours later. Second, your written record helps if you need to follow up with another provider about the same problem. Third, if your child has an emergency, the records may be critical to a nurse or doctor who doesn't know your child's medical history. Fourth, they are critical when you move and enter into a partnership with a new provider.

Always read your child's medical records yourself and ask about anything you don't understand. If your child is referred to a specialist, ask the specialist to send a report to the primary care provider so that your child's record is always complete, and make sure you get a copy, too.

Keep your records handy at home, and bring them with you to all health visits. One good idea is to assemble all the records you keep into a "passport," maintained jointly by you and your children's health care providers. Such booklets contain a range of information, from your child's height, weight, and immunization record to a complete set of health records and guidance for educating your child about health. The passport not only keeps information in one place but helps to empower you as a parent to actively participate in your child's care, in both sickness and health.

There are many types of parent-held child health records. Perhaps the most thorough is the Denver Child Health Passport. A notebook with tear-out sheets designed to fit into a diaper bag or a large purse, it covers the first six years of life and includes the family's social and medical histories, health evaluations from the neonatal examination through the six-year health visit, a summary chart documenting the dates of each preventive service, and much more.

The Denver Child Health Passports are being distributed through physicians. For more information, write to Community Child Development, Children's Hospital, 1056 E. 19th Avenue, Box B215, Denver, CO 80218.

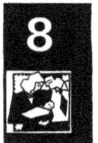

Second Opinions

Don't hesitate to seek a second opinion if you're unhappy about your child's care—or if you simply want reassurance about a diagnosis or recommended treatment. Medical providers often differ widely on the best course of treatment. Even if they do agree, a second opinion will sometimes help you understand a situation better or feel more at ease. Still, always let your primary provider know what you are doing and why you are doing it.

For more information on second opinions and specialists, turn to chapter 13.

Pages from the Denver Child Health Passport

Health Suggestions

4 Month

Nutrition
- Keep breast feeding or using formula. Babies aren't ready for cow's milk yet.
- You can start feeding solid foods now. Try one new food at a time.
- Your baby might like different foods than you. That's OK! Let your baby try different kinds of food, even those that you don't like.

Safety
- Put your baby in a car seat whenever you go in the car.
- Protect your baby from burns! Keep curling irons, clothes irons, and other hot objects out of your baby's reach.
- Keep your house safe. Put away small objects your baby could swallow.

Development
- Keep talking to your baby. Babies learn to talk by listening to other people.
- Babies like toys! Give your baby rattles, spoons, and squeeze toys to play with.
- Play games with your baby. Babies love playing games like Peek-a-Boo and So-Big!
- Let your baby look in the mirror.

Health Education
- Keep your baby healthy. Talk with your health provider about shots for your baby.
- Get to know your babysitter or child care person. It is important to feel good about the person who takes care of your baby.
- Your baby may start to get teeth soon. Babies may drool and be more fussy when their teeth come in.
- Ask your health provider if the amount of medicine you give your baby for fevers should increase.
- Ask your health provider when to call him or her for advice or information.

Your next visit to your Health Provider is on

Day/Date: _____

Time: _____

Person: _____

Phone No. _____

Poison Control Phone No.

PARTNERS IN HEALTH CARE

A health care provider fills in the information at the right before the parent leaves the office after the child's four-month visit.

Fill in this box if name, address or phone have changed. ☐

Child's Name: _____

Address: _____

Phone: _____ Message Phone: _____

Date: _____ Chart #: _____

021

Parent worries/questions: _____

What does your child drink (milk, juice, other)? _____

What solids does your child eat? _____

Illnesses/accidents since last visit: _____

Does your child reach for objects?	☐ Yes	☐ No
Does your child laugh?	☐ Yes	☐ No
Does your child grasp objects with his/her hands?	☐ Yes	☐ No
Do your child's eyes turn in or out, or are they ever not straight?	☐ Yes	☐ No

Screening: N   A   Who administered & when, if at other time
- Vision ☐ ☐
- Hearing ☐ ☐
- Development/Behavior ☐ ☐

Physical: N   A
- General appearance ☐ ☐
- Skin ☐ ☐
- Head/Fontanelle ☐ ☐
- Eyes ☐ ☐
- Ears ☐ ☐
- Nose ☐ ☐
- Oropharynx/Teeth ☐ ☐
- Neck ☐ ☐
- Nodes ☐ ☐

  N   A
- Chest ☐ ☐
- Lungs ☐ ☐
- Cardiovascular/Pulses ☐ ☐
- Abdomen ☐ ☐
- Genitals ☐ ☐
- Spine ☐ ☐
- Extremities ☐ ☐
- Neurological ☐ ☐
- Hips ☐ ☐

Describe abnormal findings above _____

Wt: ____ kg. ____ lbs. ____ oz. ____%   Head Circ: ____ cm. ____ in. ____%

Length: ____ cm. ____ in. ____%   Temp. (optional) _____

Diagnosis: ☐ Well Child (if not, specify) _____

Recommendations: _____

Immunizations: Who administered & when (if at other time), or reason if not given
(Fill in box if done)
- ☐ DPT/DT #2 _____
- ☐ Oral Polio/IPV #2 _____
- ☐ HIB #2 _____

Health Education: *(Fill in box if done)*
- ☐ Nutrition ☐ Safety ☐ Family Planning
- ☐ Development ☐ Health Education ☐ Car Seat

Next Visit: 6 months (or other) Date: _____ Person: _____

Health Provider:

Name _____

Address _____

Signature of Health Provider _____

4 Month Visit   Date: _____ | Recommendations

At the child's four-month visit, the parent fills in the information on the top of the form, and the health care provider fills in the information on the bottom half.

Priority One: Immunizations

To keep your children healthy, make sure they receive all their immunizations at the recommended times as part of their regular checkups and well-child care.

It's remarkable how many families don't take this simple step in primary care. A study published in the *New England Journal of Medicine* looked at the vaccination records of the children of 1,500 adults with health insurance. Only 55.3 percent of the children had received all recommended vaccines by the age of six. The biggest obstacle: Parents couldn't take time away from work to get to a physician.

Day care programs, schools, and colleges may require proof of immunization for enrollment. (Medical and religious exemptions are allowed.) Proof includes hospital or clinic records or an immunization booklet or other official form of documentation—but not the parent's word. It's up to you to keep copies of your children's immunization records in addition to those the provider maintains. If the school gets no written record, the child has to receive the shots again.

The federal Centers for Disease Control suggests this immunization schedule:

Age	Routine Vaccine
Birth to 2 months	Hepatitis B
2 months	Diphtheria/tetanus/pertussis (DTP)
	Polio
	Hemophilus influenza B (HiB)
2 to 4 months	Hepatitis B
4 months	DTP
	HiB
	Polio
6 months	HiB
	DTP
6 to 18 months	Hepatitis B
	Polio
12 to 15 months	HiB
	Measles/mumps/rubella (MMR)
12 to 18 months	DTP

8

Age	Routine Vaccine
4 to 6 years	DTP
	MMR
	Polio
11 to 16 years	Diphtheria/tetanus

For more information on immunizations, talk with your doctor or nurse, or contact your local department of health.

Goals for the Health Care Partnership

✔ At each age, you, your children, your health care providers, and others will collaborate to achieve certain health goals and pay attention to certain areas of development and healthy living.

Infancy (birth to 12 months)

- Forming a therapeutic alliance
- Preparing parents for their new role
- Optimal nutrition
- Satisfactory growth and development
- Injury prevention
- Immunizations
- Promoting developmental potential
- Preventing behavioral problems
- Promoting family strengths
- Enhancing parental effectiveness

Early Childhood (1 to 5 years)

- Early autonomy
- Optimal nutrition
- Satisfactory growth and development
- Establishing good health habits
- Injury prevention
- Immunizations
- School readiness
- Promoting developmental potential
- Preventing behavioral problems

Children and Rights

In most cases, parents make health care decisions for their daughters and sons. However, parents don't have unlimited rights regarding children's medical care. Besides, parents usually want to involve their children in health care choices as much as possible.

In most states, children can consent to medical care on their own for certain conditions, such as treatments associated with drug dependency, pregnancy, and sexually transmitted diseases. In addition, an "emancipated minor"—a member of the armed forces, for example—can make medical decisions without parental permission. While the laws vary from state to state, an emancipated minor must generally live apart from his or her parents and be self-supporting.

In most instances, a mature minor can consent to care if he or she can understand the nature, extent, and consequences of the medical treatment. Children may even agree to some treatments over their parents' objections, usually for simple procedures. By the same token, a child who legally can say yes to medical care can also say no. However, a parent can commit a child to mental health or chemical dependency treatment without consent.

Hospitals also have certain rights with regard to children in their care. In a life-threatening emergency, hospital staff will treat a child immediately—parental consent isn't needed. And if parents object to some types of treatment, a hospital can seek court permission to treat a child whose life is in danger. If the court sides with the hospital, it will appoint a guardian, perhaps a member of the hospital staff, to decide whether or not to proceed with treatment.

Hospitals *can't* restrict the right of parents to visit a hospitalized child—at any time of day—if the law requires them to give informed consent. Hospitals can only limit access when it would interfere with the care of other patients.

Children as Health Care Consumers

Insist that health care providers respect your child and give direct answers to her or his questions. Also, help your child to identify his or her concerns and to think about how to ask about them.

Respect Your Child's Privacy

Children have a right to privacy about medical care. Confidentiality is critical to any patient-doctor relationship, even if the parent is the person who gives consent.

If a child doesn't want certain information to reach his or her parents, doctors and other medical personnel should only tell parents what they need to know to give or withhold informed consent for treatment. If you need to discuss some topics with your child's provider in private, ask to be allowed to do so.

Privacy is especially important to teenagers. A physician with training in adolescent medicine will almost invariably keep the content of your teen's visits in confidence. On the other hand, some pediatricians are used to telling Mom and Dad everything—to the detriment of everyone concerned.

For more information on the rights of parents and children, turn to chapter 3.

Specialists for Children

At times, your child may require a specialist to diagnose or treat a specific problem or condition. Your primary care provider will refer you to specialists. The provider's office may either make appointments for you or give you the names and numbers of the specialists for you to call. Many primary care providers work regularly with certain specialists to whom they refer patients when necessary.

Large hospitals and specialized children's hospitals have pediatric specialists in many departments. In some managed care plans, such as HMOs, a wide variety of pediatric specialists are on staff or closely affiliated; other plans have few or no established relationships with these specialists. If the specialists your child needs aren't in your plan, it may be harder to get a referral to them. However, even under such plans, parents can often get the referrals they need—if they know enough to ask for them specifically. In any case, review your health plan materials or call

- Promoting family strengths
- Enhancing parental effectiveness

Middle Childhood (5 to 11 years)

- Sense of personal competence
- Sense of self-efficacy and mastery
- Active role in health supervision and promotion
- Optimal nutrition
- Satisfactory growth and development
- Good health habits
- Injury prevention
- Personal safety
- Social competence
- Promoting developmental potential
- Preventing behavioral problems
- Promoting family strengths
- Enhancing parental effectiveness
- Success in school

Adolescence (11 to 21 years)

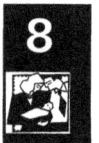

8

- Self-efficacy and mastery
- Independence
- Active role in health supervision and promotion
- Optimal nutrition
- Satisfactory growth and development
- Good health habits
- Reducing high-risk behavior
- Injury prevention

(continues)

- Promoting developmental potential
- Preventing behavioral problems
- Sense of responsibility and morality
- Promoting family strengths
- Enhancing parental effectiveness
- Educational and vocational success

Source: *Bright Futures: Guidelines for Health Supervision of Infants, Children, and Adolescents,* ed. by M. Green (National Center for Education in Maternal and Child Health, 1994)

member services to ask how to get a referral and to make sure the referral is covered.

For more information on insurance, turn to chapter 4.

If you are referred to a specialist for your child, ask about his or her experience treating your child's condition. You'll also want to know how your insurance coverage works to get access to any needed facilities, such as pediatric hospitals. If a local specialist doesn't have extensive experience with your child's specific problem, you may decide to travel elsewhere for help.

For more information on choosing and using specialists, turn to chapter 13.

Timely Questions

Some questions about providers and treatment are much easier to consider fully when you have time to plan ahead. But if your child needs emergency care, the situation may be so pressing or emotionally charged that you aren't able to investigate all your questions. In these situations, get the best care you can immediately, then go back and tackle the rest of your questions when you have more time and feel more in control.

The Specialists

People with pediatric training practice within almost every medical specialty. Their training is likely—though not guaranteed—to make them particularly sensitive to and knowledgeable about children's care. Specialists may have a private practice, either alone or with a group, or work in a community health center, HMO, or hospital.

Be sure all the specialists you work with report to your primary care provider as well as to you. And arrange to discuss these reports with the primary care provider either over the phone or in person.

The following list describes many—but far from all—of the many pediatric specialties:

Pediatric cardiologists evaluate and treat patients with congenital or acquired heart disease and symptoms related to heart disease or rhythm irregularities.

Pediatric hematologists specialize in blood disorders such as anemia, sickle cell disease, and hemophilia.

Pediatric oncologists treat cancer. Major pediatric cancer-treatment centers will have subspecialists in many fields.

Specialists in *adolescent and young adult medicine* provide care for patients twelve to twenty-three years old, often including medical, gynecological, and psychological care.

Pediatric endocrinologists treat glandular disorders that might affect a child's height, weight, and development.

Specialists in *genetics* diagnose and manage inherited diseases, such as congenital malformations and chromosomal disorders. Genetic counselors discuss with families the chance of future children being affected and methods of diagnosis.

Specialists in *pediatric allergy and immunology* evaluate and treat children with diseases such as asthma, drug allergies, insect-sting hypersensitivity, and immunodeficiency disorders.

Specialists in *pulmonary medicine* evaluate and care for children with cystic fibrosis, recurrent respiratory tract infections, chronic coughs, and other pulmonary diseases.

Pediatric neurologists evaluate and treat such problems as seizures, headaches, developmental problems, hyperactivity, neuromuscular disorders, and learning disabilities.

Pediatric orthopedic surgeons diagnose and treat congenital and acquired orthopedic conditions, such as bone fractures, cerebral palsy, and dislocated joints.

Psychopharmacologists specialize in using medicine to treat psychiatric disorders, including mood and anxiety disorders.

Child psychiatrists, trained as M.D.'s, specialize in children's emotional problems.

Child psychologists, trained as Ph.D.'s, evaluate and treat children with emotional and behavioral issues.

Specialists and Hospitalization

An important factor in choosing a specialist (as well as a primary care provider) is the hospital(s) to which he or she could send your child. If you live in an area with only one local hospital, this isn't an issue. On the other hand, ask your providers where they have admitting privileges if you live in a large city or a rural area equidistant from several medical centers, especially if you have reason to prefer a particular facility.

Hospitals differ in their attitudes about involving the family of a hospitalized child. Children and families weather hospitalizations best when they can interact as much as possible in their usual ways. Find out if a hospital allows parents to stay with their children during procedures and overnight, keeps parents fully informed about the plan of care, and helps parents take part in that care as much as they wish. Siblings and extended family members who visit can also help maintain a more normal life during these stressful times.

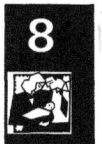

Discuss these issues with your health care providers before a hospitalization. Ideally, they'll support your views and rights—and advocate for them with hospital personnel.

For more information on hospitals, turn to chapter 6.

You, Your Child, and Hospitals

To find a hospital that's responsive to your desires, question your doctor and hospital personnel about hospital policy on parental rights *before* your child is admitted. Select the health care providers and hospitals best able to make the arrangements you seek.

For example, you may want to be present while your child is receiving a treatment. If so, be prepared to negotiate directly with a person in authority, such as the chief of pediatrics or the chief of anesthesia.

For more information, contact the Federation for Children with Special Needs or another advocacy group with experience in dealing with health care institutions and securing the rights of parents. The addresses and phone numbers are listed at the end of this chapter.

Birthing Options

Couples make many decisions in the months leading up to childbirth. Perhaps most important when preparing to have a child is your prenatal care. Seek an obstetrician or clinic with whom you feel comfortable. Locate a primary care provider for your new child, even as you prepare your home and choose a name.

In addition, you might want to check on these services and options:

Childbirth education. Parents who attend these classes gain more control over the birth and undergo fewer cesarean deliveries and other interventions. Also called birthing classes, they teach parents what to expect during labor and delivery.

Birth arrangements. If the birth will be in a hospital, does the hospital offer birthing rooms? Must your insurer certify admission in advance? Can siblings be present?

Obstetric anesthesia. What are the approaches to anesthesia? Do you want to have an epidural block to relieve the pain of childbirth? Clearly state your wishes.

Breast-feeding. Will the facility where you give birth respect your instructions about feedings? Will your baby room in, or will the newborn be brought to you for feeding at your request? Does the facility encourage breast-feeding and offer classes or instruction? Learn how to express milk with a handheld pump.

Circumcision. Once routine, this custom has joined the list of medical procedures whose necessity is being questioned. Read up on it, keep an open mind, and try to reach an informed decision. Check to see if your insurance covers circumcision.

Home birth. Physician and midwife groups sometimes offer this option.

It's important for parents to consider their own preferences and to talk these matters over with their health care providers before the mother goes into labor. Make sure you devote enough time to thinking about the options carefully. For a further discussion of these and other birthing issues, consult *Pregnancy, Childbirth, and the Newborn,* by Penny Simkin.

For more information on health care for women, turn to chapter 9.

Birth Insurance

Check your insurance coverage for its guidelines for coverage of childbirth. How long can you stay in the hospital? Are any prior approvals necessary? What services are provided when you return home, such as home visits?

Cesarean Sections

Cesarean sections, or c-sections, when infants are delivered through an incision into the mother's abdomen and uterus, are the most frequently performed unnecessary surgery in the United States. C-sections expose women to many health risks, often without any benefit.

Try to select an obstetrician and a hospital that have a low "c-section rate"—that is, they perform relatively few c-sections compared to the total number of live births they perform. If possible, use *adjusted* rates that reflect the particular mix of cases seen at the hospital. Otherwise, a high, but unadjusted, c-section rate could indicate an excellent doctor or hospital that is prepared for the most troubling cases, rather than one that opts for a c-section too readily.

When looking for an obstetrician, Public Citizen's Health Research Group suggests you ask:

- Under what conditions would the doctor perform a c-section?

- Would you have a choice?

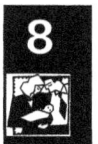

■ What is the doctor's c-section rate? Ideally, doctors dealing with high-risk pregnancies should conduct c-sections in less than 17 percent of their cases, and doctors with low-risk practices should have rates under 10 percent. The Health Research Group recommends that you try to avoid doctors with *unexplained* rates above the national average, about 23 percent.

■ If you have already had a baby delivered by c-section, would the doctor deliver one vaginally now? The answer may depend on the type of incision from the previous c-section.

For more information on c-sections, including the overall c-section rates for most states, see Unnecessary Cesarean Sections: Halting a National Epidemic. *To order a copy, send $10 to Health Research Group, Publications Department, 2000 P Street, N.W., Washington, DC 20036; tel. (202) 833-3000.*

Money Matters

Long-standing, strong relationships in which providers work in concert with one another are crucial to both primary and specialty care. However, continuity of care is hard to maintain these days. For one thing, a rapidly changing health care marketplace makes it difficult for many families to stay with the same providers. Moreover, families sometimes *want* to take advantage of an opportunity to choose a new health plan, such as when they begin a new job with better benefits or during "open-enrollment" periods that some employers offer yearly. At these times, look carefully at the providers and benefits offered by different health plans.

Responsible Employers

Parents have to pick up more of the family health-insurance tab these days. According to a 1994 study by the Children's Defense Fund, the proportion of children covered by their parent's employee insurance benefits has fallen steadily over the past fifteen years: In 1992 only three-fifths of children were covered through parents' employers. Instead, parents pay the insurance bills themselves. "Too many employers have ignored their responsibility for the well-being of their employee's families," notes CDF president Marian Wright Edelman.

Picking a Plan

Parents are making more decisions than ever before about health-insurance coverage for their children. As a mother or father, you probably need health insurance that covers all your children until they are twenty-one years old, perhaps longer if they're still in school. Along with the questions you ask of insurers you consider for your own care, the American Academy of Pediatrics recommends you check each plan's coverage for:

- Family-planning services
- Well-care, including immunizations
- Pregnancy services, including prenatal care, prenatal consultation with a pediatrician, and care for the pregnancy of a single dependent daughter
- Care of newborn infants, including a pediatric specialist to attend high-risk pregnancies, exams and health checks from the time of birth, and treatment of birth defects and other illnesses and injuries
- Services to help a child recover from an illness or injury, including physical therapy, speech therapy, and occupational therapy
- Long term care, *and*
- Hospice care for a terminally ill child

Talk with your pediatrician about your children's health care needs for the coming year. Are his or her services covered by the insurance plan you're considering? If not, do you want to change pediatricians, pay for your pediatrician's care out of pocket, or change plans? How many preventive visits can the family foresee in the coming year and what will they cost? The American Academy of Pediatrics recommends six well-child visits in the first year, three visits the next year, one yearly visit for ages three to six, and one every other year for ages seven and up. And don't forget other charges, such as lab tests, prescription drugs, and immunizations.

No matter what health-insurance plan you choose, learn how it works for children. When comparing plans and deciding on options, find out:

- What are the basic costs associated with the plan?
- Is your choice of providers limited?
- Are affiliated pediatricians board certified?
- How many pediatricians are available to you? Who are they?
- Can your child see the same pediatrician for most visits?
- What limits are placed on referrals to subspecialists, such as pediatric cardiologists or pediatric allergists?
- Can your child go to a special hospital that treats children, if need be?

Also consider coverage for children's mental health when buying insurance:

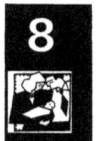

TIP

Insurance Help

Medicaid, a state/federal program, covers some health care costs for low-income people, including many children with special health needs.

For more information on Medicaid, turn to chapter 4.

Children with Special Needs

Even as health care costs soar, perhaps 40 million people have no health insurance, and an additional 59 million find their coverage inadequate to meet family needs. Families whose children have serious ongoing health needs are disproportionately represented in both groups.

Children with special health needs or chronic health conditions are heavy users of health care. Their families spend a great deal of effort trying to understand what special care their children need, what services are available, and how to pay for it all. Solutions often require a complicated mix of private health insurers and public programs. Families need immediate help with the

Some Typical Fees

	Well-Baby Checkup	Normal Delivery of a Baby
Boston	$69	$2,825
New York City	$100	$3,843
Washington, D.C.	$68	$3,239
Phoenix	$52	$2,166
National Average	$47	$2,037

Source: Medirisk, Inc.

■ Does your health plan pay for the mental health services your family may need, such as outpatient therapy, day-treatment programs, hospital treatment, and treatment programs for alcohol and other types of drug abuse?

■ Will it allow you to choose an expert: a qualified child and adolescent mental health professional to provide and direct your child's treatment?

■ Does the plan provide broad enough coverage to permit an adequate period of treatment in a setting appropriate to the disorder?

For more information on choosing a health plan, turn to chapter 4.

Two Plans?

Many health-insurance plans have special payment methods if both parents are insured. Find out in advance which plan will be the one with the main responsibility for your children's coverage and how the two plans would coordinate payments.

Insurance and Immunizations

One sign of a health plan that pays attention to preventive care for children is the percentage of enrolled children that have received all their recommended immunizations. Ask the members services of the plans you are considering for this information. Check the percentages for the past several years. Are they improving?

Your Teenagers and Health Insurance

When planning your family's health care coverage, keep in mind the distinct needs of your teenage children. Many teens aren't covered after a specific age—typically eighteen or twenty-one, or twenty-five if your son or daughter is a full-time student. If your teen is in college and isn't covered under your plan, a school policy may cover his or her health care. If so, check the extent of coverage.

Even if your family policy covers your teenager, he or she may want and need confidential services. A few insurance companies will make arrangements for your teenager, not you, to receive the bill.

Choosing an HMO as your insurer results in significant benefits for teenagers, particularly in terms of coverage for preventive services. However, HMOs also have shortcomings. They typically exclude or provide poor coverage for specific teen illnesses, such as anorexia nervosa. In addition, an HMO might steer you away from particular options you'd prefer. For example, an HMO could save money by prescribing birth control pills that you'd pay for rather than Norplant or another long-acting birth control that would be fully covered.

complex, long, and confusing process of assembling a package of caregivers and payers.

Many organizations and parent education centers advocate on behalf of children with special needs and their families. For information and referrals on special-education rights and laws, issues related to children with special health care needs, and workshops on special-education issues, call the Federation for Children with Special Needs at (617) 482-2915. For information on health issues, call Family Voices at (505) 867-2368.

Resources
Organizations

American Academy of Child and Adolescent Psychiatry
3615 Wisconsin Avenue, N.W.
Washington, DC 20016
(202) 966-7300
Call or write for a list of publications and resources, including a series of pamphlets called "Facts for Families" with information on topics such as children and grief, bed-wetting, day care, children and divorce, lead exposure, discipline, and conduct disorders. Also available is a free brochure with recommended insurance coverage for children's mental health services. For free copies of individual pamphlets, send a self-addressed, stamped envelope to AACAP Public Information, P.O. Box 96106, Washington, DC 20090.

American Academy of Husband-Coached Childbirth
P.O. Box 5224
Sherman Oaks, CA 91413
(800) 423-2397
Write for information on preparing for natural childbirth.

American Academy of Pediatric Dentistry
211 E. Chicago Avenue, #700
Chicago, IL 60611-2616
(312) 337-2169
Call or write for referrals and for pamphlets on safety, sealants, regular dental visits, dental care for babies, care for teens, and other topics.

American Academy of Pediatrics
141 NW Point Boulevard
Elk Grove Village, IL 60007

8

(800) 433-9016

Free brochures are available on allergies in children, child sexual abuse, day care, diaper rash, family health insurance, immunization schedules, managed care for families, temper tantrums, tobacco abuse, and many other topics. Send a stamped, self-addressed envelope for any of these brochures or a publications list.

American College of Nurse-Midwives
818 Connecticut Avenue, N.W., #900
Washington, DC 20006
(202) 782-9860
Send $6.95 for the *Directory of Nurse-Midwifery in the United States.*

American Society for Psychoprophy-
    laxis in Obstetrics (ASPO/Lamaze)
(800) 368-4404
Call for information about prepared childbirth and referrals to ASPO/Lamaze childbirth educators.

Association for the Care of Children's
    Health
7910 Woodmont Avenue, #300
Bethesda, MD 20814
(301) 654-6549
This organization has a number of educational booklets available at a small charge on such topics as "Caring for Your Child in the Emergency Room" and "For Teenagers: Your Stay in the Hospital." Call or write for a resource catalogue. The association also operates the National Information Clearinghouse for Infants with Disabilities and Life-Threatening Conditions, serving family members and health care providers. For a list of services and fact sheets, call (800) 922-9234, ext. 201.

Association of Maternal and Child
    Health Programs
1350 Connecticut Avenue, N.W., #803
Washington, DC 20036
(202) 775-0436

Call to get the phone number of your state's program for children with special health care needs.

Birthright
P.O. Box 98363
Atlanta, GA 30359-2063
(800) 550-4900
With offices throughout the country and abroad, Birthright offers free services for pregnancy counseling, pregnancy tests, prenatal support, reproductive health services, and complete support services.

Cesarean/Support, Education and Con-
    cern
22 Forest Road
Framingham, MA 01701
(508) 877-8266
Parents and professionals can write or call for information and support on cesarean birth, prevention, and vaginal birth after a cesarean (VBAC).

Children in Hospitals
31 Wilshire Park
Needham, MA 02192
(617) 482-2915.
Contact this nonprofit organization of parents and health care professionals for information about the needs of children in hospitals and other health care settings.

Disability Rights Education and De-
    fense Fund
2212 Sixth Street
Berkeley, CA 94710
(510) 644-2555
ADA Hotline: (800) 466-4232
Contact DREDF for technical assistance, information, and referrals on disability rights laws and policies. Parents of children with disabilities can call for training, information, and legal advocacy. Call the ADA Hotline for information and assistance in connection with the Americans with Disabil-

ties Act. DREDF is a national law-and-policy center dedicated to furthering the civil rights of people with disabilities.

Family Voices
P.O. Box 769
Algodones, NM 87001
(505) 867-2368
e-mail:FAMV01RW@wonder.em.
cdc.gov
Call or write this national grassroots network to receive a free bimonthly publication on state and federal issues affecting children with special health care needs and to order fact sheets on a number of health and insurance topics in English and Spanish.

Federation for Children with Special Needs
95 Berkeley Street, #104
Boston, MA 02116
(617) 482-2915
Call for referrals to organizations in every state that advocate on behalf of children and families with special needs.

Informed Birth and Parenting
P.O. Box 3675
Ann Arbor, MI 48106
(313) 662-6857
Call or write for a publications list and information and referrals on childbirth education training.

International Childbirth Education Association
P.O. Box 20048
Minneapolis, MN 55420
Write for information on family-centered maternity care and freedom of choice based on knowledge of alternatives.

La Leche League International
P.O. Box 1209
Franklin Park, IL 60131-8209

(800) 525-3243
Call or write for information and support on breast-feeding, as well as referrals to local groups.

March of Dimes Birth Defects Foundation
1275 Mamaroneck Avenue
White Plains, NY 10605
(914) 997-4701
Write or call to get the number of your local chapter as well as information on prenatal care and healthy pregnancies.

National Association of Children's Hospitals and Related Institutions
401 Wythe Street
Alexandria, VA 22314
(703) 684-1355
Contact NACHRI for free pamphlets for parents on choosing a health care plan for your child and managed care.

National Health Information Center
U.S. Public Health Service
P.O. Box 1133
Washington, DC 20013-1133
(800) 336-4797
(301) 565-4167 (in Maryland)
This national toll-free service puts people with health questions in touch with organizations best able to provide answers. Call or write for a publications list and the "Health Finder" list of toll-free numbers.

National Information Center for Children and Youth with Disabilities
P.O. Box 1492
Washington, DC 20013-1492
(800) 695-0285
Contact NICHCY to receive information on disabilities, disability-related issues, child care, special education, transitions, and education rights.

National Maternal and Child Health Clearinghouse
2070 Chain Bridge Road, #450

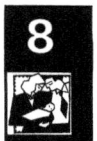

8

Vienna, VA 22182-2536
(703) 821-8955
Call or write for information and a publications catalogue. You can also view the publications catalogue on the World Wide Web: http://www.uchp.ufl.edu.

Parents Choice Book Center
57 Stevens Street
Stoneham, MA 02180
(800) 722-2939 or
(617) 438-8791
Call or write for a mail-order catalogue of childbirth and parenting books.

Publications

Bright Futures: Guidelines for Health Supervision of Infants, Children, and Adolescents. Order from NMCHC, 2070 Chain Bridge Road, #450, Vienna, VA 22182-2536; tel. (703) 821-8955, ext. 254. $20 plus $2.35 shipping and handling.

Caring for Your Baby and Child: Birth to Age 5 (1991), $15.95; *Caring for Your Adolescent: Ages 12 to 21* (1991), $19.95; *Caring for Your School-Age Child* (1995), $13.95. To order any of these books, call the American Academy of Pediatrics at (800) 433-9016.

Fighting Back Health Insurance Denials, by Robert Peterson, with David Tenenbaum. Order from the Center for Public Representation, 121 South Pinckney Street, Madison, WI 53703; tel. (800) 369-0338. $14.95.

Home Care for the Chronically Ill or Disabled Child: A Manual and Services Book for Parents and Professionals, by Monica Loose Jones (Harper and Row, 1985), $12.95.

Ourselves and Our Children, by the Boston Women's Health Book Collective (Random House, 1978). Out of print but available in many libraries.

Pregnancy, Childbirth, and the Newborn, by Penny Simkin (Simon and Schuster, 1991), $12.

Special Needs/Special Solutions: How to Get Quality Care for a Child with Special Health Needs, by Georgianna Larson and Judith A. Kahn (Life Line Press, 1990), $7.95. Order from Life Line Press, 2500 University Avenue, St. Paul, MN 55141.

"SSI: New Opportunities for Children with Disabilities," pamphlet by Joseph Manes and Lee Carty, $3.00. Order from Mental Health Law Project, 1101 15th Street, N.W., Washington, DC 20005; tel. (202) 467-5730.

Take This Book to the Pediatrician with You, by Charles B. Inlander and J. Lynee Dodson, $14.95 plus $3.00 shipping and handling. Order from People's Medical Society, 462 Walnut Street, Allentown, PA 18102; tel. (800) 624-8773.

9 Women as Health Care Consumers

Martha Snyder Taggart

Martha Snyder Taggart is a medical writer in the Washington, D.C., area, specializing in women's health issues. Her readership includes consumers, physicians, and health policymakers.

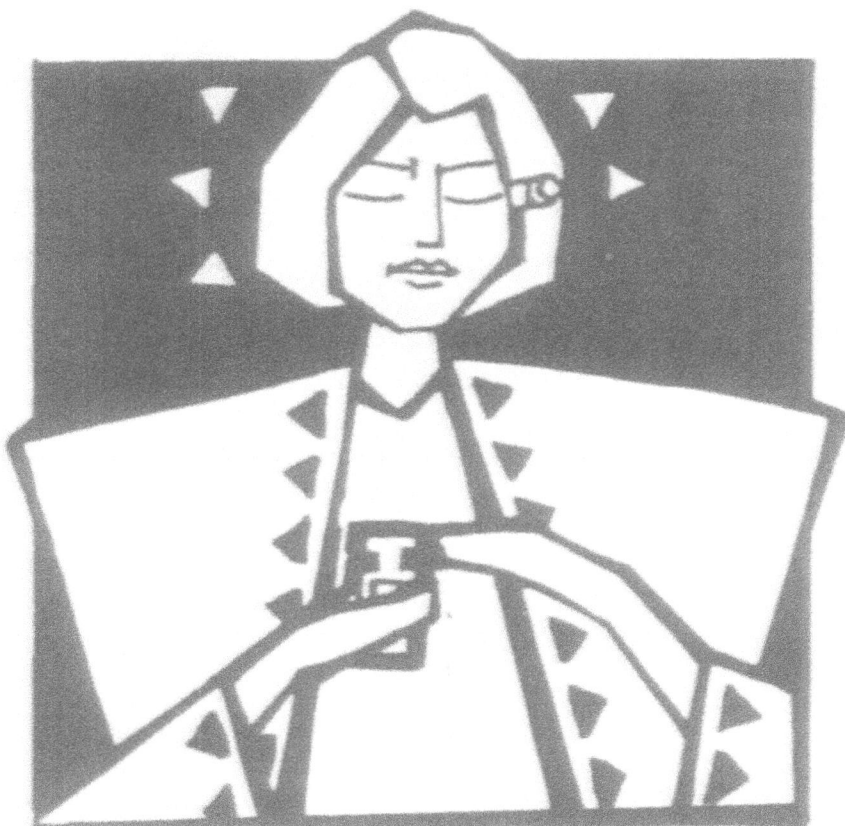

Women have reached a crossroads in their quest for good health care. At the start of the twentieth century, they were lucky to live through their childbearing years. Now many live well into their ninth decade, thanks in part to antibiotics, birth control, and sterile medical procedures. Women have also learned to speak up about the kind of health care they want—and good providers are listening.

Today, the health care that women seek is consumer-oriented, women-centered, and based on a "wellness model" of staying healthy. A woman can reasonably expect health care providers to view her as a whole person, not a sum of body parts or medical conditions.

Women: The Primary Consumers of Health Care

Women live an average of seven years longer than men. Women also:

- Suffer more from chronic illness
- Use health care services more frequently
- Represent a greater proportion of the uninsured
- Are prescribed drugs more often
- Are less likely to be included in clinical research trials
- Are much more likely to be the caretakers for parents and dependent children, *and*
- Spend more of their income on health care

Building the Health Care Relationship

Trust and mutual respect characterize good relationships with health care providers. You want to be able to trust your providers to be open-minded, knowledgeable, competent, and responsible. And you want providers to respect *your* knowledge, welcoming the challenge an informed patient represents.

In general, strive to engage your providers in two very different modes:

■ For *wellness counseling,* the ideal is a "health mentorship" with providers who educate you about your body, emphasize ways to prevent illness, and help you set independent health goals.

■ *When your health is threatened,* you want a wise, reassuring presence. A good provider will believe what you say about your symptoms and investigate the causes by taking a medical history, conducting a physical exam, and drawing on his or her prior experience in treating you. Next should come options for treatment and help in reaching a decision based on the best information available.

Healthy or ill, exercise your right to ask questions, however complicated or simplistic. Insist on a response. And as you travel through the health care system, take pride in the time and knowledge *you* devote to your own health and to caring for others.

A good basis for judging your relationship with your provider comes from the steady contact required to stay in good health—things like physical exams and yearly Pap smears to screen for cervical cancer. Arrive at these tests with questions you'd like to ask.

Don't expect unlimited time, but insist that providers give you their complete attention. If someone cuts you off, gets impatient, or listens poorly, you can't form a real bond. Nor will you be comfortable with a person who condescends to you or takes an oversimplified approach. Your provider should take your concerns seriously and offer referrals to specialists when you ask for help with such problems as depression, substance abuse, and domestic violence.

If you have trouble communicating with your current provider, you might want to consider these three options:

1. Try to improve the relationship by becoming more outspoken and assertive about your health care. Write down your questions before your next appointment. Bring along someone who can ask them if necessary.

2. Redirect the relationship. If the provider's reputation or expertise impresses you, you may want to see someone else in the practice or clinic with whom you can talk more directly, perhaps a nurse practitioner or a physician's assistant. That way, the expert is available for consultation, yet you can form the partnership you want.

3. Switch providers.

Consumer Alert: Less Care?

Health care providers often treat women much less aggressively than men. A study published in the *Annals of Internal Medicine* found that a man with an abnormal initial heart test is much more likely to get further treatment than is a woman: 62 percent of men had additional tests; only 38 percent of women received them. (Of course, *more* isn't always the same as *better,* even with health care.)

Continuity of Care

You want health care that is ongoing and long term. That allows you to build a foundation of communication, familiarity, and trust.

Look for continuity of care in a number of ways. For example, do you get reminders for a follow-up Pap smear at a particular date? If you need a specialist, does your record from the primary care provider reflect all necessary information, including your medical history, risk factors, and recent test results? Many doctors complete a preprinted form that centralizes vital prenatal information.

Office and computer systems that link information about you, your providers, and all your medical visits are helpful. HMOs, women's clinics, and even hospitals and other acute-care settings can enhance continuity of care in other ways as well—for example, by using case managers, taking a team approach to caregiving, and encouraging frequent staff communication.

Counseling and Prevention

Avoiding health risks—smoking, poor nutrition, physical inactivity, substance abuse, injuries, and so on—holds the greatest promise of improving your overall well-being. Even though it's important for doctors and other health care providers to examine you regularly and screen for early disease, such conventional medical activities ultimately may prove of less value to you than counseling and education on what *you* can do for yourself.

You can gauge health care providers on this measure. Does your doctor or nurse:

- Counsel you in ways appropriate to your age, race, sex, income, and personality?
- Connect behavior and health by explaining the health risks of smoking, lack of exercise, poor nutrition, and other lifestyle factors?
- Work with you to develop and act on plans to foster healthy behavior?

For more information on wellness, turn to chapter 2.

Consumer Alert: The Difference

In a 1993 Commonwealth Fund study, dissatisfaction led two in five women to change physicians at some point. One in four men did so.

A third of the women cited communication problems as the leading reason.

Health care providers are more apt to condescend to women than to men. One in four women—versus one in eight men—said the physician talked down to her or treated her like a child. The physicians told 17 percent of women that a medical condition was "all in her head." Only 7 percent of men were insulted in this way.

The Field of Providers Caring for Women

Your best choice of a primary medical provider depends partly on your age and your state of health. For example, if you have a special condition, such as diabetes, you may get regular care from a physician who can treat that and also take care of your routine health needs. That would probably be an internist. If you are nearing menopause, you may benefit from seeing a gynecologist with specialized knowledge of reproductive hormones.

Women with relatively basic health care needs can choose among several types of providers. They all have strengths and weaknesses. Bear in mind that any individual may be an exception to the rule.

For more information on primary care, turn to chapter 5.

Women's Health Specialty

The American Board of Medical Specialties doesn't recognize women's health as an "official" specialty in which physicians can acquire certification. Advocates for such a specialty argue that it would benefit women by creating a pool of experts who can treat most of women's health needs, emphasizing the whole person, not just the reproductive system. Training would cover internal medicine, gynecology, psychiatry, endocrinology, nutrition, orthopedics, and sports medicine, with obstetrics as an option.

Opponents of a women's health specialty argue that it would marginalize the care of women and maintain the mainstream focus on men. They propose that women's health be integral to the training for all physicians.

Family Physicians

Family physicians train in several different fields that prepare them to deliver general medical and surgical care to people of all ages: internal medicine, pediatrics, obstetrics/gynecology, surgery, psychiatry and

TIP

Collaborative Care

Many ob-gyns work collaboratively with nurse-midwives, nurse practitioners, physician assistants, or other non-physician providers. They often employ these caregivers in their private practices. As a result, you may benefit from more time with a provider and from the collective skills and experiences of more than one person.

neurology, and public-health medicine. They are among the rare doctors with specific training in preventive medicine.

Their comprehensive training predisposes family physicians to treat the whole person, not just conditions and symptoms that relate to a narrow specialty. Using one person for a wide range of services can be very convenient, lessening the time and expense of referral care. Another advantage is that a family physician may care for your entire family, thus gaining insight into individual and collective health problems.

Specialists in family medicine often profess that women are people first and that much of medical care is asexual. Many women disagree and feel that medical care must take their gender and special needs into account. The growing numbers of women in training to become family physicians could translate into more emphasis on women's health in the future.

Obstetricians and Gynecologists ("Ob-Gyns")

Obstetricians and gynecologists treat only women. The typical gynecologist has in-depth knowledge of the female reproductive system, urinary system, and endocrine system (which involves reproductive hormones), and a background in screening and treating cancers particular to women. Obstetricians specialize in maternity care. These closely related specialties are taught together and usually are practiced together, although ob-gyns are evolving from doctors who mainly deliver babies to ones who provide lifelong care for women. Many in the specialty have even dropped obstetrics altogether in favor of general gynecology, some emphasizing adolescent gynecology, others treating primarily older women.

Of all physicians discussed here, ob-gyns most consistently ensure that women receive regular Pap smears and screening mammograms. And obstetricians *at their best* take to heart many of the premises of primary care practice, including an emphasis on wellness over disease and a low-tech, holistic approach that favors counseling and prevention over procedures.

Ob-Gyns and Primary Care

Their relative inexperience in treating other parts of the person—the heart and the emotions, for example—is probably the greatest drawback of using ob-gyns as primary care providers. Even if you dutifully see an ob-gyn for a yearly Pap smear and pelvic and breast exams, don't assume you're getting primary care.

If you receive your regular medical care from an ob-gyn, keep track of whether he or she screens you for hypertension and cholesterol, asks about your moods, and broaches topics like diet, exercise, smoking, and alcohol use. If the ob-gyn doesn't, you may need to clarify your relationship or seek a provider trained in primary care.

For more information about primary care, turn to chapter 5.

Internists

Internists, or internal medicine specialists, are known as expert diagnosticians—the "Sherlock Holmeses" of medicine. They do not perform surgery and instead draw on training in microbiology, pharmacology, and chemistry to find out what's going on inside you. In situations in which other doctors might conduct tests or exploratory surgery, internists pride themselves on doing more thinking and less cutting or testing.

Because internists like to employ deductive reasoning, they often excel at cases that frustrate and puzzle other doctors. They are good at treating several health problems simultaneously, which makes them an excellent choice for women with complicated and chronic health problems, particularly ones that don't involve the reproductive tract. Prescribing and adjusting drugs—along with taking into account such factors as potential interactions among medications—is another strength of internists.

The internist's "high-powered" reasoning and ability to integrate the diagnosis and management of different systems of the body can be reassuring for both women and men. Look for a general internist with a stated interest in health maintenance, preventive care, and women's health, unless you have a serious problem requiring a subspecialist.

Advanced Practice Nurses

Advanced practice nurses are gaining favor as an alternative to physician-centered health care for women. They have completed graduate-level education or are certified in a specialty. Their technical skills tend to equal those of physicians for the services they offer, and their fees are significantly lower.

Some advanced practice nurses practice independently or in conjunction with individual physicians. Most work in clinics, hospitals, and HMOs.

Three types of advanced practice nurse are of particular interest to women:

TIP

Internists and Tests

If you are under the care of an internist for specific health problems, make sure you also get regular screening tests, including Pap tests, breast exams, and referrals for mammograms. These tests are especially important for older women.

9

Nurse practitioners (NPs) typically do almost everything physicians do: examine patients (including conducting gynecological and breast exams), take medical histories, diagnose and treat minor illnesses and injuries, order and interpret lab tests and X rays, and counsel patients. They refer patients to physicians if more expert medical attention is required. Many states allow NPs to prescribe medications.

Nearly 50,000 NPs practice in the United States, many in such specialties as adult health, family health, gerontology, ob/gyn, and community health. The congressional Office of Technology Assessment has found that the quality of NP care is as good or better than physician primary health care—and that NPs may have better communication, counseling, and interviewing skills.

Clinical nurse specialists (CNSs) are registered nurses with master's or doctoral degrees in specialized areas, such as mental health, maternal and child health, gerontology, cancer, diabetes, and cardiac care. About 58,000 are in practice—traditionally in hospitals but increasingly in HMOs and clinics, where they often provide mental health services. A CNS can provide primary care and psychotherapy, conduct health assessments, and diagnose and treat illnesses.

Certified nurse-midwives (CNMs) supervise labor, perform routine deliveries, and provide gynecological exams and prenatal and postpartum care. They deliver about 4 percent of babies in the United States.

If you prefer a natural birth, a CNM is an excellent choice. They are more apt to allow labor and delivery to progress naturally, with less use of electronic fetal monitoring and fewer procedures. CNMs attend births in all settings—primarily in hospitals, but 11 percent do so in birth centers and 4 percent in homes. They usually collaborate with obstetricians and refer patients with complications. If you plan to deliver outside a hospital, find out how you will be transferred if an emergency arises.

CNMs are trained and practice according to guidelines set by the American College of Nurse-Midwives. They can practice legally in all fifty states. Lay midwifery, on the other hand, is illegal in most states. Insurance usually doesn't cover the services of lay midwives. Many plans do pay for CNMs who are affiliated with an obstetrician.

Birth Centers

Birth centers offer prenatal care, up through delivery, under one roof. The cost is lower than in traditional settings: about $3,268 versus $5,436 for a hospital-based birth in 1993 (including all prenatal and postpartum care). Nurse-midwives usually attend the birth, and there are fewer restrictions than elsewhere. You can relax in a Jacuzzi during labor, for example, and your children or other family members may be present for the birth. Most women are discharged within twelve hours.

Consider this option only if you have an uncomplicated pregnancy. No anesthesia or emergency surgery are provided (although pain medication may be administered). Ask if the facility is licensed (a majority of states require this) and where you will be transferred in the event of an emergency. Also check your insurance policy: Fewer than one-third of the estimated 135 birthing centers are accredited, which may be required.

For more information on birth centers, contact the National Association of Childbearing Centers at (215) 234-8068.

For more information on childbirth, turn to chapter 8.

Making Your Choice

A successful health care relationship depends largely on three factors: the provider's qualifications, the quality of your personal interaction, and convenience. No selection process is foolproof in predicting your relationship with a particular provider. Still, you can proceed methodically.

Step 1: List Your Needs and Requirements

What type of provider and what setting is best for you? List the factors that matter to you in order of importance; you undoubtedly will have to compromise on some items.

For many women, the top considerations are the provider's training, specialty, licenses and certification, and hospital privileges. Beyond that, a good match will probably be determined by whether your personalities are compatible.

Other factors to consider: Where is the practice located? Does it offer evening and weekend hours? Is free parking available? Do you want a female physician or nurse? Do you prefer an individual practice, a group, or a clinic setting? Do you want to see specialists who focus only on women or people in your age group? Does your health plan allow you the option of signing up for more than one provider (for example, an ob-gyn and another a primary care provider)?

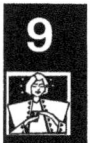

Women's Health Centers

The "women's health center" has joined the health care scene, with more than three hundred facilities across the country. A center may be a clinic or a group of programs for women. Most are attached to or affiliated with hospitals, but some are freestanding. Examples of the latter include family-planning clinics.

The focus of women's health centers varies from obstetrics and reproductive health care to a full range of primary care and mental health services. Advantages include convenience and continuity of care, with services from many different providers coordinated under one roof.

At their best, women's health centers empower women to become partners in their own care by offering educational programs and resource libraries in addition to counseling, screening, and diagnostic and treatment services. At their worst, they amount to a marketing ploy by some hospitals and other providers to attract more business.

In other words, apply the same standards, and ask the same questions, that you would for any health care provider.

Step 2: Begin Your Search

Create a list of providers who meet your criteria. To do this, you can:

- Seek referrals from pediatricians, nurses, and other health care providers you know.
- Talk to friends and acquaintances about their care and their providers.
- Ask your last provider to recommend a person near your new home, if you recently moved.
- Contact local women's organizations and speak with a person involved in health care issues.
- Ask women's health centers and Planned Parenthood clinics for referrals.
- Check local newspapers and magazines for recent features on women's health care.
- Seek referrals from medical societies and other provider organizations.
- Consult the county medical society.
- Contact other referral agencies.

Your choice of provider may seem unlimited at this point; keep your criteria in mind to narrow the field.

Next, pick up the phone and call the practices. Tell them that you're searching for a personal caregiver and would like to ask some initial questions. Is the practice taking new patients? Mention your health insurance.

If you've gotten a green light so far, ask more questions. If the person at the other end of the line acts harried, ask if there's a better time to call or if someone from the practice can call you back. With luck, you'll soon speak to a nurse or office manager.

Start with open-ended questions. These encourage the person at the other end to give a full description rather than one-word answers. In general, seek:

Information about the provider. What is the person's training and certification? Does he or she have any special interests in practice? Does his or her general philosophy about medical care include a strong role for you as a partner in your own health care?

What surgical procedures is the doctor qualified to perform? Has she or he had any special training? Does the doctor routinely counsel patients about diet, exercise, alcohol and drug use, and smoking? Does he or she deliver babies? Perform abortions or sterilizations (or refer to providers who do)?

Information about the practice. How many providers are in the practice? What are their specialties? If your own doctor were unavailable, would someone else in the practice see you? Does the practice offer educational materials for patients? Does the practice specialize in women of your age or with your health problems?

With which hospital is the practice affiliated? Are out-of-hospital births an option? Are infertility patients treated or referred elsewhere? Do appointments tend to run on time, making working-day visits more feasible? Are mammograms and ultrasound testing performed on site? Are test results delivered by phone? What guidelines are followed for preventive health screening—mammograms, Pap smears, and so on—and are reminders issued to patients?

For more information on primary care providers, turn to chapter 5.

For more information on medical specialists, turn to chapter 13.

Step 3: Interview Candidates

Say Doctor X or Nurse Y has the qualifications you seek, and the practice seems to offer the right features. It's time to meet. Ask whether the prac-

At the Interview

As you consider different people as your primary care provider, consider the following as suggestions to guide your thinking:

■ If your initial appointment included a physical exam, did you get a chance to meet the doctor or nurse before an assistant ushered you into an examining room and asked you to remove your clothes?

■ If you declined to undress before meeting the doctor or nurse, was this request accepted and treated as normal?

■ Did the doctor or nurse make eye contact? Did he or she ask permission before calling you by your first name?

■ Did the doctor or nurse seem comfortable answering your questions? If not, did he or she offer any explanation, such as a crisis with another patient?

■ Did he or she volunteer information about practice style or beliefs?

■ Did he or she seem genuinely interested in you?

tice has a special way of handling the first appointment. Some doctors will set aside time to meet with prospective patients at no charge. If not, and if you're fairly confident this provider is for you, perhaps schedule a routine physical examination. This allows you and the provider to get to know each other while you're healthy. As an added benefit, it allows time for the provider to take a thorough medical history, which is critical for your ongoing care.

At this first meeting, determine the level of care the provider can offer. Will this be a primary care provider? Will he or she handle your childbirth needs? Follow you beyond your reproductive years and into menopause?

Pursue any unanswered questions, and zero in on aspects of care that are important to you. If you're interested in stopping smoking, for example, ask if the provider has helped patients to do that successfully. Has he or she routinely cared for women with your needs? Had experience with treatments you're considering?

In general, get a sense of this person's practice style and experience. For example, you may want to know about his or her attitude toward cesarean sections and how often he or she delivers babies this way. Does the provider believe in postmenopausal estrogen replacement? How does her or his hysterectomy rate compare to the national average of about six per one thousand women? How would he or she manage a problem such as abnormal uterine bleeding or uterine fibroids, two common reasons for performing hysterectomies?

For more information on hysterectomies, turn to page 175.

For more information on estrogen replacement, see bottom of page 174.

Discuss your future needs for maternity care, birth control, weight control, or smoking cessation. You might also seek this person's views on a hysterectomy. Usually, practitioners who are overeager to perform this surgery will assure you it makes no difference—or even stands to improve your quality of life. Be wary if they don't also explain the drawbacks.

Ask about "on-call" schedules. This is particularly important if you're interviewing a physician or nurse-midwife for childbirth. Are you apt to be delivered by someone else in the practice? At what point in your labor will the provider appear?

After this first meeting, you'll form an overall impression of the provider and the practice. Certain considerations will be more important to some individuals than to others.

Step 4: Make a Decision

You know the type of health care relationship you seek. Is it possible with this individual? Trust your instincts to tell you yes or no.

If your answer is yes, nurture the relationship. Assert yourself and become an active partner in your care. If your instincts tell you no, continue the selection process with another candidate on your list.

A third option is to delay your decision, particularly if extenuating circumstances at the first appointment may have made it impossible to judge. You can wait and see how you feel after your *next* appointment. In the meantime, however, you risk continuing in the care of someone who may be unsuitable.

Women's Health throughout the Life Cycle

Most women are cared for by several providers—simultaneously or sequentially—over the course of their lives. Rarely will any one of them see that a woman gets *all* the counseling, tests, and procedures she needs at any given moment, let alone throughout her life. As a result, many vital aspects of preventive care—referral for mammograms, for example—tend to slip through the cracks.

These gaps in continuity of care are narrowing. Within the past five years, all the specialty groups traditionally serving women have issued lifelong health-screening guidelines for women. These guidelines are available from the American College of Obstetricians and Gynecologists, the American College of Physicians (representing internists), and the American Academy of Family Physicians.

It takes time for recommendations to filter down from professional organizations to individual practices, however. This makes the partnership approach to care all the more essential. Women must actively question their providers to ensure that nothing is overlooked.

Start by learning about your own health. Don't think that the task is too difficult or the information too complicated. A foray through your local library or the health section of any bookstore can fill your arms with excellent books, some of them listed at the end of this chapter. Once you begin your research, you will realize how satisfying and empowering it is to have direct access to information about your health.

The pages ahead will introduce you to some of the major health challenges facing women at different stages in their lives, as well as a few

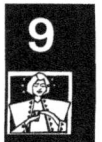

TIP

Levels of Care

Women's health care, as provided by conventional medical specialties, is too often fragmented among a variety of caregivers, and some problems slip through the cracks. To keep this from happening, start by letting a provider know if you are interested in seeing her or him in a *primary care capacity,* not just as a specialist. That is, will he or she take care of all your health needs? You want to be confident that the provider will comfortably assume this role.

health conditions all women must consider. These are the concerns you and your health care providers will address and keep in mind.

Young Womanhood: The Teen Years

Parents should steer teenage daughters toward lasting, one-on-one relationships with providers. As a parent, encourage your daughter to speak openly about her health concerns, and even to rehearse or write down questions. And it's best if the mother and father aren't always in the examining room.

Puberty, which usually arrives between age ten and age fourteen, is an especially critical time for individualized health counseling. Early maturing girls are most at risk for a number of problems, including the early onset of sexual activity, poor body image, and depression.

Health care providers, along with parents, should discuss menarche and puberty to prepare a girl for the physical and emotional changes that are in store for her. Menstrual hygiene and the risks of tampon use should be explained. If you worry that your daughter may become sexually active soon, discuss her contraceptive options and provide information about how she can protect herself from sexually transmitted diseases. Even if her health care provider handles this topic, it's essential for her parents to be involved and supportive. Talking honestly about sex does not encourage sexual activity. Help your daughter to formulate values in this area.

You want your daughter's health care providers to address risk-taking behaviors related to the major causes of death and injury among young women—motor-vehicle accidents, homicide, and suicide. Risk-taking and impulsiveness may be linked to depression or a lack of self-esteem, and alcohol or drug use makes such behaviors even deadlier. Too few youngsters get the mental health counseling they need.

Preventive counseling at an early age can yield lifelong benefits since young women are especially prone to health risks that can have lasting repercussions. They are more likely to start smoking than any other sex/age group. There is a link between sexually transmitted diseases they may acquire and subsequent infertility, as well as a possible link with gynecological cancers. Avoiding sun exposure is important—a peeling sunburn at a young age multiplies the risk of skin cancer.

During adolescence, many young women begin to feel that they have outgrown the "baby doctors" of their childhood, and it's time for their first visit with a gynecologist. The proper time is age eighteen at the latest, and earlier if a young woman is or expects to become sexually active.

One of the most significant goals of this first visit is to serve as an "ice-breaker" between a young woman and the gynecologist who could meet many of her health needs for years to come. Parents and health care providers should encourage the young woman to speak candidly, be it about her sexuality, body image, eating habits, health fears, or complexion.

For more information on children, turn to chapter 8.

Teenagers and Privacy

Adolescent patients deserve the same confidentiality that protects the adult physician-patient relationship. Anything less is unacceptable. The earlier a young woman can discuss her health concerns and learn responsible behavior, the better she can protect her health and well-being in the years to come.

Early Adulthood

A woman's twenties, thirties, and early forties are her reproductive years. Not every woman gives birth, but the ebb and flow of reproductive hormones, particularly estrogen, have a great impact on health at this time.

Your health care providers will watch for signs of heart disease, AIDS, stroke, and breast and uterine cancer, all of which are among the top ten mortality risks for adult women. Now is the time to take steps to prevent many diseases that typically appear later in life. A good health care provider will recommend simple preventive health strategies, such as exercise, diet, and screening for risk factors.

Birth control and sexual activity (including risk prevention) are other important topics. Women who desire children later can combine contraception with barrier methods to protect their fertility from the onslaught of opportunistic infections and sexually transmitted diseases. Infertility can also be caused by endometriosis, a disorder in which uterinelike tissue grows outside the uterus and causes painful scarring. Particularly because women today are attempting to have babies at a later age, when they are less fertile, infertility is sometimes called the disease of the modern age.

For more information on childbirth, turn to chapter 8.

9

The Infertility Workup

About 15 percent of couples don't conceive after 12 months of trying, which is usually considered the time to seek help. Basic tests done on both partners determine such things as whether you are ovulating, whether you might be producing antibodies to your partner's sperm, and his sperm count and sperm motility (or ability to swim).

Depending on the cause of the problem, such interventions as artificial insemination, drugs to induce ovulation, or alterations in the timing, technique, or position of intercourse may be recommended. Surgery to correct blocked tubes and/or in vitro fertilization are more extreme measures. Be sure you are in the hands of a qualified clinic and provider.

For more information, contact Resolve or the American Society for Reproductive Medicine, both listed at the end of this chapter.

Middle Age

Middle age is said to begin in the years surrounding menopause, which for most women occurs around age fifty. These years are a window through which you can view the last third of your life. If you take the right steps, you can enjoy these years in relative health and vitality.

The risk of most gynecological cancers, as well as colorectal and breast cancer, multiplies for this age group. Once ovaries cease to function and estrogen levels in the blood fall, women begin to develop heart disease in proportions equal to men, and that becomes the leading cause of death for women by their mid-sixties. The loss of estrogen also leads to the threat of osteoporosis, a weakening of the bones that makes a person more prone to fractures and other ailments. It afflicts 50 percent of women over age forty-five and 90 percent of women over age seventy-five.

Women at heightened risk of either heart disease or osteoporosis may face a decision about hormone replacement therapy (HRT). Women who undergo HRT after menopause have half the rate of fatal heart attacks as those not undergoing HRT. Estrogen also protects against osteoporosis and alleviates unpleasant symptoms of menopause—which often is the reason why women opt for treatment.

Only about 15 percent of eligible postmenopausal women take estrogen in the United States. This low percentage is due to fears about a slightly increased risk of breast cancer and a sixfold increase in the risk of endometrial cancer. To protect against cancer, progestin is added routinely to estrogen preparations for HRT, but the therapy remains a source of controversy.

If you are a postmenopausal woman, particularly if you have highly elevated cholesterol or a family history of heart disease, the benefits of estrogen may outweigh the risks. If you elect to undergo HRT, make sure you're in the care of a physician who has extensive experience managing this therapy, and be prepared to experiment with dosages and the right combination of medications.

Hormone Debate

Health professionals disagree about using combined hormone replacement therapy for relieving menopause symptoms. Some people object to using drugs to manage a natural occurrence in women's lives. Also, HRT isn't for everyone, and it may be twenty-five years before researchers know the long term effects of the combined therapy.

There are also alternatives that help reduce the risk of heart disease and fractures for postmenopausal women, such as moderate exercise and quitting smoking. Explore the risks, benefits, and alternatives to HRT.

For more information, call the National Women's Health Network Clearinghouse at (202) 347-1140.

Consumer Alert: Hysterectomy Options

Hysterectomy, or surgical removal of the uterus, is the second most frequently performed surgery on women in the United States. One of the few clear-cut indications for it is advanced cancer. For other diagnoses, alternative treatments may work, including special exercises, drug treatments, or new, localized surgical techniques that don't involve removing the uterus.

A hysterectomy *can* have an emotional impact. Ask your doctor to repeat the diagnosis. Read up. Get a second opinion. With the help of your doctor, explore all your options.

The Later Years

Optimistically, you will be in good shape when old age arrives, but no one can postpone health problems forever. Anticipate your health needs before they arise.

A very real threat facing older women is widowhood. The loss of a spouse, partners, relatives, and friends can cause loneliness and isolation. Physicians caring for older women should be alert for normal and abnormal grieving.

The loss of friends and family members may also lead older people to place exaggerated trust in health care providers. As a good health care consumer, you'll do just the opposite. Ask many questions and be assertive. Older women tend to be underscreened and undertreated for

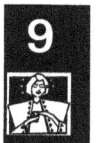

Breast Cancer Genes

A small number of women have a high risk of developing breast cancer at a young age. These are women with mutations on the recently discovered "breast cancer genes," BRCA1 and BRCA2. Carriers of these genes have an 85 percent probability of developing breast cancer over their lifetime and also a greater than average risk of developing ovarian cancer.

Your doctor will be suspicious if your mother, sister, or daughter has had breast cancer. If so, you might be advised to undergo breast cancer screening earlier or more frequently than usual. You can also reduce your risk of breast cancer by exercising regularly, avoiding obesity, eating a low-fat diet, and having children earlier rather than later in life, if possible.

A test for BRCA1 and BRCA2 mutations will be available soon. However, testing could create problems if it leads to some women being denied health insurance. The rapid pace of genetic research makes this scenario frightening not only for breast cancer, but for other diseases. A federal task force has recom-

cancer and other major health problems, including urinary incontinence, osteoporosis, and heart disease.

Urinary incontinence is too often tolerated in old age, despite the fact that health care providers can treat it. More older women might talk to their doctors about this condition if they knew that incontinence makes the move to a nursing home more likely. An estimated half of individuals experiencing urinary incontinence don't get appropriate care. The actual treatment approach depends upon the cause of the problem and varies from surgery to drug therapy to biofeedback.

At any time in your life, make sure that your providers justify the trust you place in them—that you base your trust on good care and not merely on familiarity. As you age, your health care needs grow. Keep a sharp eye on your health care providers—and find new ones if your current providers seem indifferent or reluctant to treat you.

For more information on the health concerns of elders, turn to chapter 11.

High Consumption

At all ages, women make one-quarter more visits to physicians than men do. Women sixty-five years and older see physicians the most, averaging 8.8 visits per year, versus 6.1 visits for reproductive-age women.

Ironically, more visits don't necessarily mean better care. Older women are most apt to go without preventive services.

Special Health Concerns of Women

Some health concerns for women are particularly important and span many ages. Obviously, it's impossible to do justice to all of them here. Enlist the help of your local librarian, check in bookstores, or consult the resources listed at the end of this chapter. In addition, turn to other chapters in this book for information, in particular on such topics as mental health—depression strikes women at twice the rate of men—birthing, dental and vision care, workplace health and safety, and a fuller discussion of primary care.

Urinary Incontinence

Three times as many women as men suffer from urinary incontinence. With treatment, it may be significantly improved or cured in about 80 percent of cases.

Unfortunately, half of all victims are too embarrassed to discuss their problem with a doctor, and wind up severely curtailing their activities and independence instead. Speak up.

Breast Cancer

Most women have a one-in-eight chance of developing breast cancer by age ninety-five. At younger ages, the risks are much smaller (one in twenty-five hundred at age thirty, and one in two hundred at age forty). It is not until age fifty that your risk increases sharply. By then you should be getting regular mammograms (if not earlier, as some groups recommend).

Most breast cancer can be treated successfully if discovered early enough. For tumors found in early, localized stages, the survival rate is up to 95 percent. Mammograms detect breast lumps when they are mere specks on film—up to two years before they can be felt by hand.

The cost of a screening mammogram ranges from $50 to $200. Facilities doing the highest volume usually offer the best quality at the lowest price. Your local branch of the American Cancer Society can refer you to an accredited facility and also provide information about low-cost or free programs that might be available in your area. For insurance reimbursement, however, you may have to be referred by your doctor.

Before you get a mammogram, find out when and how the results will be conveyed to you. If anything suspicious is found, additional steps may be required for diagnosis—another higher powered mammogram, ultrasound, or fine-needle aspiration to see whether the lump is fluid-filled. A lump that does not appear malignant may be observed with regular follow-up mammograms for a period. More suspicious lumps may require a surgical biopsy, where the lump is actually removed and examined under a microscope.

Your doctor should discuss your treatment options in advance, including your preferences for a mastectomy or lumpectomy, breast reconstruction, and follow-up therapy. Adjuvant therapy (drugs or radiation administered after the malignant tissue is removed) help prevent any recurrence.

All of these tests and procedures can be confusing, frustrating, and downright inconvenient if they aren't coordinated in some fashion. Some centers offer all these services in one facility and may place you under the care of an integrated team of doctors and specialists who provide counseling, treatment, follow-up care, and moral support. Aside from sheer "medical" concerns, breast cancer can have a tremendous impact

mended prohibiting insurers from using genetic information to deny or limit coverage, and from establishing differential premium rates based on genetic information. Some states have passed laws to protect individuals, but no federal legislation is in place.

For more information on genetic testing, call the Office of Policy Coordination at the National Center for Human Genome Research at (301) 402-0955.

Questions About Cancer?

The National Cancer Institute's Cancer Information Service is staffed by 250 specially trained experts who are willing to answer questions, mail information to you, and refer you to hospital treatment programs. Dial (800) 4-CANCER on weekdays from 9 A.M. to 7 P.M. EST.

Through CancerFax, also run by the Cancer Information Service, you can have information faxed to you almost instantly. Dial (301) 402-5874 at any time.

on your lifestyle and emotions—from the initial suspense of waiting for your mammogram results to the coping skills required to do battle with the disease. Trusting in and relying on a team could help.

Needless Consequences

The five thousand women who die each year in the United States from cervical cancer do so needlessly, according to a National Institutes of Health panel of experts. Mortality could be prevented with safe sex (to prevent spread of human papilloma virus, which is associated with virtually all cervical cancer), and annual Pap smears leading to earlier, life-saving treatments. Pap smears detect abnormal cells in the cervix before they become cancers. Half the women diagnosed with cervical cancer in the United States have never had a Pap smear.

Safe and Legal Abortion

All sexually active women need to take precautions against unintended pregnancy and sexually transmitted diseases. If you err at some point, however, the right combination of oral contraceptives, taken within 72 hours of intercourse, can provide "emergency contraception." The pills prevent pregnancy by altering the uterine lining so it will not allow a fertilized egg to implant. Most doctors consider this to be safe and effective method of birth control, and many will prescribe it even if they do not perform abortions. If not, *place a call to the Emergency Contraception Hotline at (800) 584-9911 for a referral.*

If you believe you might wish to consider an abortion, the National Abortion Federation refers women to its member clinics and abortion providers through a toll-free hotline: (800) 772-9100.

The federation suggests that you ask the following questions when seeking a safe, legal abortion:

■ Are the facility and its physicians licensed and experienced?

■ Does the provider have admitting privileges to a nearby hospital (no more than twenty minutes away) in the event of an emergency?

■ What is included in the flat fee? Are pregnancy screening, anesthesia, and follow-up visits extra?

■ What is the complication rate? The National Abortion Federation advises looking for providers with a rate of less than 3.0 percent to 5.0 percent for minor complications, less than 0.1 percent for major complications during first trimester procedures, and less than 0.5 percent for second trimester procedures.

■ Is laminaria (a seaweed product that naturally dilates the cervix) used? It must be applied the night before and therefore requires an extra office visit, but it does reduce discomfort and complications.

Battering and Abuse

Women are frequently the target of physical violence, often within the home. An estimated one-fourth of all American women have suffered physical abuse from an intimate partner at some time. It is the leading cause of injury to women—exceeding auto accidents, muggings, and rapes combined. The American Medical Association reports that woman abuse leads to 100,000 days of hospitalization, 30,000 emergency room visits, and 40,000 visits to doctors' offices every year.

A doctor's office or clinic represents one of the few safe havens an abused woman can turn to when she is cut off from the rest of the world. All health care providers should respect your confidentiality and do nothing to jeopardize your safety. For example, they should hold all discussions about abuse out of earshot of your partner.

Good caregivers are alert to bruises and other signs of unexplained injury and emotional distress. While not apt to intervene directly, they may question you about the nature of the abuse, refer you to sources of help in the community, and assist you in formulating a plan to leave the abusive relationship.

The consequences can be devastating if you don't seek help. Abuse travels through generations. An abused child is much more likely to be part of a violent family in the future, in part due to impaired self-esteem and difficulty in managing anger and forming intimate relationships. Treatment involves the whole family working with teams of professionals—psychologists, social workers, nurses, school officials, law-enforcement officials, and community agencies.

Health care providers may be legally required to report cases of child abuse to authorities. Women are the perpetrators of child abuse just as often as men.

Age and Cancer

Older women need Pap smears and mammograms as much as younger women, but half of all women over age sixty-five don't get them. As a result, cancers tend to be detected at later stages and are more apt to prove fatal. Only one-fifth of U.S. women are over age sixty-five, but two-fifths of all deaths from cervical cancer occur in that age group.

Some health care providers are reluctant to treat early cancers aggressively in older women, out of fear of complications. Their fears may be unwarranted. When older women receive hysterectomies for early cervical cancer, their survival rate is comparable to that of younger women.

Medicare will pay for one mammogram every two years for women over age sixty-five. Unfortunately, too few women take advantage. The incidence of disease peaks in women at age seventy-five.

9

Preventing Domestic Violence

The most effective way to prevent domestic violence is the arrest and prosecution of the abuser. Call the police if you are in danger.

Safer Abortions Ahead?

Two drug regimens that appear safe and effective for early abortion await approval in the United States. Either regimen would greatly expand women's access to first trimester abortions. About half of this country's 1.5 million annual clinical abortions are performed within nine weeks of gestation, when drug regimens would be effective. Many ob-gyns who don't perform surgical abortions would prescribe drugs for that purpose, and a large pool of providers in private offices—family physicians, nurse practitioners, and others, in addition to ob-gyns—would also be able to prescribe the regimens.

Mifepristone (RU-486), available in a pill form, is widely used in France. However, it's unavailable on the U.S. market pending Food and Drug Administration approval.

The other regimen consists of a methotrexate injection and a misoprostol suppository—both available here as cancer and ulcer medications. Doctors have some discretion in prescribing them for abortion, but malpractice protections

In most states, the police must write a report and have you and your children taken to a safe place for medical care. You may also be eligible for protection for you and your children.

For more information and help in breaking the cycle of violence, contact:

- *National Women's Health Resource Center,* 2440 M Street, N.W., #325, Washington, DC 20037; tel. (202) 293-6045
- *National Council on Child Abuse and Family Violence,* 1155 Connecticut Avenue, N.W., #400, Washington, DC 20036; tel. (202) 429-6695
- *National Coalition Against Domestic Violence,* P.O. Box 34103, Washington, DC 20043-4103; tel. (202) 638-6388

Insurance Issues for Women

Don't take it on faith that your insurance policy offers "comprehensive" coverage for a woman's health care needs. The definition of comprehensive varies under the insurance regulations for each state. Some states mandate that all policies must include certain benefits, such as maternity or well-baby care. But if your state has no mandate, these benefits may be unavailable to you or subject to a surcharge. Read the fine print and consult your insurance agent about the following areas:

Preventive health benefits. Mammograms and Pap smears are sometimes excluded unless they are used to confirm a diagnosis (for example, if you have felt a lump or are experiencing some symptoms of disease). Make sure screening mammograms and Pap smears are covered.

Outpatient mental health benefits. Depression is a common illness in women. Will your insurance plan cover outpatient counseling? Does it place a cap on the amount reimbursed per visit, or on the number of visits allowed? Will it cover marriage counseling?

Lifetime benefit caps. You may need hundreds of thousands of dollars to battle or recover from a catastrophic illness such as stroke or cancer or to have an organ transplant. What are your policy's lifetime caps and are they sufficient?

Double coverage. If you are covered by two insurance policies (you and your spouse's, for example), you may have more benefit options. The secondary policy may reimburse for testing or procedures not allowed by the primary carrier, or may help cover copayments—such as the cost of going out of network for care.

Infertility treatment. Costs vary depending on the method or procedure used. They can range from hundreds of dollars for fertility drugs to tens of thousands for in vitro fertilization. (At a cost of about $8,000 per treatment cycle, it usually takes two tries.) Will your plan cover a basic infertility "workup" (preliminary diagnostic tests for you and your partner)? What treatments are covered?

Maternity care. The medical cost of having a baby in 1991 averaged $4,720 for a normal vaginal delivery and $7,826 for a cesarean delivery.

Prenatal diagnostic testing. Amniocentesis and chorionic villi sampling are costly and will be recommended if you are over thirty-five years old.

Well-baby care. Healthy babies require about six medical checkups in the first year. With immunizations and testing, these visits can run over $100 apiece.

For more information on health plans, turn to chapter 4.
For more information on insurance and parenting, turn to chapter 8.

Do You Have a Choice?

Women typically see ob-gyns for maternity care, Pap smears, and gynecological exams, and family physicians or internists for acute and chronic illnesses. In surveys, most women say they like having these choices.

Many health plans do let you choose an ob-gyn as your primary care doctor or allow you to see an ob-gyn regularly in addition to a primary care doctor. Some plans allow unlimited visits ("open access") to ob-gyns, while others may limit the number of times or reasons for which you can see them.

Your health plan's policy in this area is based in part on the insurance regulations in your state. Slightly fewer than one-third of states have laws specifying that ob-gyns can serve as primary care doctors or guaranteeing women direct access to ob-gyns for a variety of conditions, such as well-woman exams, routine and acute gynecological care, and all care related to pregnancy.

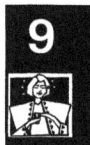

or health insurance coverage may be denied.

Currently, ob-gyns are virtually the only practitioners trained to do surgical abortions, and the number of U.S. ob-gyns willing to perform them is declining, according to a 1995 Kaiser Family Foundation survey. About 40 percent of gynecologists in the Northeast and West now say they are willing to provide abortions, but only 25 percent in the South and 16 percent in the Midwest.

9

Home Safe

"Early dis-charge"—sending new moms and babies home twenty-four hours or less after birth—has created a furor around the country. Some states are passing legislation to restrict the practice.

Early discharge need not be unsafe as long as the proper protocols are followed. Most insurers require doctors to follow specific criteria in deter-mining which women (and babies) can be dis-charged early. There should be follow-up visits at specified intervals to ensure that your wounds are healing properly, that your newborn is not jaundiced and is eating properly, and to check for any other problems. Under some health plans, a home-health nurse may visit you within a couple days.

If you are breast-feeding, you insurance may cover the cost of a breast pump obtained in the hospital. Ask a hospital nurse to observe to see if the infant is positioned prop-erly and latching on. At home, watch for any signs of dehydration. Some hospitals offer twenty-four-hour breast-feeding and infant care hotlines to answer new parents'

How Women Are Faring under Managed Care

In 1995 the Commonwealth Fund, a nonprofit health research organiza-tion, asked women about their experiences under both managed care and fee-for-service arrangements (where you see your doctor of choice and the insurance company pays the bill).

In general, women in managed care programs tend to be less satis-fied, particularly about such items as choice and ease in changing doc-tors, access to specialty care, communication, time spent per visit, and appointment waiting times. Women who had no choice in their plan expressed the most dissatisfaction.

Women in both types of plans make about the same number of vis-its to the doctor. Managed care plans are more likely than fee-for-service plans to cover such things as a complete physical exam, mam-mogram, and Pap smear. Despite that, roughly one-third of women in both types of plans went without complete physical exams and mam-mograms in the previous year, and about one-quarter went without Pap smears and pelvic exams. This suggests that even when cost isn't an issue, many other problems prevent women from gaining access to care.

Another problem with all types of health insurance is a lack of con-tinuity in care. About half of all insured adults have been enrolled in their current health plan for less than three years, according to the survey. Three-quarters of them had to change plans involuntarily due to a change in employment or because their employer selected a new plan.

The Cost of Typical Services

	Mammogram	Gynecological Exam	Pap Smear
National average	$104	$ 78	$13
Boston	$109	$115	$17
New York	$120	$197	$16
Washington	$131	$114	$15
Phoenix	$101	$ 80	$14

Source: Medirisk, Inc.

Resources
Organizations

American College of Nurse-Midwives
818 Connecticut Avenue, N.W., #900
Washington, DC 20006
(202) 289-0171
Call for their directory of nurse-midwife practices and to get help locating a certified nurse-midwife in your community.

American College of Obstetricians and Gynecologists
409 12th Street, S.W.
Washington, DC 20024-2188
(800) 673-8444
(202) 638-5577
Call or write for information and literature on over 150 general and reproductive health topics.

American Society for Reproductive Medicine
1209 Montgomery Highway
Birmingham, AL 35216-2809
(205) 978-5000
Call or write for information on a variety of reproductive health matters, including in vitro fertilization and other reproductive technologies.

Association of Reproductive Health Professionals
Birth control information and an Emergency Contraception Hotline: (800) 584-9911

Boston Women's Health Book Collective
240A Elm Street, 3rd floor
Somerville, MA 02144
(617) 625-0271
Call for a literature list and information on a wide variety of health subjects. Send questions and messages through e-mail to bwhbc@igc.apc.org.

The collective or its members are the authors of *The New Our Bodies, Ourselves* (Simon & Schuster, 1992), $20 and *The New Ourselves, Growing Older: Women Aging with Knowledge and Power* (Touchstone Books, 1994), $18.

FDA Breast Implant Information Line
(800) 532-4440
(301) 881-0256 in Maryland
Call to report problems or to get updated information about breast implants.

HERS Foundation (Hysterectomy Educational Resources and Services)
422 Bryn Mawr Avenue
Bala Cynwyd, PA 19004
(215) 667-7757
Call or write for free telephone counseling, referrals, and a list of publications. A quarterly newsletter is available for $20 per year, and a free lending library of books, audiotapes, and videotapes circulates by mail.

Susan G. Komen Breast Cancer Foundation
(800) IM-AWARE
Call for information on breast health and breast cancer.

National Abortion Federation Hotline
(800) 772-9100
Call for facts about abortion and referrals to member clinics.

National CDC/STD Hotline (Sexually Transmitted Diseases)
(800) 227-8922
Call for information on sexually transmitted diseases, as well as for local and national referrals.

National Women's Health Network
514 10th Street, N.W., #400

questions. If not, request the name and number of a lactation consultant to contact at any sign of a problem. Considering what you're saving in formula, it could be well worth the cost.

Washington, DC 20004
(202) 347-1140
This national public-interest membership organization provides free or low-cost information on a wide variety of topics in women's health. Call or write for information and a publications list.

National Women's Health Resource
   Center
2425 L Street, N.W.
Washington, DC 20037
(202) 293-6045
A subsidiary of the Columbia Hospital for Women Foundation, the center provides information to women interested in preventive care and making informed decisions about their health. The *National Women's Health Report,* a bimonthly newsletter, is available with the $25 membership fee. Information packages are available on autoimmune diseases, breast cancer, hysterectomy, urinary incontinence, sexually transmitted diseases, breast implants, infertility, osteoporosis, PMS, hormone replacement therapy, menopause, and cardiovascular disease ($10 each/ members; $15 each/nonmembers). Information searches on health topics are free to members, $5 to nonmembers.

Planned Parenthood Federation of
   America
810 Seventh Avenue
New York, NY 10019
(800) 829-7732
(212) 541-7800
Call or write for information on family-planning issues and referrals to local Planned Parenthood clinics. Planned Parenthood publishes *Women's Health Letter* ($24.95 per year).

Resolve, Inc.
1310 Broadway
Somerville, MA 02144-1731
Helpline: (617) 623-0744

Call for information on infertility and referrals to physicians, IVF clinics, local chapters, and support groups.

Women's Cancer Resource Center
P.O. Box 11235
Oakland, CA 94611
(510) 548-9272
A hotline offers information and referrals on specific types of cancer, support groups, and mainstream and alternative treatments. Volunteer lawyers offer workshops, free consultations, and referrals. Also, call or write for information on receiving a newsletter and a wide variety of educational resources.

WMM—Women: Midlife and Menopause
7337 Morrison Drive
Greenbelt, MD 20770
This mutual-help group offers information, referrals, and help in starting local groups. Send $5 for a materials packet.

Y-Me National Association for Breast
   Cancer
212 W. Van Buren
Chicago, IL 60607-3908
(800) 221-2141
Call for information, support, counseling, and advocacy.

Publications

The Black Women's Health Book: Speaking for Ourselves, edited by Evelyn C. White (Seal Press, 1994), $14.95.

Dr. Susan Love's Breast Book, by Susan M. Love, with Karen Lindsey (Addison-Wesley, 1994), $15.95.

Harvard Women's Health Watch. Monthly newsletter from Harvard Medical School.
Call (800) 829-5921, or write to P.O. Box

420235, Palm Coast, FL 32142. $24 for an annual subscription.

Men, Women, and Infertility: Intervention and Treatment Strategies, by Aline P. Zoldbrod (Lexington Books, 1993), $29.95

The Menopause Self-Help Book: A Woman's Guide to Feeling Wonderful for the Second Half of Her Life, by Susan M. Lark. (Celestial Arts, 1990). Write to P.O. Box 7327, Berkeley, CA 94707.

Planning for Pregnancy, Birth, and Beyond, by the American College of Obstetricians and Gynecologists (Dutton, 1995), $23.95.

Take This Book to the Gynecologist with You, by Gale Maleskey and Charles B. Inlander (Addison-Wesley, 1991) and *Take This Book to the Obstetrician with You,* by Karla Morales and Charles B. Inlander (Addison-Wesley, 1991). Each book is $9.95 and can be ordered from People's Medical Society, 462 Walnut Street, Allentown, PA 18102; tel. (800) 624-8773.

Trusting Ourselves: The Complete Guide to Emotional Well-Being for Women, by Karen Johnson (Atlantic Monthly Press, 1991), $12.95. Mental self-help from a feminist, and historical perspective.

Women and Doctors, by John M. Smith (Atlantic Monthly Press, 1992), available in many libraries.

Women's Health Alert, by Sidney M. Wolfe (Addison-Wesley, 1991), $7.95. Send check or money order to Public Citizen Books, 2000 P Street, N.W., Washington, DC 20036.

9

10 Men as Health Care Consumers

Jeffrey Kellogg

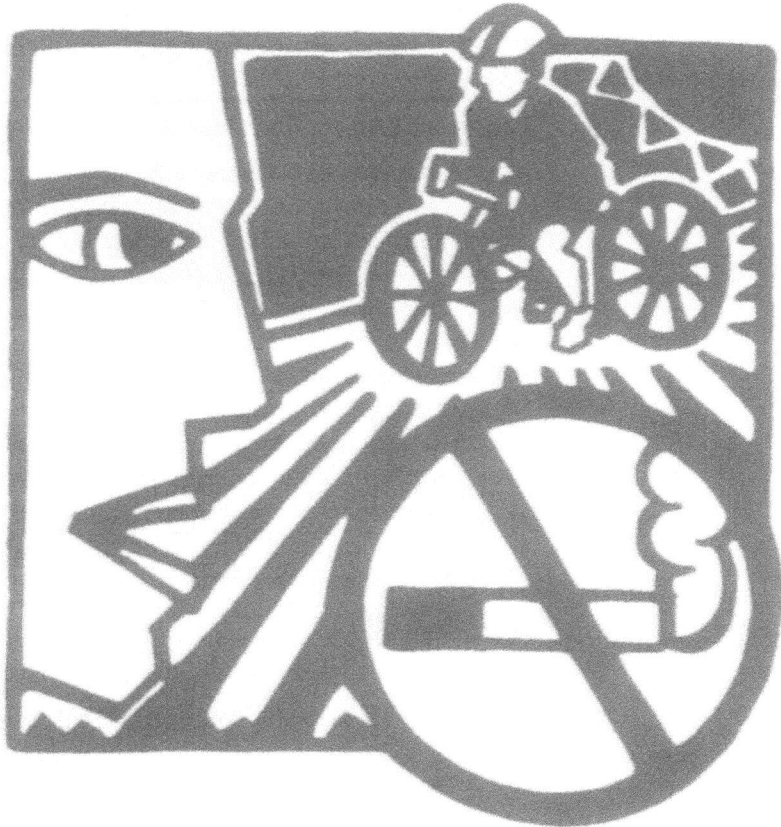

Jeffrey Kellogg is executive director of the Men's Health Network, a national coalition of health care providers and support groups for men founded in 1992. He has worked in the public interest on many health issues, including the environmental implications of biotechnology and genetically engineered foods, the health effects of transportation pollution, and the impacts of emerging employment trends and corporate downsizing on health. He has researched and written about men's health issues extensively and works closely with men's organizations and individual men regarding male health concerns and needs.

American men are in the midst of a growing—but predominantly silent—health crisis. Their well-being is slowly yet steadily deteriorating relative to that of women, who generally take a far more proactive approach toward their own health care. In 1920 men and women had roughly the same life expectancy. Today, men's average life expectancy is over seven years, or 10 percent, less than that of women.

The lag in men's health is mainly a result of two factors: First, this century's elimination of infection as the primary cause of death has lent increasing prominence to illnesses that are selectively afflicting men earlier in life. These illnesses include cancers (both those that affect men in particular and those that strike both sexes equally), heart disease, stress-related diseases such as ulcers and hypertension, sexual diseases and dysfunction, depression and other mental conditions, destructive addictions, and violence-related injuries.

Second, and much more important, is the pervasive lack of health awareness among men and their health care providers. This deficiency is the result of both poor education about health matters and culturally induced behavior patterns that harm men's health at work and in their personal lives.

Pay Attention to Your Health

In 1995 a survey of 1,500 physicians, sponsored by the Men's Health Network, a national coalition of male health care providers and men's support groups, revealed that men pay far too little attention to their own health. They fail to take necessary actions to prevent illness and injury, and they seek professional care or assistance far too infrequently. In other words, men aren't taking a proactive stance toward their own physical and mental well-being.

According to the survey, men make 150 million fewer visits per year to physicians than do women. Yet men account for two-thirds of the patients admitted to emergency rooms, and their hospital stays are longer because their conditions are more severe.

Health Care for Men

The total damage from men's low level of health awareness, poor information on preventing male-specific diseases, and insufficient psychological help is especially tragic because *virtually all the major killers of men are preventable.* Simple changes in lifestyle, eating habits, and workplace environments, combined with disease prevention and early detection, could save millions of men's lives each year and alter the negative stereotypes that plague men and reinforce their poor health patterns.

Breaking the Silence

Men can consciously and effectively address one major threat that surrounds them daily: the cultural message that they shouldn't react to pain in their bodies or their souls. Many men fear the risk of appearing unmanly if they change their behavior or their environment in life-preserving ways. The unfortunate consequence is that men continue to be at greater risk for many of the top killers of Americans.

A tragic side effect accompanies this same cultural message: the lack of health care information and programs for male-specific disorders. Numerous programs actively and appropriately alert women to such dangers as breast cancer and cervical cancer, encouraging women to examine themselves for these diseases and get regular checkups. In addition, many clinics are devoted solely to these important goals. However, depending upon the disease, few to zero programs or clinics target male-specific diseases.

This situation puts the burden for proper male health care directly on the shoulders of each individual man himself. Start taking a stronger proactive stance toward your own health care. As you do, you'll discover that many resources are available to help you avoid the leading killers of men, even if these resources don't explicitly target men. Take advantage of resources, and you'll learn more about your health care needs and how to stay healthier. You'll also become a catalyst in the vital work of promoting better health awareness for all men.

Finding the Right Doctor

In *How Men Can Live As Long As Women,* Dr. Kenneth Goldberg, founder and director of the Male Health Center in Austin, Texas, outlines seven steps for you and your health care providers to follow toward maintaining proper male health.

1. Take charge of your own health.
2. Be better informed.
3. Find the correct doctor.
4. Eat and exercise properly.
5. Confront the ten leading killers of men.
6. Attend to your sexual health and behavior.
7. Connect with your family, friends, and community.

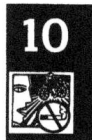

10

Male Wellness

No natural curse dictates a shorter life for men. No studies have ever borne out the existence of the so-called testosterone tax. While heart disease and other selective illnesses may strike men earlier in life than women, detection and proper attention can prevent their occurrence or development.

The most important step you can take to improve your own health care is to care for yourself on a daily basis. In general, to live longer and enjoy a better life:

- Drink no more than two alcoholic beverages per day—one is better.

- Don't smoke cigarettes.

- Keep your weight under control.

- Sleep a comfortable seven to eight hours per night.

- Get sufficient and appropriate exercise, both aerobic and muscular, *and*

- Eat low-fat, primarily vegetarian, diets and high-fiber breakfasts regularly.

For more information on wellness, turn to chapter 2.

All seven steps require a great deal of initiative on your part, coupled with real concern for your own well-being. Such personal responsibility is all too rarely found among most men's personal health care practices. This chapter can help you address many of the most critical tasks. Use the resources here to get started on the right paths. You'll improve your own health awareness, and you'll gain access to many other resources as well.

This is not an easy assignment. Consider the search for the right doctor. Traditionally, men are reluctant to talk about personal health problems, even with their own physician; but open discussion is the only way you can make your symptoms fully known. When choosing a doctor, look for trust, compassion, and understanding. You must be able to speak freely with your doctor about any problems you might have, including sexual issues, personal lifestyle habits, and physical problems that may be embarrassing. For example, if a man can't tell the doctor about sensations in his testicles that have bothered him for weeks or months, there is no chance of curing the problem, much less preventing the development of a possibly fatal disease that could be treated easily when caught early.

If you find it difficult to talk with your doctor and other health care providers about personal issues, or the physician doesn't seem to be interested, try to find out why. Is it the physician's manner or your own reluctance to discuss private matters, or both? Perhaps you can improve the relationship, or you may want to try other physicians until you feel comfortable with one.

If you decide to look elsewhere, let prospective providers know that you are searching for the right person for *you*. Make sure they realize you want a person who'll discuss *all* aspects of your health as part of your regular health care, even those that may not be strictly physical or disease-oriented, such as your sexual life, family life, social life, work life, and personal habits and behaviors.

Remember, you are looking for a long-term relationship, a health care partnership. Establish a rapport that satisfies you as it relates to your health *and* your identity as a caring and feeling man; you're not just a patient.

For more information on choosing and using a primary care provider, turn to chapter 5.

Real Men

Changing how men think of themselves is essential to wellness, and an effective way to extend and improve the quality of men's lives.

In *The Masculine Mystique,* author and lawyer Andrew Kimbrell points out that parenting, nurturing, stewardship, husbandry, mentoring, and creativity are truer qualities of the male psyche and character than the socially stigmatized stereotypes of masculinity, including competition, mechanization, power, and the pursuit of profit.

A cofounder of the Men's Health Network, Kimbrell recommends that men learn to break out of the masculine mystique. He calls on men to alter their personal habits and lifestyles to reinforce the positive traits of male well-being and protective health, both for themselves and for their fellowmen.

TIP

Good Habits

Work with your health care providers to develop habits that will help you prevent unnecessary fatal diseases. Learn to detect the symptoms early, when they are easier and less costly to treat and cure.

Confronting the Top Killers of Men

According to Dr. Louis Sullivan, former Secretary of Health and Human Services, about 900,000 of the 2.2 million deaths in the United States each year are preventable, including deaths from ten of the top eleven leading killers of men—heart disease, cancer, accidents, stroke, lung disease, pneumonia, influenza, HIV infection, suicide, homicide, and diabetes. Only death by homicide is not directly preventable through actions you can take entirely by yourself. Even so, you can make it far less likely.

Heart Disease

More than 350,000 men die each year from heart disease, the leading cause of death for men. One in every five men suffers a heart attack before the age of sixty-five. Between the ages of twenty-five and seventy-five, men die from heart disease at two to three times the rate of women. Over three-quarters of all heart disease relates to diet and stress.

Diet. As Hippocrates observed more than two thousand years ago, food is the best medicine. American men are traditionally voracious meat eaters, especially of beef and other red meats, but these foods contain extremely high levels of fats, lipids, and cholesterol, all of which contribute significantly to the development of heart disease.

The key to preventing heart disease is reducing the blood cholesterol level. Many men can do this easily by eating the proper foods, although in more extreme cases you may want to consult a physician or other health care professional about the possible need for medications as well as proper diet.

A vegetarian diet is ideal for reducing cholesterol. Provided you consume enough high-protein vegetables such as beans and legumes, you

10

can get all the nutrients necessary for proper health from a vegetarian diet alone. Perhaps one of the simplest and best ways to lessen your likelihood of suffering from heart disease (and many types of cancer as well) is to avoid fast-food chains, stop eating processed hot dogs, hamburgers, and sirloin steaks, and start eating more vegetable and fruit salads. The U.S. Department of Agriculture recommends five servings of fruits and vegetables each day. Follow this recommendation strictly, and you'll go a long way toward living longer and better. You might choose to eat a very small amount of meat to make it easier to obtain certain amino acids and proteins. If you do decide to eat meat regularly, however, organically raised cattle, chicken, and other livestock or poultry are much healthier to consume than those raised by mass production.

Diet References

Two organizations can provide you with free information on proper eating habits:

- American Dietetic Association, tel. (800) 366-1655
- Food and Nutrition Information Center of the National Agricultural Library, tel. (301) 504-5719

Two excellent books on the subject are

- *Controlling Cholesterol* by Kenneth Coopers (Bantam Books, 1988), $6.50
- *Eat More, Weigh Less* by Dean Ornish (HarperCollins, 1994), $14

Stress. As the second major factor contributing to heart disease, stress has reached unprecedented levels in contemporary society. Whether at work or at home, learn how to minimize stress as much as possible. Take relaxing and revivifying breaks whenever necessary. Avoid unnecessary conflicts with co-workers and family members. Seek out comforting and supportive friendships that provide relief from routine daily pressures. And find meaning in life that broadens experience beyond the workplace, while increasing your self-esteem and enjoyment of life.

Stress contributes not only to heart disease but also to cancer and a variety of other disorders, including hypertension, high blood pressure and peptic ulcers. Contemporary male stress and its implications may be the most pervasive factor affecting lower life expectancy among men.

For more information on handling stress, see Men's Health Advisor by Michael LaFavore (Rodale Press, 1992), $14.95.

Tips for a Healthy Heart

If you smoke, stop. When smokers give up the habit, their risk of heart attack drops 50 to 70 percent within five years.

Try to keep your blood pressure within a healthful range of systolic 120 and diastolic 80. A diet low in cholesterol and salt, along with proper exercise, will help achieve proper blood pressure.

For more information, call the Office on Smoking and Health of the U.S. Centers for Disease Control at (800) CDC-1311.

Aspirin: Prevention for Heart Disease and Cancer

Taking aspirin every other day helps prevent heart disease in men, according to a well-publicized Harvard Medical School study. Aspirin thins the blood slightly, reducing pressure on the heart.

For many men, aspirin taken once every other day can also help prevent the development of cancers. Aspirin helps mitigate the physiological consequences of stress and inflammation.

Consult your doctor about using aspirin properly as a preventive measure against heart disease or a cancer-preventive measure. For most people, aspirin has no side effects other than the possibility of slight stomach irritation.

For more information on preventing heart disease, call the American Heart Association at (214) 706-1179.

Cancer

More than 270,000 men die of cancer each year, with lung cancer accounting for about one-third of the fatalities. The other major cancer killers of men are prostate cancer, colorectal cancer, pancreatic cancer, non-Hodgkin's lymphoma, and testicular cancer.

All cancers, including both those that affect only men (testicular and prostate cancer) and those that affect men and women alike, are reaching epidemic proportions among men. One man in eleven will develop prostate cancer at some point in his life, and by the age of seventy-five men are dying from all forms of cancer at twice the rate of women. Black men are especially at risk: their cancer death rate is twice that of white males.

A healthy lifestyle is the best approach to preventing cancers of all types. This includes the traditional healthy habits of eating right, exer-

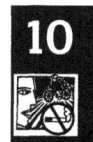

Prostate Disease

Prostate cancer takes the lives of 34,000 American men each year, and the numbers are increasing rapidly. While this disease is a painful killer, it responds well when diagnosed and treated early.

Learn to recognize symptoms of prostate cancer: restricted flow of urine and pain in the prostate region or perineum (between the scrotum and anus). As the disease progresses, sexual dysfunction can occur.

To detect prostate disease, make sure you get a simple digital examination. If you are over forty years old, get an exam at least once every three years. If you are over fifty, one every year is recommended.

Hundreds of thousands of unnecessary deaths occur each decade simply because only about 15 percent of men aged fifty and over are examined. This is the most frequently avoided or overlooked test in a general health examination.

In addition to prostate cancer, *prostatitis*—infections of the prostate gland—is more prevalent today than in former decades. According to the Prostatitis Foundation, 50 to 80 percent of all men get prostatitis, usually

cising properly, and getting regular physical checkups. Above all, the single most immediate and beneficial action you can take to reduce the threat of death by cancer is to *stop smoking*. Men who have never smoked in their lives (especially cigarettes), and who aren't killed by violence or other diseases related to mental health or stress, generally live on average as long as women, seventy-eight years. In addition, as with heart disease, stress is a major factor in the development of cancer in men. You can greatly decrease the chance of developing cancers by altering your lifestyle to reduce stress.

You will also be less likely to develop cancer if you take these other preventive measures:

■ Reduce your alcohol consumption to no more than two beverages per day. One drink per day—but no more—may even relieve stress.

■ Avoid environmental pollutants, such as air pollution, herbal pesticides, and toxins in the workplace, as well as unprotected exposure to sunlight.

■ Go easy on salty and fatty foods, and consume lots of dietary fiber that dilutes and expels cancer-causing substances from your digestive tract.

■ Learn about, and test yourself for, the warning signs of various types of cancer to facilitate early detection and effective treatment.

For more information on cancer prevention, call the American Cancer Society at (800) 227-2345 and the Cancer Information Service of the National Institutes of Health at (800) 422-6237.

Testicular Cancer

Testicular cancer, a leading killer of men from ages fifteen to forty, is the most common cancer in men between those ages.

Fortunately, testicular cancer can be detected in its early stages by a simple self-examination, checking the testicles, with delicate pressure between the fingers, for tiny lumps. In the early stages, testicular cancer can be treated and cured easily before it becomes malignant.

Strokes

Strokes kill more than 56,000 men each year. Yet even this number does not fully suggest the prevalence of strokes, which is the number-one crippling disease in the United States. More than 270,000 men suffer strokes each year.

Unlike heart attacks, which can physically inhibit your actions, strokes are more damaging to your general ability to function because they affect the brain. You can become paralyzed or lose sensation, memory, or the capacity to speak and understand speech. Stroke victims are often completely dependent on others for survival.

Because more than 80 percent of all strokes result from causes similar to those that lead to heart attacks, many of the same preventive steps can help prevent stroke. For example:

- Regular exercise cuts risk of stroke by 40 percent.
- Aspirin every other day reduces risk of stroke by 25 percent.
- Eating vegetables and fruits high in beta carotene (an antioxidant vitamin) decreases risk of stroke by 40 percent.
- And, of course, *don't smoke.*

Lung Disease

Lung diseases result directly from inhaling bad air, whether from smoking, from pollution and toxins, or from particulate matter. About 50,000 men die of lung diseases each year. Besides lung cancer, emphysema is the most fatal lung disease.

Emphysema is one of the simplest diseases to prevent, which is particularly significant since there is no cure for it:

- Once again, don't smoke.

- Avoid heavily polluted areas, such as busy streets and industrial toxic regions.

- Avoid other areas with bad air or wear a protective mask when in areas that are strewn with particulate matter or contain dust; sand dust; sawdust; car, truck, bus, or diesel exhaust; asbestos; or lead paint.

For more information, call the American Lung Association at (800) 586-4872.

Pneumonia and Influenza

Although infection is no longer the dominant cause of death for Americans, pneumonia and influenza infections still take the lives of over 36,000 men every year. As you grow older, these infections are progressively more difficult to shrug off. Older men therefore need to take special care not to become sick.

during midlife, and as early as twenty-seven years of age. Symptoms include discomfort in the testicles and scrotum, slight pain in the bladder region or lower anal area, and pain in the perineum.

While prostatitis can be difficult to cure, there is no reason to endure its pain for extended periods of time. As part of treatment arranged with your health care providers, a few weeks of antibiotics should cure prostatitis.

If symptoms occur, see a urologist and discover the problem as soon as possible. Warm baths, a good diet, and adequate exercise will also help keep the prostate in proper working order.

For more information on prostate cancer, call the American Prostate Society at (800) 308-1106. For more information on prostatitis, call the Prostatitis Foundation at (309) 664-6222. For information on finding a urologist, turn to chapter 13.

If you are over sixty-five, get vaccinated for influenza virus and pneumococcus bacteria. In addition, avoid exposure to people who have the flu or pneumonia. Eating well and getting regular exercise boosts your immune system, helping you fend off life-threatening illnesses as well as to recover from them more quickly and easily.

Multivitamins can be beneficial in warding off these infectious diseases, too. According to a Johns Hopkins University study, people who took one multivitamin a day got sick less than half as often as those who took no vitamin supplement.

Antibiotic Resistance

Take antibiotics only when absolutely necessary, because you can develop resistance to them. Were an emergency situation to arise that required antibiotics to fight an infection (for example, after an operation), they might not work properly. The number of in-house hospital deaths as a result of antibiotic resistance has risen substantially.

Personal Injury and Violence-Related Deaths

Deaths by suicide, homicide, and accidents are predominantly a male phenomena: 60,000 men die of accidents each year; 24,000 of suicide; and 20,000 of homicide. This is an inexcusable tragedy.

Suicide. Four out of five deaths by suicide are men. Men between the ages of twenty and twenty-four are over six times more likely than women to commit suicide. Above the age of eighty-five, men are over eleven times more likely to take their own lives. Veterans and divorced men have suicide rates even higher than those of other men.

Depression, the primary cause of suicide, is severely underdiagnosed for men compared to women. Consequently, even though women are twice as likely to suffer from depression, they are only one-fourth as likely to take their own lives. The reason is that they receive some kind of treatment much more often than do men. It's vital to pay close attention to your psychological state and act in ways that serve to heal emotional wounds and establish supportive living situations.

For more information on suicide, call the American Association of Suicidology at (202) 237-2280 or the American Suicide Foundation at (800) ASF-4042.

Homicide. Homicide kills more than 20,000 men each year. Of the top ten killers of men, only homicide can't be directly prevented by your own actions, although you can severely lessen your risk of becoming a murder victim.

Most homicides happen on a moment's impulse. Avoid dangerous and violent situations, especially those that involve guns and weapons. Remember that how you behave will influence how others behave toward you. Don't provoke a fight or argument that may lead to the use of a weapon out of instantaneous rage. Learn to dispel violence and make friends rather than promote violence and make enemies.

Accidents. Accidents, including workplace accidents, are the third leading killer of men, after heart disease and cancer. Many of these occur at the workplace: 98 percent of the employees in the ten most dangerous professions are men, and 94 percent of those who die in the workplace are men. Over 90 percent of fatal workplace accidents occur to men.

Start taking a good hard look at your workplace environment and your behavior at work. Don't take any work situation for granted, but rather analyze each activity and the way you perform it from a health perspective. Avoid any dangerous or threatening activities.

Do the same outside of work, whether at home or on vacation. If you incorporate healthy approaches and observations into your everyday life, you will greatly reduce the risk of accidents that needlessly and recklessly kill men.

For more information on workplace health and safety, turn to chapter 12.

Diabetes

Diabetes, the body's inability to properly process sugar, kills more than 20,000 men annually. There are two types: Type I, insulin-dependent diabetes, usually occurs during youth, but can develop at any age, and requires insulin throughout a person's life. Type II, non-insulin-dependent diabetes, typically occurs after age forty and may come on gradually. Symptoms of diabetes include regular or constant thirst, frequent need to urinate, fatigue, and unexplained weight loss.

Experts estimate that only half the people who have type II diabetes even know it. Nonetheless, their bodies are deteriorating, and they're risking blindness, heart attack, kidney failure, loss of a limb, impotence, and even death.

Steps you can take to prevent diabetes include:

- Maintaining your weight within the recommended range
- Exercising aerobically—regular exercise can reduce the risk of diabetes by 40 percent

Male Impotence

Men rarely talk about impotence because of the intimate nature of the problem. Consequently, those who have potency disorders can become severely depressed, traumatized, and emotionally isolated. In our efficiency-driven society, performance by men—in bed or on the job—is often taken to be the indicator of worthiness. When the machine stops, men often feel useless.

While the best solution is to alter these self-destructive stereotypes, you need not suffer the emotional embarrassment, guilt, or shame of impotence. Nearly all types of sexual impotence can be prevented or cured. If you experience difficulty obtaining an erection, see your doctor and don't be afraid to discuss the situation openly and candidly. This is the only way to address and solve the problem.

Embarrassment, guilt, or shame are horrible emotions to bear, so learn to understand impotence and don't go it alone. Impotence is not just a man's disease; it includes your partner as well. Both partners working together can usually solve the problem.

- Eating regularly—steady blood-sugar levels help the body's sugar-processing system to cope
- Reducing saturated fats in your diet, *and*
- Consuming foods rich in chromium, such as mushrooms and broccoli

For more information, call the American Diabetes Association at (800) 232-3472.

HIV and Other Sexually Transmitted Diseases

Sexually transmitted diseases (STDs) are a major concern for men, as for women. In particular, the AIDS pandemic is taking a frightening toll on young men, who are its primary victims. Men represent more than three-quarters of the 14 million people worldwide who are infected with HIV, the virus that causes AIDS. Over the past two and a half decades, tens of thousands of people have died of AIDS in the United States, making it one of the leading causes of death.

HIV. You don't give up your right to make your own health care decisions if you are HIV-positive. The first step is to educate yourself about the services that are available. A wide number of agencies and organizations offer a variety of programs both for people with HIV and to prevent the spread of this disease. These services range from medical care to emotional counseling to legal assistance for people who suffer discrimination because they are HIV-positive. Take advantage of them, and you can live a longer, healthier life.

For services and referrals to other public and private AIDS agencies, contact your county health department's HIV/AIDS programs. Many of these offices provide free, anonymous HIV/AIDS testing and counseling.

AIDS Resources

For information on HIV/AIDS, call:

- *National AIDS Hotline,* U.S. Centers for Disease Control: (800) 342-AIDS (English); (800) 344-7432 (Spanish); (800) 243-7889 (TDD)
- *AIDS Information Office,* U.S. Centers for Disease Control: (404) 329-2891
- *HIV/AIDS Treatment Information Services:* (800) 448-0440 (Spanish or English)

Other sexually transmitted diseases. Discussion about STDs other than HIV infection is taboo in our social discourse, yet these diseases are quite rampant. They include genital herpes, gonorrhea, chlamydia (the most commonly reported STD, with 4 million new cases each year), syphilis, chancroid, human papillomavirus, trichomoniasis, urethritis, ureaplasm urealyticum, genital warts, and hepatitis B. Of all STDs, you have the *least* likely chance of contracting HIV through unprotected sex. The risk of HIV infection when having sex without a condom is only 1 percent; for genital herpes it's 30 percent. If you sense any discomfort or experience any pain when urinating, see your doctor immediately.

For more information on male STDs and male sexual health concerns, see The New Male Sexuality, *by Bernie Zilbergeld (Bantam, 1984), $6.99. You can also contact the Sexually Transmitted Disease Hotline at (800) 227-8922.*

Kenneth Goldberg's *How Men Can Live As Long As Women,* thoroughly discusses the various techniques and approaches to overcoming sexual impotence and provides many resources. Other good resources are *The New Male Sexuality* by Bernie Zilbergeld, *Superpotency* by Dudley Danoff, and *The Potent Male* by Irwin Goldstein and Larry Rothstein.

For more information, call the Impotence Institute of America at (800) 669-1603.

Protect Yourself

Safe sex in not an option, it is a must. The use of a condom is imperative if you have had more than one partner in recent years.

You have no choice. You are virtually guaranteed to contract some kind of sexually transmitted disease if you don't use a condom when having sex with multiple partners or with people you haven't known for very long.

Men's Mental Health

Mental health for men today, when traditional roles of work and family are rapidly changing, is of prime importance to your overall health. Although many men may believe otherwise, there is nothing unmanly about taking care of your mental health. What is unmanly is pretending that no problems exist when the signs say that they do.

Wellness of the Mind

You can strengthen your inner self and discover outer support structures that help you deal more effectively and healthfully with work, family, friends, and community. Heed your intuitions and feelings closely, rather than denying or dismissing them. Act in ways that show concern for and attention to your true emotions, rather than repressing or resisting them.

10

Young Men's Health Crisis

The men's health crisis begins early in life.

School years are especially difficult and damaging for many boys. Thousands of elementary children are treated with drug therapy each year for hyperactive behavior in the classroom. The vast majority of these children are boys.

Teenage boys represent over 90 percent of those taking steroids and growth hormones to build up their bodies. The results are devastating, including leukemia, enlarged hearts, and immune response failure.

School sports take a toll on boys. Over 300,000 young men are injured every year in high school and college football, with over 15,000 requiring surgery.

Over 60 percent of high school dropouts are boys.

Boys aged ten to eighteen are four to five times more likely than girls to commit suicide.

New health programs are needed at all grade levels to raise the consciousness of schools about male physical and mental health. These programs should actively instruct

Therapy: A Vital Link

Men are chronically underdiagnosed for depression and other mental diseases. As a result, men are both far more likely than women to be admitted to psychiatric hospitals *and* less likely to seek mental and emotional health assistance for themselves. Many of the tragic deaths of men from causes such as suicide and addictions result from this lack of effective psychological help.

Men overwhelmingly are the primary victims of health-destroying addictions due to mental disturbances, often as a result of cultural demands, unrealistic expectations of themselves, and stressful work and living situations. Over two-thirds of alcoholics are men, as are over 80 percent of those suffering from fatal, alcohol-induced liver disease. The male death rate for drug abuse reflects this same percentage.

Mental therapy is essential for coming to grips with this pervasive and destructive situation. An effective forum for men to address contemporary mental health problems adequately is a supportive and comforting atmosphere, where you can feel you aren't alone in your predicaments and can discuss personal issues with like-minded and sympathetic individuals.

For many men, therapy is vitally important to confront, understand, and heal past or current emotional wounds. Among other things, therapy can help you come to terms with traumatic experiences so they don't ruin your life. And it can be an antidote to the adversarial and unsympathetic relationships among men that are ingrained into the social system, based on competition and the masculine mystique.

For more information on mental health services, turn to chapter 14.

Seek Support

For many men under psychological distress, men's support groups can provide emotional help and encouragement. For referrals to men's support groups in your area, call the Men's/Father's Hotline at (512) 472-DADS.

For more information on support groups, turn to chapter 22.

For men and women with alcohol addictions, Alcoholics Anonymous is a well-established and effective self-help organization. Others sources for help dealing with alcohol abuse include:

- The National Council on Alcoholism and Drug Dependency, tel. (800) 622-2255
- The American Council on Alcoholism, tel. (800) 527-5344

Fatherhood as a Health Issue

More and more men are facing the challenge of being the single parent after a divorce. Fathers now head 21 percent of single-parent households, and the trend of fathers gaining custody is growing slowly. Many of these new single-parent fathers need encouragement and other forms of assistance as they seek to cope with expanding financial and personal responsibilities.

How you treat your children often reflects how you treat yourself. If you are a father, learn to see your family role as health supporting and health promoting. Incorporate active health awareness and mentoring into your household. Besides benefiting your children, this will boost your own health awareness and improve your emotional and psychological inner life as a man.

For more information on fatherhood health issues and child custody for fathers, call the Children's Rights Council at (800) 787-KIDS, the National Center on Fathers and Families at (215) 573-5500, and the Men's/Father's Hotline at (512) 472-DADS.

young men on such critical topics as diet, violence, sports injuries, and substance abuse, including the abuse of steroids and hormones.

Child Custody and Mental Health

About 90 percent of all custody cases in the United States grant child custody exclusively to the mother. In many instances, the legal and emotional barriers following divorce prevent fathers from interacting with their children, leading to even greater psychological devastation. The suicide rate for men after divorce is four times that of women, and the rate of alcohol abuse is six times that of women.

Resources
Organizations

AIDS Clearinghouse
P.O. Box 6003
Rockville, MD 20850
(800) 458-5231
Call or write for information on HIV/AIDS.

National AIDS Hotline
(800) 342-AIDS
TDD: (800) 243-7889
Call for information and referrals on HIV/AIDS.

American Association of Suicidology
4201 Connecticut Avenue, N.W. #310
Washington, DC 20008
(202) 237-2280
Call for information on suicide.

American Cancer Society
1599 Clifton Road, N.E.
Atlanta, GA 30329
(404) 320-3333
(800) 227-2345
Call or write for referrals to local chapters and information on cancer prevention.

10

American Council on Alcoholism
5024 Campbell Boulevard
Baltimore, MD 21236
(800) 527-5344
Call for information on alcohol abuse.

American Diabetes Association
1660 Duke Street
Alexandria, VA 22314
(800) 232-3472
Contact the ADA for information on diabetes.

American Dietetic Association
Consumer Nutrition Hotline
216 W. Jackson Boulevard
Chicago, IL 60606
(800) 366-1655
Contact the ADA for pamphlets containing basic dietary guidelines, general health, and maintaining or achieving a healthy weight.

American Foundation for Urologic Disease
300 W. Pratt Street, #401
Baltimore, MD 21201
(800) 242-2383
(410) 727-2908
Call for information on urologic disorders, prostate cancer, incontinence, infertility, urinary tract infections, and referrals to support groups.

American Heart Association
7372 Greenville Avenue
Dallas, TX 75231
(214) 706-1220
(800) 242-8721
Contact the AHA for information on preventing heart disease and strokes.

American Lung Association
1740 Broadway
New York, NY 10019-4374
(800) 586-4872
Call or write for referrals and for information on lung cancer and smoking.

American Prostate Society
(800) 308-1106
Contact the society to receive a package of information on prostate cancer.

American Suicide Foundation
1045 Park Avenue
New York, NY 10028
(800) ASF-4042
Call for information on suicide.

Children's Rights Council
220 I Street, N.E., #200
Washington, DC 20002
(800) 787-KIDS
Contact the council for information on fatherhood health and child-custody issues.

Food and Nutrition Information Center
National Agricultural Library
(301) 504-5719
Contact the center for information on proper eating habits and on preventing heart disease.

Impotence Institute of America
10400 Little Patuxent Parkway, #485
Columbia, MD 21044
(800) 669-1603
Contact the institute for information on impotence and a list of Impotence Anonymous chapters.

Men's/Father's Hotline
807 Brazos, #315
Austin, TX 78701
(512) 472-DADS
Men's Healthline: (888) MEN-2-MEN
Call the hotlines for crisis assistance and referrals to providers, resources for family health, legal concerns, and men's support groups. Contact the Men's Healthline for information about male-specific diseases and referrals to health care providers and other resources for men. On the Internet,

you can reach the Men's Hotline at men@menhotline.org and the Father's Hotline at dads@fathers.org.

Men's Health Network
310 D Street, N.E.
Washington, DC 20002
(202) 543-6461
mensnet@capaccess.org
Contact the MHN for general information referrals to its national network of men's health care providers and men's organizations.

National Center on Fathers and Families
Box 58
Philadelphia, PA 19104-6216
(215) 573-5500
Contact the center for information on fatherhood health and child-custody issues.

National Council on Alcoholism and Drug Dependency
(800) 622-2255
Call for information on alcohol and drug abuse.

National Institutes of Health
Cancer Information Service
Building 31, Room 10A24
Bethesda, MD 20892-3100
(800) 4-CANCER (422-6237)
PDQ by fax (301) 402-5874
WWW site: http://www.nci.nih.gov/
Contact the CIS for general information on treatments, services, and provider referrals.

Office on Smoking and Health
U.S. Centers for Disease Control
(404) 488-5701
Contact the office for information on stopping smoking.

Prostatitis Foundation
Information Distribution Center

Parkway Business Center
2029 Ireland Grove Road
Bloomington, IL 61704
(309) 664-6222
Contact the foundation for information on prostatitis.

Sexually Transmitted Disease Hotline
U.S. Centers for Disease Control
(800) 227-8922
Call for information, free pamphlets, referrals, and counseling on STDs.

Publications

Controlling Cholesterol: Preventive Medicine Program, by Kenneth H. Coopers (Bantam Books, 1988), $6.50.

Eat More, Weigh Less, by Dean Ornish (HarperCollins, 1994), $14.

Fatherhood, by Bill Cosby (Berkley Books, 1987), $11.

How Men Can Live As Long As Women, by Kenneth Goldberg (The Summit Group, 1993), $22.95.

Iron John, by Robert Bly (Vintage Books, 1992), $11.

Knights Without Armor, by Harold Kipnis (Tarcher Books, 1991), $12.95.

"The Man's Cancer," by Leon Jaroff, *Time,* April 1, 1996.

Man-to-Man: Surviving Prostate Cancer, by Michael Korda (Random House, 1996), $20.

The Masculine Mystique, by Andrew Kimbrell (Ballantine Books, 1995), $23.

Men's Health Advisor, by Michael LaFavore (Rodale Press, 1992), $14.95.

The Myth of Male Power, by Warren Farrell (Simon & Schuster, 1993), $6.99.

The New Male Sexuality, by Bernie Zilbergeld (Bantam, 1984), $6.99.

The Prostate: A Guide for Men and the Women Who Love Them, by Patrick Walsh and Janet Worthington (Johns Hopkins, 1984), $15.95.

Prostate and Cancer: A Family Health Guide to Diagnosis, Treatment, and Survival, by Sheldon Marks (Fisher Books, 1995), $14.95.

"The Sex-Bias Myth in Medicine," by Andrew Kadar, *Atlantic Monthly,* August 1994.

"Staying Strong: For Men Over Fifty, A Common Sense Health Guide," December 1993, Washington, D.C., American Association of Retired Persons.

11

Elders as Health Care Consumers

Lou Glasse and Mal Schechter

Lou Glasse is a consultant on aging policies and services. She is President Emerita of the Older Women's League and former director of the New York State Office for the Aging.

Mal Schechter is a consultant on population aging and public policy. He is former associate director of the International Longevity Center (U.S.) and assistant professor of geriatrics and adult development at the Mount Sinai School of Medicine in New York City.

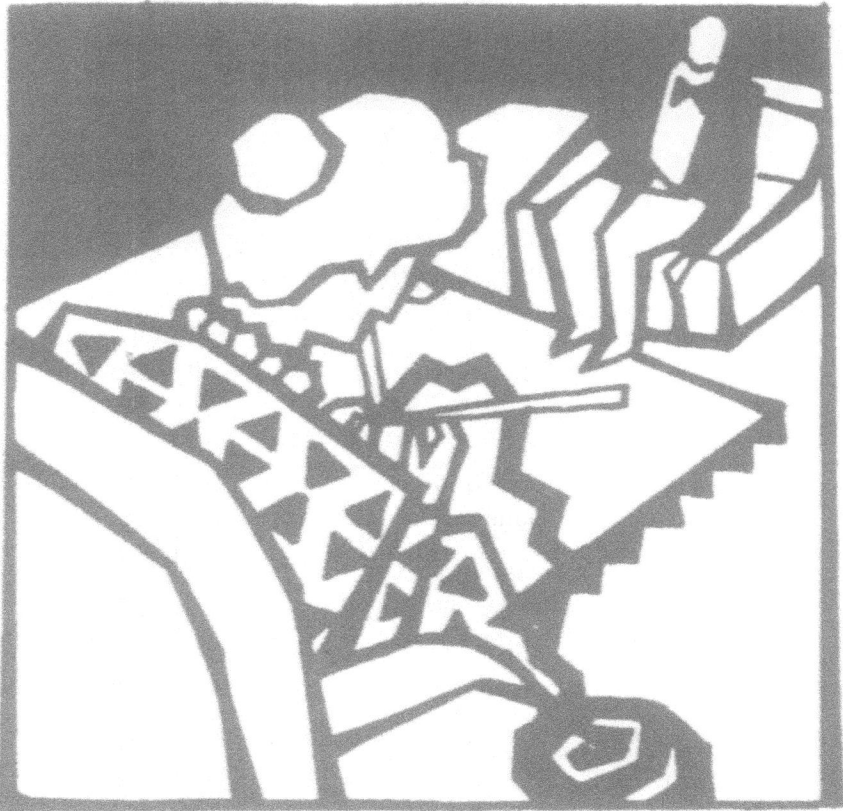

About 20 million women and 13.5 million men in the United States are sixty-five or older—about 13 percent of the total U.S. population—and the number grows by over a thousand each day.

When the twentieth century started, the average life expectancy at birth was forty-five years or so. Later, half of newborns could expect to live into their sixties, thanks to improved public health, living conditions, and medical care, especially for infants, children, and mothers. Today, men who reach age sixty-five will live, on average, another fifteen years; women, another seventeen years.

About 3.6 million Americans are over eighty-five years old. This is one of the fastest-growing age groups and, largely female. Because women live longer, after age eighty-five there are 259 women for every 100 men. And the current estimated 54,000 centenarians will number 81,000 in the year 2000 and 834,000, if not more, by 2050.

These population expectations—more people living longer—represent a triumph. They also pose a wide-ranging—but hardly impossible—challenge to our innovative society.

Unfortunately, America is far less developed in the field of geriatrics and long term care than it should be, considering these demographic trends. There are far too few geriatricians, organized arrangements for care in the community, reliable residential care (including nursing homes and assisted living units), or affordable, reliable, and geriatrically smart insurance policies covering long term care in coordination with Medicare, which is chiefly designed to support acute care. All of this makes it tough for older health care consumers and their adult children who may represent them.

Still, most older people are relatively healthy and functional. Today, about 1.2 million of the 33 million older Americans are in nursing homes. Perhaps another 2 million live at home with a severe disability; several million more have a less severe disability. And about half the population age eighty-five or older is relatively healthy and functional. Generally speaking, rates of death and disability do rise with age, but such statistics don't say how *individuals* will function in the future—the same, better, or worse.

It's important for you, your health care providers (chiefly doctors, nurses, social workers, hospital officials, nursing home officials, home health care agency personnel) and your family to recognize that:

■ The U.S. health care system tends to deny or misinterpret the many needs of older people—or simply isn't geared to handle all of those needs.

■ Older people respond in distinctive ways to drugs, foods, stress, infections, and wounds.

■ Elders are far more likely to need long term care, which represents their largest out-of-pocket health care expense.

■ Elders are more likely to have a variety of both single and combined health problems. And they are more likely to take one or more prescription drugs regularly, constituting their second-largest out-of-pocket expense.

■ A federal insurance system—Medicare—pays for a significant portion of the health care of almost all people sixty-five and older; on the other hand, elders spend more out of their own pockets today for health care than they did before Medicare began, and they also devote far more of their income to health care than do younger adults.

If you have been a careful health care consumer in the past, you've probably acquired talents applicable at any stage of life to finding the right doctor and services. However, if you are an older person or acting with or for one, you also need knowledge about normal aging as well as diseases that become more common in later years. This chapter introduces you to this information. It covers the nature of the medical system, the medical and psychological and social characteristics and needs of older people, and the financial resources to cover costs of professional care, principally Medicare, Medigap, and Medicaid.

Elders and Others

This chapter summarizes the health care needs of elder consumers. But elders share many concerns—and services—with people of all ages, so you'll find important information throughout this book. In particular, refer to chapter 3 on rights, chapter 15 on long term care, chapter 16 on home care, and chapter 20 on death with dignity.

Rising Costs

A 1994 study by the American Association of Retired Persons and the Urban Institute projected that retirees would spend an average of $2,803 in out-of-pocket health costs during that year, more than twice as much as in 1987.

11

Aging, Health, and Well-Being

If you are over sixty, the most disturbing aspect of the health care system may well be the lack of providers with training for certain circumstances that occur more and more often at the later ages. Organs and tissues change with age, as does your ability to move and think. You respond to infectious diseases differently from the way you did as a young adult, and diseases may appear differently and take different courses. You may have a heart attack without experiencing any chest pain. Infection may not be accompanied by much fever. Moreover, very old patients tend to have more than one disease or chronic condition at a time, complicating care significantly.

The essence of geriatrics is the care of older persons with several simultaneous problems or disabilities. Psychological and social factors as well as physical disabilities may complicate treatment of chronic diseases, as seen in such questions as:

- Is the patient too depressed to take medication without supervision?
- Can a family helper assure the patient's cleanliness, nutrition, and correct drug taking?
- Is the home environment safe?

To design and implement a treatment or care plan, the geriatrician has to be a coordinator of medical specialists and other services or work with a team of experts.

A geriatrics-trained doctor may not be able to prevent or cure you of chronic conditions, but he or she can help you live as well as possible at home. And, when the time comes, this doctor and colleagues can assist you in finding a nursing home or other kind of living arrangement. Such a doctor knows about rehabilitation therapy, control of pain, and terminal care. At the same time, recognizing that long term care at home involves a family member, the doctor will take this caregiver into consideration in describing your options.

Your present physician may be such a doctor or have the connections to make geriatrics consultants quickly available. Find out. Any primary care physician should be able to tell you what will happen if you need geriatrics.

Unfortunately, however, health care providers trained to work with older Americans are in critically short supply. Geriatrics is not yet a popular field for doctors, in part due to society's unwillingness to confront age and death, but also because geriatrics offers physicians lower average incomes than do many other specialties. A severe shortage of teachers and teaching programs in geriatrics means that consumers can expect this state of affairs to last for the foreseeable future.

This makes it all the more important for you to educate yourself and take an active role in fostering your own well-being.

Provider Shortage

With far too few people fully trained in geriatrics, don't rule out a provider who lacks such credentials. But look more favorably on a person who has a certificate from a geriatrics course, participates in a group practice with access to a geriatrician, or belongs to a relevant professional group, such as the American Geriatrics Society or the Gerontological Society of America.

Not everyone over age sixty-five has to have, or can find, a fully schooled geriatrician. A sophisticated consumer can be served by physicians who know basic geriatrics and have access to geriatricians for consultation. Some internists and family and other practitioners hold a certificate of added competence in geriatrics, which means they have taken short courses in geriatrics and have passed an examination.

However, there is no board certification in geriatrics as there is in internal medicine, psychiatry, gynecology, and other medical fields. For this reason, *geriatrician* is an unofficial term and any practitioner may use it. Don't accept the label without questions about training, experience, and skill.

Habits and Health

Your chances of living a long life depend on a number of variables, of which the supply of trained medical personnel is only one. Perhaps even more so than for younger people, you can reap rewards by paying attention to your health and living in ways likely to preserve your physical, psychological, and social well-being:

- Don't smoke or abuse alcohol or drugs.
- Wear seat belts.
- Eat a diet rich in fruits, vegetables, and grains. Avoid a diet based on convenience and fast foods.
- Exercise regularly. Don't be a couch potato.
- Check your home and workplace for environmental hazards such as dangerous chemicals, poor lighting, and rough floors.

11

Pre-Medicare: Younger Elders

The least-insured group of older Americans are people out of work, whether due to job loss or early retirement, but too young for Medicare. According to the American Association of Retired Persons, "50- to 64-year-olds are more critical of the U.S. health care system than any other age group." About 55 percent of men and 50 percent of women of this age rate it as poor, compared to about one-third of men and women ages 18 to 49 and over 65. More than 40 percent of 50- to 64-year-olds believe that the quality of their health coverage will decline in the future or that they will lose coverage entirely.

For more information on workplace health, turn to chapter 12.
Your mental and social health can affect not only the length but the quality of your life as well:

- Socialize regularly with friends and family.
- Participate in stimulating activities such as part-time work, hobbies, public affairs, volunteer services, travel, and education.

In addition to these "lifestyle" factors, you and your primary care provider and other health care personnel should pay attention to your family's medical history for clues to your own future health. Your genes may predispose you to certain maladies, such as cancer, and also to certain strengths, such as a freedom from major mental decline. Knowing your family medical history can help you avoid particular kinds of behavior that increase your risk.

Avoiding Inherited Ills

Gladys, a fifty-year-old woman, knew that both her mother and grandmother had suffered from severe osteoporosis, a painful and disabling bone disease. She realized that she might have the same fate.

In consultation with her physician, Gladys adopted a diet rich in calcium and an exercise regimen that helps strengthen her bones. She considered hormore replacement therapy. She and her physician will monitor her condition so they can identify the disease early if it occurs and begin treatment.

The Health Care Spectrum

At any age, but particularly late in life, your care agenda should include several components:

Health promotion and disease and accident prevention. This includes sound nutrition, exercise, vaccinations, vision and hearing correction, and avoiding drug abuse, alcohol abuse, and smoking. *Sources:* your doctor, hospital programs, books, newspapers, magazines, television programs, voluntary associations, retirement groups, mutual-help groups, the Internet.

Acute medical care. You must have access to emergency and other medical services when your life and limb are at stake. *Sources:* hospitals, ambulance services with emergency medical technicians, your doctor, surgeons, telephone-alert services.

Rehabilitation. These services aim at minimizing losses of function and restoring your ability to do as much for yourself as possible. *Sources:* hospitals, outpatient facilities, nursing homes, rehabilitation centers, physical, speech, and occupational therapists.

Custodial or long term care. This refers to personal assistance to meet your needs for bathing, eating, moving from bed to chair, grooming, and going to the toilet. *Sources:* family members, friends, volunteers, home-health agencies, skilled nursing homes, adult day care centers, public or private social service agencies, private professional nurses, and aides.

Social support services. If you lose some physical or mental abilities, your health and independence may depend on someone's helping you with such needs as housekeeping, shopping, paying bills, getting to the doctor's office, and completing official forms for financial help, meeting bills for heating, or low-cost housing. You also may need assistance for family conflicts or making complaints about essential services and physical or mental abuse. *Sources:* social workers, counselors, lawyers, accountants, volunteers, religious and fraternal organizations, senior centers, professional advocates and care coordinators, and social service and housing agencies.

This short list may help you find your way to services and care you need. Ideally, an organized system of providers, coordinators, volunteers, and others should be available to meet needs comprehensively; however, you're unlikely to find such one-stop shopping. Organizations that cover a spectrum of medical, nursing, social work, long term care, housing, and other services are few and far between. You or a family member or friend may have to put together a tailored set of services with as much professional and volunteer help as you can muster. Keep in mind that people with chronic illnesses and disabilities may experience sudden acute illnesses, and that acute and long term care require close coordination. Ask your doctor, hospital, HMO, nursing home, and home-health agency about finding "integrated acute and long term care."

Chronic Illness

You can't be sure how long you'll live, what chronic diseases may arise, how much they'll interfere with your activities, and how much you'll be able to compensate for any losses of function. Even if you avoid major diseases and trauma, you can't be sure of the exact extent to which your physical and mental functioning will change. Keep in mind that half of all eighty-five-year-olds lead independent lives.

Elder Abuse

One million to 2 million elders are victims of abuse every year, and millions more fear it.

Abuse takes two basic forms: physical or emotional injury and financial exploitation. According to the National Center on Elder Abuse, neglect by caregivers accounts for 37 percent of abuse cases; 26 percent are cases of physical abuse; 20 percent result from financial exploitation; 11 percent are psychological abuse; and 6 percent result from other causes.

Among the situations that could make you vulnerable to abuse are a lack of family support, the reluctance of caregivers to provide care and their frustrations in giving care; a lack of knowledge and professional guidance that would enable caregivers to deal with frustrations and tensions; disharmony among caregivers who share responsibility; overcrowding in the home or facility; isolation and mental decline; marital conflict; and financial, job, and family pressures on caregivers.

Most elder-abuse victims are women. Most abusers within the family are spouses or children, usually male.

In general, people become more prone to a chronic illness or disability as they age. The list of conditions they face includes arthritis, osteoporosis, diabetes, and incontinence, as well as heart disease, stroke, cancer, and dementia. Be aware that chronic illnesses are likely at some point to affect your ability to carry out your normal activities of life. The self-sufficiency you now take for granted may be reduced. In 1993 one American in seven faced major limitations on his or her activities as a result of chronic illness, including about two-fifths of all elders.

You can improve your chances of avoiding or minimizing these spoilers and killers through steps you can take throughout your life. Keep in mind two opposing forces. Physical aging means that the peak performance of your body's organs and tissues will gradually decline, even without disease or trauma or any noticeable effect on your ordinary activities. On the other hand, you have good resources to adjust to, or compensate for, losses. These resources are both internal and external: You can learn how to use an impaired arm or leg. You can rely on people as well as mechanical and other aids to help you do things. And you and your friends can watch out for and avoid problems.

To prepare for—or respond to—any declining abilities, you, your relatives and friends, and your primary care physician and other health care providers should consider some basic questions:

■ Can family members and good friends assist you if you can't care for yourself? Do these people live nearby?

■ Will you need help in your home? What community services could help you remain in your own home? If you can't climb stairs or walk to the bathroom in your home, can you modify your home, or should you move to a new living environment?

■ How will you decide if you need a nursing home? How will you select one? How much will it cost? Do you have the financial resources to pay for nursing-home care?

For more information on long term care, turn to chapter 15.

■ Do you have access to health care providers who can help you define and meet your evolving needs as you age?

■ Do you have insurance or other financial resources to cover the health care services you may need?

■ Have you made personal and legal arrangements in case you become mentally or physically incapable of making health care decisions and handling your financial affairs?

For more information on planning for future incapacity, turn to chapter 20.

For more information, contact the National Center on Elder Abuse, 810 First Street, N.E., Washington, DC 20002; tel. (202) 682-2470.

Caregiving/Caregivers

Nine out of ten disabled elders who aren't in nursing homes depend on their families and friends for help. This assistance may be for a few weeks, or it may extend for many years. The need may vary from handling financial matters and running errands to around-the-clock care, seven days a week. Most families willingly aid aging relatives and adjust their other commitments to do so.

Depending on the complexity of the care and the duration of your infirmity, family and friends may not be able to provide all the needed assistance in your home or the home of a relative. To prepare for this possibility, you and your family may need to consider two general types of alternative arrangements for long term care:

- Paying for services in your home and community, *and*
- Moving to another living arrangement where services are provided

Use It or Lose It

Lying in a bed without exercise may be damaging, whether in a hospital, a nursing home, or your own home. Doctors and other professionals should know the amount and kinds of exercise safe for a person.

If you need long term care after a hospital stay, your physician, consulting specialists, and the hospital social-work unit should help in making the arrangements before you leave the hospital.

Share the Load

In almost three out of four families, the role of caregiver falls to women: wives—often elders themselves—daughters, and daughters-in-law. Husbands are also important caregivers if their wives become chronically ill. If families share this responsibility among sons as well as daughters, grandchildren, and other relatives, the burden of care is spread. This reduces the likelihood of overburdening one person.

Long Term Care and the Consumer

Long term care means services that help you with activities you must do every day. Though they relate to health, these services don't necessarily

11

TIP

Mix and Match

Specialists trained to help you develop a plan for long term care may be hard to find, especially in rural areas and inner cities. Check with your local Area Agency on Aging and senior advocacy organizations such as the American Association of Retired Persons, the Older Women's League, and the Alzheimer's Association.

require a physician or a skilled nurse. Services are provided in the home, in the community, or in a variety of residential settings.

As the U.S. population ages and the need for services in both homes and institutions expands, more organizations are providing long term care. Both for-profit and nonprofit agencies are responding to the growing demand. Fortunately, government regulation of nursing homes that participate in Medicare and Medicaid has been strengthened over the years. If you're paying the bill yourself, nursing-home and home-care charges may be higher than under the government programs. You may need professional help in judging these prices and evaluating the quality of the services offered. Official standards for quality of home care, in particular, are in their infancy.

Given the choice, most people choose to live at home even if they require ongoing, around-the-clock services and can no longer care for themselves. About one-third of older Americans—mostly women—live alone. If no family member is immediately available to provide care, certified or trained home-care providers are available in many communities.

For more information on home care, turn to chapter 16.

Still, it can be difficult and expensive to arrange a complete set of home-care services. People who have major care needs and live alone—one-third of seniors (mostly very old women)—should consider an assisted-living facility, if they can afford it. Most such facilities accept only residents who can walk, aren't demented, and don't pose behavioral problems. For the greatest support needs, a nursing home may be essential. While Medicare covers medically related services in a skilled nursing home after hospitalization, long term care in a nursing home, as well as round-the-clock home care, are unaffordable for most older persons. The older consumer and family may have to resort to Medicaid. Qualifying for Medicaid requires tests of income, wealth, and disability status, and plenty of documentation.

Long term care is frequently called *custodial care,* which means that the patient needs only basic maintenance of a kind that an unskilled outsider or family member can provide on a daily basis, such as help with eating, hygiene, dressing, and moving about. A confused or depressed person may need simple supervision. Even an opportunity to socialize with someone else may be therapeutic for a person who otherwise is alone at home most of the time. Absent such mundane help, the frail or disabled person, sooner or later, would probably need acute care by a doctor or in a hospital. In this context, long term care is a set of essential preventive services.

The goal of long term care is to provide just enough support for you to be as independent as possible. "Oversupport" works against self-reliance.

However, self-reliance involves a degree of risk: In trying to help yourself, you may fall. How much to expect yourself to do, reasonably, can be determined with professional help by a geriatric assessment or evaluation and incorporated into a plan of care. Many people live for decades, enjoying activities despite disabilities.

Even when you draw on professional expertise, keep in mind that long term care should center on *your* concerns and resources. Explore options in your community in terms of types of care, service providers, and the available facilities. It's important that you and your advocates clearly understand your preferences. At the same time, educate yourself about the purposes and methods of the various professionals and facilities you employ. This knowledge is a key to managing an important part of your life with disability or frailty.

For more information on long term care, assisted living, and nursing homes, turn to chapter 15.

The End of Life

As you enter the last phase of your life, you and your family will encounter a new set of critical issues concerning health.

First of all, both you and your caregivers must take another look at dying as a part of life. Even more than death, many people in their last months fear isolation and pain. Communication with family and friends and pain control are essential, whether you are at home or in an institution. You may want to consider hospices, which are organizations devoted to helping people die at home or in a homelike facility, free of pain and without futile, extreme medical interventions.

Second, you retain all the rights of an adult. Exercise these rights. For example, *you* decide what medical option is best for you, and you can refuse any treatment for any reason.

Third, when you are healthy, prepare for the possibility of a time when you can't understand the information needed to make an informed decision about health care. You can authorize your guardian or next-of-kin to act for you. The next-of-kin or guardian should have your written authority to act in your best interest. If you can, decide now on a health advocate or provide a durable power of attorney to someone you trust and with whom you have discussed your wishes.

For more information on end-of-life decisions, turn to chapter 20.

11

The Elements of Geriatric Care

Geriatrics encompasses the special knowledge and skills applied through medicine, nursing, social work, and other areas to help elders stay independent, despite impairments. Geriatric care isn't confined to long term care. It covers care for acute and chronic illnesses in a hospital, your own home, your community, or a nursing home.

Geriatrics is concerned principally with:

- Your ability to function as independently as possible
- You as a whole person, including your emotions, values, interests, and physical, mental, and social functioning
- Your capacity for physical and mental rehabilitation and for emotional growth
- Helping you compensate for limitations
- Involving you and your family in planning care
- Adjusting your physical and social environment to make it easier for you to function, *and*
- Using the appropriate team of professionals and paraprofessionals to address the needs of you and your family

With far too few health care practitioners schooled in geriatrics, your knowledge of what constitutes a comprehensive approach can help you—and the caregivers available to you—assemble a better plan for care.

The basic components of organized geriatric care are

- *Diagnosing* (or assessing) your social, nursing, and medical problems
- *Developing* a care plan
- *Implementing* the plan, *and*
- *Adjusting* it periodically as problems and conditions change

Individual Treatment

The comprehensive approach of geriatrics requires practitioners to have a thorough understanding of you and your background. Your doctor, nurse, and social worker should be thorough, taking little for granted, and they can't rely on stereotypes. As people grow older, treatments must become more individualized. Elders are a highly diverse group, and statements about averages, typical situations, and general trends don't necessarily describe your current or future situation or that of siblings, spouses, and parents, if you are aiding them.

The Geriatric Assessment

You, your family, and professionals collaborate in developing a plan of care. Together, you'll develop a sense of your potential, resources, and limitations as they relate to possible courses of treatment.

The process rests on a geriatric assessment that may take over two or three hours, including fact gathering with relatives of the patient. Ideally, this assessment looks at your:

- Ability to function in maintaining yourself and doing preferred activities
- Medical problems, whether or not they impair your basic functioning at the moment
- Environment (where you live), *and*
- Socioeconomic status

A geriatric assessment differs from a younger person's assessment. First of all, it takes longer. Simply recording your medical history takes longer. Some older people move slowly, hear poorly, take longer to recall and express themselves precisely; some are lonely and stretch the encounter. Some may not be clear about facts and problems or afraid to present them in a straightforward manner. Despite these hurdles, the interviewer must still take all your symptoms seriously because they may be clues to a problem. Your social, sexual, and medication histories as well as a physical examination are all important in establishing a diagnosis. All this requires patience on the part of providers and family members.

To answer your needs, geriatricians are versed in understanding the unusual ways illnesses manifest themselves in elders, especially when other factors mask the main symptoms or when symptoms occur in confusing combinations. For example, diseases may have different signs and symptoms in older and younger adults. Elders are especially likely to have medical, physical, and functional problems at the same time. Because fatigue, low sodium concentrations in the blood, and depression may not indicate precisely what is wrong, the doctor may have to order many tests and ask more questions.

A frequent cause of an older person's declining ability to function is malnutrition, in part because of isolation, depression, and less enjoyment of food due to decreased smell and taste perception. Malnutrition can contribute to pressure sores, infections, muscle wasting, ambulatory weakness, and slow recovery from an illness.

TIP

Autonomy Is Healthy

The more self-reliant you are, the more likely you will be to survive a disease and regain your health. A wise practitioner knows when to push you to do more. A wise patient knows when to take it easy.

11

Drug Use and Abuse

Geriatric specialists discourage self-medication and a hasty resort to prescribed drugs: 90 percent of elders take at least one medication; most take two or more. Adverse side effects of drugs account for a substantial proportion of elders' problems with memory, attention, and mood, as well as constipation, incontinence, depression, male impotence, appetite changes, dizziness, and many other conditions. Doctors who aren't trained to work with elders may not realize that many side effects are common in older people though they're rare in younger people taking the same drugs.

Make sure that your caregivers consider all your prescribed or over-the-counter drugs. Their use may be hazardous to you and can complicate treatment of an illness or disability. Elders are two to seven times more likely than younger adults to react badly to drugs. Moreover, the consequences of taking the wrong drugs and taking the right drugs in the wrong amounts are much more severe in elders. The misuse of drugs includes forgetting or omitting a dose, changing

Your Plan

Together with professionals, make sure you participate in making a plan of care that:

- *Integrates* acute care and long term care
- *Provides* services for mental health, rehabilitation, and prevention
- *Integrates* medical and other services—for example, assisted housing, adult day care, and social services
- *Coordinates* paid and unpaid—and formal and informal—caregivers, *and*
- *Checks* on the quality of the service system you use and of direct services

Geriatric Discharge Planning

If you are completing a stay in a hospital or nursing home, you should receive help in preparing for the move home. This "discharge planning" aims to

- Prevent your condition from worsening and requiring a readmission to the hospital or nursing home
- Lessen your need for visits to the emergency room, *and*
- Speed your recovery

Like geriatric-care assessments in general, part of discharge planning is a *nursing and social-work assessment* to determine the supports needed and available to you and your family in the community and at home. The discharge plan may cover steps you have to take to pay rent and other bills and the availability of insurance and income to cover health care. The assessment may determine what follow-up examinations you'll need to check on your response to therapy.

A *physical therapy evaluation* is also part of discharge planning in some cases. The physical therapist identifies physical problems that make living at home difficult for you. Exercise may be prescribed so you can regain the strength, flexibility, and sensation for general movement, particularly walking, climbing, and rising from a chair or bed. Physical therapy that begins in the hospital or nursing home may continue at home.

A *nutritional evaluation* may be included in discharge planning. Nutritionists explore problems that might interfere with eating, swallowing, and chewing. One result might be a referral to a dentist—for a denture fit, for example.

Money Matters

$ Despite federal health insurance, the average older American pays almost $3,000 a year for health care; the average person over eighty-five pays over $5,000. Moreover, elders spend six times as much of their income on health as do younger people.

For more information on health care insurance, turn to chapter 4.

Medicare

Medicare and supplemental private insurance pay a significant portion of the bills for acute medical care for almost all older Americans. Medicare is a federal health-insurance program available to most older Americans and also to many adults with disabilities. The more you understand about how Medicare works, the better you'll do at getting its full benefit for you or a family member.

Medicare has two parts: Part A covers inpatient care in a hospital or a skilled nursing facility, home-health care, and hospice services. Part B covers physicians' services, outpatient hospital care, durable medical equipment, laboratory tests, X-ray therapy, mental health care, and ambulance services.

Medicare is available to you—regardless of income—if you meet one or more of the following criteria:

- You are sixty-five or older and eligible for Social Security or Railroad Retirement benefits
- You receive Social Security Disability Insurance payments for at least twenty-four months, *or*
- You have end-stage renal disease

If you are eligible for Social Security retirement benefits but don't take them at age sixty-five—for instance, if you're working after age sixty-five—you can still receive Medicare benefits. At sixty-five, spouses or former spouses of people who are eligible for Social Security retirement benefits as dependents are eligible for Medicare as well. United States citizens and permanent legal aliens who have resided in the United States for five years and who are sixty-five or older and aren't eligible for Social Security or Railroad Retirement benefits can buy into Medicare.

Signing Up for Medicare

Medicare coverage begins when you turn sixty-five. If you're still employed, you may choose job-based insurance as your first-line cover-

the dosage without consulting the doctor, taking a medicine for an unintended purpose, using outdated prescriptions, or using prescribed drugs in improper combinations with over-the-counter medicines.

For all these reasons, *pharmacists* often play a central role in developing and implementing a geriatric plan. In collaboration with your doctor, the pharmacist takes account of physiological and psychological changes that influence drug metabolism, ability to swallow pills of given sizes, sensitivities to drugs, drug interactions, and the possibility of combining pills to make taking medications easier at home.

The bottom line? Make sure all your doctors know all your drug intake, and don't rush to conclude you need a prescription.

For more information on medications, turn to chapter 7.

11

Health and Income

Good health, higher education, and higher income are interconnected. As people age, income tends to decline. They use up assets and can't replace them. Income from Social Security reflects the lower living costs of yesteryear. The median income for people over eighty-five is substantially below that for people in their sixties and early seventies. Perhaps one-third of older Americans are in or near poverty levels.

The very old may need more care when they are least able to afford it. Long term care, prescription drugs, and other out-of-pocket health care expenditures eat up savings. Some older people can't afford the high cost of prescription drugs or long term care services.

The federal government offers two programs for low-income people over age sixty-five and for the disabled:

■ The Qualified Medicare Beneficiary Program (QMB) applies to people with incomes at or below the federal poverty level and with limited savings or other resources. Your state picks up the cost of the Medicare Part B premiums and coinsurance, as

age for hospital care. You can defer Part B coverage *and having to pay the Part B premium.* If you're retired, you can add Part B coverage by allowing an automatic deduction from your monthly Social Security check.

It is important to contact the Social Security office to make sure coverage is in place—call (800) 772-1213. You can file an application with your local Social Security office within three months before or after your sixty-fifth birthday.

You may also enroll in Part B between January 1 and March 31 of any year after you turn sixty-five, although you may have to pay a penalty for the postenrollment.

Consumer Alert: Spouses

Medicare doesn't cover dependent spouses under age sixty-five. Many younger spouses lose their private health insurance as dependents when the working spouse turns sixty-five and switches to Medicare. This is especially important to consider as more companies cut back or eliminate coverage for retirees and their families. Check with your employer benefits counselor on COBRA provisions before you switch to Medicare. Still, a dependent covered through your former employer usually has the right to buy the group insurance for three years.

What Medicare Covers

Medicare covers most reasonable and necessary medical and hospital services but not most preventive care, dental services, long term care, or experimental procedures. It also doesn't pay for prescription drugs, unless you are hospitalized.

Covered under Medicare Part A

Inpatient hospital care: Medicare Part A covers medically necessary hospital costs for up to sixty days in a benefit period. The hospital must be a Medicare-participating institution, accredited, and meet federal desegregation requirements. (Medicare also usually pays for bona fide emergency care in a nonparticipating hospital if it's the closest hospital to you.) You pay a deductible ($736 in 1996). If you need up to thirty more days in the hospital, you pay coinsurance ($184) for each day. If you need even more time in the hospital, you can draw on a reserve of sixty "lifetime" days and pay a higher coinsurance ($368) per day. Most Medicare stays are under two weeks.

Skilled nursing facility care: Medicare Part A covers up to one hundred days of care in a Medicare-certified skilled nursing facility per benefit period. There are key conditions: (1) The patient must require skilled nursing seven days a week or rehabilitation services five days a week, and (2) the care in the skilled nursing facility begins within thirty days of discharge from a hospital, and the care is for the same condition treated in the hospital during a stay of at least three days. This care is usually for convalescence after hospitalization.

Nursing Homes and Prepayments

A skilled nursing facility can't require you to prepay anything for services as a condition for admission unless it's clear at the start that Medicare or Medicaid won't cover the services.

The facility can ask you to pay for services in advance if it informs you in writing that Medicare may deny coverage as "not medically necessary" *and* you agree to pay privately. But you can demand that the facility bill Medicare anyway if there's a chance Medicare will cover the care. Such a demand will prevent the home from charging you until Medicare formally decides to deny coverage.

Home-health care: Medicare Part A covers the full cost of home-health care if your physician prescribes it for you and it's provided by a Medicare-certified agency. Your physician tells Medicare that you need skilled nursing at home intermittently. Your physician may also certify that you need speech, physical, or occupational therapy at home. In addition, the plan may justify the use of a home-health aide as long as your need for skilled services continues. The plan also may call for medical social services, medical equipment and supplies, and certain outpatient services arranged through the Medicare-certified home-health agency.

For information and referrals on Medicare-covered home-health care, consult your local Area Agency on Aging.

Hospice care. Part A covers hospice services for individuals who are diagnosed as terminally ill.

For more information on hospice care, turn to chapter 20.

Other Part A benefits. These include care in psychiatric hospitals for up to 190 days in a lifetime and payment for inpatient blood transfusions after the first three pints per year. Note that you can't be charged if people replace the blood in your name or if the blood expense is part of the

well as the Part A hospital deductible and coinsurance.

■ The Specified Low-Income Medicare Beneficiary Program (SLMB) assists people with incomes 20 percent above the federal poverty level. The state pays the Part B premium. You are responsible for the Medicare deductible, copayments, and related charges.

For more information, call (800) 638-6833 for the number of your state's health-insurance counseling program, or contact your county department of social services. You can also call that 800 number to receive a free copy of Your Medicare Handbook.

11

TIP

When Medicare Does Not Pay . . .

Even if you or a doctor assume that Medicare won't cover a service, file a claim. You can ask for a review if the claim is denied. Medicare patients who appeal denials receive additional payments more than half the time. To seek a review, send a copy of the denial back to Medicare with a signed note asking for a review.

Part B deductible. When collected by the American Red Cross, there is no charge for the blood itself. There are special arrangements for inpatient hospital and skilled nursing facility services received in a Christian Science sanitarium.

Covered under Medicare Part B. Most reasonable and necessary physician services, durable medical equipment, physical therapy, hospital outpatient services, laboratory tests and X rays, mental health services, and ambulance services are covered under Medicare Part B.

Physician services: Medicare Part B covers 80 percent of the approved charges for reasonable and necessary physician services. This doesn't include routine checkups or most kinds of preventive care. It *does* cover annual flu shots, pneumococcal vaccines, mammograms every other year, and Pap smears every third year.

Durable medical equipment: Medicare Part B covers 80 percent of reasonable and necessary medical equipment purchased from Medicare-certified suppliers. It doesn't cover nonmedical items even if they are necessary for medical purposes—air conditioners or humidifiers, for example. For certain supplies, Medicare-certified suppliers who don't agree to abide by Medicare payment schedules may not charge you more than 115 percent of Medicare's approved amount.

Physical therapy: Medicare Part B pays 80 percent of Medicare-approved services provided by Medicare-certified physical therapists in their offices, up to a total of $900 a year. (If the care is received at home, there is no limit.)

Hospital outpatient services: Medicare Part B pays 80 percent of the approved charge for medically necessary emergency-room services and outpatient-clinic services, including rehabilitation and physical therapy.

Laboratory tests and X rays: Medicare Part B covers reasonable and necessary laboratory tests, as well as X rays required for medical diagnosis.

Mental health services: Medicare Part B pays 50 percent of the approved charge for outpatient mental health services.

Ambulance services: Medicare Part B pays 80 percent of the approved charge for medically necessary transportation to or from a hospital or skilled nursing facility.

Blood: Medicare Part B pays for blood except any charges for the first three pints if not replaced by someone else. Medicare covers the costs of processing blood.

For a summary of Medicare-covered services, turn to the chart on page 227.

Medicare "Assignment"

Medicare providers and other providers who accept "assignment" can't charge patients more than Medicare's approved charge for services. *Ask providers if they take assignment.*

By "participating" in assignment, the provider submits streamlined bills (even electronically) to Medicare and gets paid faster. For these advantages, the participating provider agrees to accept the Medicare-approved fee as the whole fee. Medicare pays 80 percent and the patient pays the remaining 20 percent coinsurance. If the Medicare patient is also on Medicaid, the provider must take assignment and the state Medicaid program pays the coinsurance.

By law, a *nonparticipating* provider can't collect more than 115 percent of Medicare's approved fee for the services billed. Medicare pays 80 percent of the approved fee and sends the check to you, the beneficiary. You pay the difference between that check and the provider's lawful charge to you. The nonparticipating provider, by the way, now has to fill out your Medicare form and send it in for you, wiping out a difference between the two provider classes.

Keep in mind: Physicians don't have to accept you as a Medicare patient. But if they do, they may not collect more than Medicare permits.

What Medicare Costs

You and your employer have prepaid for Medicare Part A by contributions over your working years. All you have to pay now for covered services is a deductible, which was $760 in 1997. Anyone not automatically eligible for Medicare, including permanent legal residents and United States citizens who worked fewer than forty quarters, may be able to obtain Medicare Part A coverage by paying a monthly premium. In 1997 this monthly premium is $311 for those who worked fewer than thirty quarters, and $187 for those who worked between thirty and thirty-nine quarters.

Medicare Part B is available for a monthly premium. The Part B premium is $43.80 in 1997; people who don't enroll when initially eligible must pay 10 percent more for the premium for each year they delay their enrollment.

Consumer Alert: What Medicare Doesn't Cover

Medicare will pay for many of your health care expenses—but not all of them. In particular, Medicare doesn't cover long term care in

1997 Medicare Benefits

Part A

	Beneficiary Pays	Medicare Pays
Inpatient Hospital Care Per Benefit Period*		
Day 1 to 60	$760 deductible	Balance
Days 61 to 90	$190 per day	Balance
Days 91 to 150†	$380 per day	Balance
All additional days	Everything	Nothing
Skilled Nursing Facility Care Per Benefit Period*		
Days 1 to 20	Nothing	Everything
Days 21 to 100	$95 per day	Balance
All additional days	Everything	Nothing
Skilled Home-Health Care		
As long as needed	Nothing	Everything
Hospice Care		
As long as needed	Small copayments	Balance

Part B

Beneficiary Pays
$43.80 per month
$100 annual deductible
20 percent of Medicare's approved charge for most services
Excess charges to the extent permitted by law

*A benefit period begins upon admission to a hospital and ends when a patient is out of the hospital or skilled nursing facility for sixty consecutive days.

†These sixty "lifetime reserve days" are not renewable. They apply after a beneficiary exhausts Medicare coverage through day ninety. They don't need to be used all at once.

the home or nursing home or prescription drugs outside a hospital. Even though disability, frailty, and memory loss may heighten your need for services, such chronic conditions don't normally require a hospital stay or the daily attention of a doctor or skilled nurse. If a medical problem isn't acute, Medicare probably won't pay for it.

Medicare also won't pay your bills for private-duty nursing, cosmetic surgery, a hospital telephone and television, care outside the United States (except in certain border areas of Canada), a private hospital room, acupuncture, hearing aids, routine eye exams and glasses, experimental procedures, most preventive care and routine physical exams, dental care, routine foot care, or most chiropractic services.

Medicare *will* pay for flu shots and pneumococcal vaccine without charge to you. Get the flu immunization each year before the flu season starts.

Medic*aid* and Seniors

Medicaid can help pay for doctors, hospital care, drugs, and long term care at home or in a nursing home. To qualify, your income and assets must be below certain limits.

Medicaid may cover part or all of the Medicare deductibles and copayments, home-health services, and some other services not covered by Medicare such as private nursing care.

For more information on Medicaid, turn to chapter 4. For more information on SSI, contact your local Social Security office.

Consumer Alert: How Medicare Patients Are Bilked

To extract more money from Medicare patients, some physicians engage in questionable, if not illegal, practices that make patients pay more than they should. Three to watch out for are overcharges, retainers, and waivers.

■ *Overcharges:* In 1993 doctors overcharged nearly 1.5 million Medicare beneficiaries a total of some $101 million. It's illegal under federal law for a doctor who accepts Medicare assignment to collect more than the Medicare-approved charge for a service.

11

■ *Retainers:* Some doctors require new Medicare patients to sign a retainer agreement obligating them to pay hundreds of dollars for a package of services, implying that Medicare doesn't cover these. These retainers may be illegal. They also duplicate provisions in Medigap policies.

■ *Waivers:* Doctors must submit their bills to Medicare; you don't fill out or send in any forms. However, many doctors ask patients to waive the "right" to have the doctor bill Medicare directly for his or her services. The only legal waiver is one that lists a specific uncovered procedure, such as cosmetic surgery. Doctors may also ask patients to pay separately for telephone advice, medical conferences, and prescription refills—all services Medicare considers part of the fees it pays physicians.

—Excerpted from *Consumer Reports,* August 1994

Beyond Medicare: Medigap and More

A variety of private insurance policies can help you pay for health care expenses that Medicare covers only partly or not at all. There are several basic types of policies:

■ Medicare supplement policies—*Medigap insurance*—pay some of the amounts that Medicare doesn't pay for covered services.

■ *Managed care plans,* including HMOs, provide health care services directly for a fixed monthly premium. These are also called coordinated care plans.

■ Some employers allow retirees to continue *employer-provided policies,* although sometimes the retired person has to pay more—or all—of the monthly premium.

■ *Long term care insurance policies* pay up to maximum amounts for each day of covered care in a nursing home or each day of home care.

■ *Hospital indemnity policies* pay fixed amounts for each day of inpatient hospital services.

■ Some policies provide *coverage for specified diseases.*

The most important option is Medigap insurance. For the premium you pay, some Medigap policies cover Medicare's deductibles; most cover the coinsurance amount. Some also pay for health services not covered by Medicare at all. The coverage for physician services anywhere in the United States is particularly valuable if you travel often or live in another area for part of the year.

Consider buying Medigap insurance if (1) you need and can afford it, *and* (2) you aren't covered by a former employer's health-insurance plan. People with serious health problems who are sixty-five should definitely apply for Medigap during the open enrollment period that ends six months after you first enroll in Medicare Part B. During this period, insurance companies can't deny coverage to you based on your medical history.

In most states, you can choose among ten standard Medigap plans, labeled *A* through *J*. This makes it easier for consumers to compare coverage and premiums. *Don't* purchase more than one Medigap policy. It's illegal for insurance agents to sell consumers duplicate policies. They can't use scare tactics to frighten consumers into dropping existing policies or purchasing policies they don't need or can't afford. And if you join a Medicare HMO, you usually don't need Medigap.

The Ten Medigap Plans

All ten plans include the basic group of benefits: Coverage for the Medicare Part A coinsurance for days 61 to 90 in a hospital, the Medicare coinsurance for lifetime-reserve days 91 to 150, 100 percent of the cost of 365 additional lifetime hospital days after all Medicare hospital benefits are exhausted, the reasonable costs of the first three pints of blood, and the Part B coinsurance. These benefits together constitute Plan A.

Additional Benefits	Plan A	Plan B	Plan C	Plan D	Plan E	Plan F	Plan G	Plan H	Plan I	Plan J
Skilled nursing home coinsurance (days 21 to 100)			Yes	Yes	Yes	Yes	Yes	Yes	Yes	Yes
Part A hospital deductible		Yes	Yes	Yes	Yes	Yes	Yes	Yes	Yes	Yes
Part B physician deductible			Yes			Yes				Yes
Part B excess physician charges						100%	80%		100%	100%
Foreign travel emergency			Yes	Yes	Yes	Yes	Yes	Yes	Yes	Yes
At-home recovery				Yes			Yes		Yes	Yes
Prescription drugs								*	*	†
Preventive screening					Yes					Yes

*Basic drug benefit with a $250 annual deductible, 50 percent coinsurance, and a $1,250 maximum annual benefit
†Extended drug benefit containing a $250 annual deductible, 50 percent coinsurance, and a $3,000 maximum annual benefit

11

Which Medigap Is for You?

$ According to *Consumer Reports*, for most people, the important Medigap options to consider are coverage for Medicare's hospital deductible, the coinsurance required for a stay in a skilled nursing facility, and coverage for at-home recovery services, a potentially useful although limited benefit.

Plans B, C, and D cover most basics with few frills. Unless you live in a state where you face a high risk of running into claims from providers who don't accept Medicare assignment, you'll save money if you skip Plan F and its higher-priced cousins, Plans G, I, and J. The plans with drug coverage (H, I, and J) don't appear to be worth the added cost.

Plan B, if you can find it, is a better choice than Plan C. It covers most of the important gaps and is about 16 percent cheaper on average than Plan C.

Plan D, a better value than Plan C, is just as hard to find as Plan B. Plan D omits coverage for the $100 deductible for Medicare physician and outpatient services; covering the deductible sometimes adds more than $100 to the pre-

Shop carefully before deciding on the best policy to fit your needs. Except in states with waivers, all new Medigap policies conform to one of the standard benefit plans—*although not at the same price*. In fact, the costs vary significantly. Compare benefits and premiums. Satisfy yourself that the insurer is reputable before buying. And in selecting Medigap benefits to meet your needs, remember that Medicare pays only for services it determines to be medically necessary and only the amount it determines to be reasonable. If Medicare won't pay for a particular service, Medigap usually won't pay either.

Note that special Medicare reimbursement rules apply if you have health insurance through your job or your spouse's job. If you accept the employer plan *and* join Medicare Part B, Medicare supplements your private insurance. If the employer plan pays less than Medicare would have paid as primary payer, Medicare pays the difference. If you reject the employer plan, Medicare is the primary payer.

Medigap Frauds

Some insurance companies and agents have thwarted the best intentions of Congress when it mandated uniform Medigap policies. They may:

- Steer you to only one or two plans and strongly disparage the others, instead of offering you a choice of the full range of available policies
- Fail to give you price information as required by law
- Urge you to buy benefits you don't need, using misleading sales pitches, *and*
- Play pricing games that will mean nasty surprises for you later on. Different insurance companies charge premiums that vary by hundreds of dollars for the same set of benefits in the same city.

If you suspect fraud or abuse of the Medicare or Medigap programs, call your state Medicare carrier, your state department of insurance, or either of two federal government hotlines: (800) 638-6833 or (800) 368-5779.

—Excerpted from *Consumer Reports*, August 1994

Medicare and HMOs

Most Medicare beneficiaries receive care on a fee-for-service basis: You are billed for each visit or procedure, and you go to the doctor of your choice. In some locations, prepaid health care is available to Medicare beneficiaries through approved HMOs and other managed care organizations. The HMO receives a guaranteed monthly payment from Medicare for each beneficiary it has enrolled. From this pool of funds, the HMO provides all the usual Medicare benefits and any additional services at its option and possibly at no charge to the beneficiary. An HMO may even relieve enrollees of having to pay a Part B premium. Among the additional benefits may be outpatient prescribed drugs, dental care, routine physicals, routine vision and hearing checkups, eyeglasses, and hearing aids.

HMOs may offer significant additions to Medicare benefits on the expectation that managed care will produce savings over traditional Medicare by controlling costs, including physician charges, hospital admissions, lab and specialist services, and office procedures. From Medicare payments, for-profit HMOs also expect to reward stockholders, administrators, and staff.

Many beneficiaries find HMO coordinated coverage more comprehensive than, and preferable to, standard Medicare with solo practitioners and fee-for-service payment. However, unless your physicians belong to the HMO you are considering, you will have to pick another set of doctors. Most HMOs restrict enrollees to their affiliated physicians and hospitals. An HMO may allow a member to go outside the plan—a "point of service" option—but the member will have to pay for the option. It may carry a $400 annual deductible and a 20 percent coinsurance, for example.

Medicare uses three types of managed care organizations:

1. *Risk-contract HMOs* are most common. Medicare pays the HMO a monthly sum to provide all your Medicare-covered health care. Depending on the plan, you may have to pay a monthly premium, deductibles, and copayments or coinsurance for certain services. The term *risk contract* means that the plan assumes the financial risk for providing your health care. If the plan spends more than it receives from Medicare under the contract, the HMO absorbs the difference.

If you join a risk-contract HMO, *learn and follow the plan's rules.* If you don't use plan-affiliated providers, you—not Medicare—pay the bills, except in the case of an emergency or urgent care away from the plan's service area.

Risk-contract HMOs must take all applicants who are Medicare beneficiaries, except people with end-stage kidney disease and those already in a Medicare hospice program. These HMOs are especially valuable to people with "preexisting" serious medical problems.

mium. Instead, Plan D covers some at-home recovery services that could be useful.

Plans C and F, the darlings of the insurance industry, are nearly identical. Attractive for *insurers*, Plan F covers the amounts physicians can bill above Medicare's approved charges. Because these "excess" charges are increasingly a thing of the past, insurers seldom have to pay off.

Consumer Reports has ranked over seventy Medigap policies by price. It lists the best policies in many states. To receive a copy, send a check or money order for $5 to Consumer Reports Back Issues, P.O. Box 53016, Boulder CO 80322. Ask for Reprint RO138.

11

2. *Cost-contract HMOs* receive a fee from Medicare to provide all Medicare-covered services. As a member, you may have to pay the usual Medicare copayments, deductibles, and extra physicians' charges. You may use medical services outside the plan's network and receive Medicare reimbursement, subject to the usual Medicare copayments. You may also pay the HMO a monthly premium to cover Medicare deductibles and copayments. Because cost-contract HMOs must take all Medicare enrollees who apply, they are another good option for people with a serious medical condition.

3. With *health care prepayment plans,* Medicare pays the plan to provide physician visits, X rays, lab tests, and other diagnostic tests. Other medical services may be included. You can go outside the plan and still have Medicare benefits.

Medicare risk-contract HMOs, promoted by the federal government, are growing rapidly in many places. In California enrollment accounts for about 15 percent of the Medicare population—over half a million enrollees. One-fourth of all southern California Medicare beneficiaries are in risk-contract HMOs.

The Center for Health Care Rights, a nonprofit organization that provides free education, counseling, and legal assistance to Medicare beneficiaries in Los Angeles County, conducted a study of risk-contract HMOs and found them to be "a cost-effective, high-quality provider of medical services to Medicare beneficiaries." However, the center points out, Medicare HMOs have advantages and disadvantages for elder health care consumers.

On the plus side:

■ HMOs can save members money. For example, enrollees don't pay the Part B deductible or 20 percent coinsurance. Thus, HMO enrollees don't need a Medigap insurance policy that would cost $700 to $2,000 a year in premiums.

■ HMOs often provide additional benefits such as outpatient prescription drugs, optometry, and preventive care at little or no added cost.

■ Your HMO primary care physician should coordinate the work of specialists and other professionals who serve you.

■ HMOs have no financial incentive to provide unnecessary—and potentially harmful—medical care.

■ Enrollees don't have to complete any paperwork for Medicare-covered services unless they use out-of-plan providers for emergencies.

On the down side:

■ Enrollees in risk-contract and cost-contract HMOs are not covered unless they use plan-affiliated health care facilities and physicians except in emergencies.

■ Enrollees must obtain approval in advance to see a specialist, to have elective surgery, or to obtain durable medical equipment or other medical services.

■ HMOs have incentives to economize on services to stay within budgets and, if they are for-profit companies, maximize profits and bonuses.

■ You can usually receive care only within the HMO's service region. This is especially an issue for people who might winter outside this area.

A Medicaid recipient who is also eligible for Medicare can join an HMO that contracts with Medicare. If you are eligible for Medicare *and* currently receive Medicaid benefits, the state Medicaid program may pay the Medicare Part B premium and, where necessary, the Medicare Part A premium. Contact your local Medicaid office.

Medicare beneficiaries who join a Medicare HMO can quit at the end of any month and resume standard Medicare coverage. To quit, Medicare patients need only submit a written notice to the HMO or the local Social Security office.

HMOs in the Medicare program can't deny enrollment to Medicare beneficiaries, and Medicare HMOs have no waiting periods before they cover preexisting conditions. Moreover, during the open-enrollment period, they'll accept all Medicare beneficiaries who wish to enroll, except people who are already in a hospice or an end-stage renal disease program.

For more information on HMOs, turn to chapter 4.

Consumer Alert: When You Join an HMO

When you sign up for an HMO, in most cases you are signing up to receive all your Medicare services through that HMO. This means you no longer have traditional Medicare. You may still have your Medicare card, but Medicare will not cover your care unless you go through the HMO.

Consumer Alert: Quitting the Plan

It can take up to thirty days to quit a Medicare HMO. If you decide to quit, you don't have an automatic right to resume your Medigap

11

insurance. The insurer may take into consideration any illnesses that occurred since you left and either raise the premium or refuse to accept you.

The SHMO

A new type of Medicare HMO, the Social HMO, is being tested in Boston, Brooklyn, Minneapolis, Portland, Oregon, and Long Beach, California. The benefits of a SHMO include coverage for a modest amount of long term care and integration of acute, preventive, and long term care.

HMO Misinformation

Consumer Reports has detailed significant abuses by some HMOs that seek elder members whose bills are paid by Medicare. For example:

■ Some sales representatives mislead customers about the HMOs and even Medicare itself. They often fail to explain that Medicare won't pay for service outside the plan. This failure could be financially devastating.

■ Some sales people employ high-pressure tactics.

Your HMO Rights

As a Medicare enrollee in an HMO, you have the right to:

■ All the services you would be entitled to if you only had traditional Medicare coverage, except hospice care
■ Receive appropriate health care for your condition
■ Receive timely health care
■ Receive quality care, *and*
■ Be discharged from a hospital only when you are medically ready to leave and only to a safe and supportive site

If you think your rights have been denied, ask your HMO to resolve the problem. If the HMO doesn't do so to your satisfaction, contact your state's peer review organization or health insurance counseling program.

For more information on receiving assistance with complaints, turn to page 233.

Consumer Alert: Follow the Rules

If you join a risk-contract HMO, *follow the plan's rules*. If you don't use plan-affiliated providers, you—not Medicare—pay the bills.

For example, in most Medicare managed care plans you must choose a primary care physician for your basic medical care and for all referrals to specialists. If you see a specialist without a referral or a specialist who isn't in the HMO's network—or even in the particular medical group of your primary care provider—you probably will have to pay the bill yourself. Before you join an HMO, if you already have a primary care physician and specialists you want to continue to use, make sure that the HMO will cover their services.

Insurance Assistance

A number of organizations and agencies can help elders and their families with a wide variety of questions about health insurance and other matters.

Medicare oversight. The federal government contracts with a peer review organization (PRO) in each state to ensure that Medicare beneficiaries receive care that is reasonable, medically necessary, provided in the most appropriate setting, and meets professionally accepted standards of quality. Directed by physicians, PROs review all written complaints from beneficiaries and their representatives concerning quality of care. They also respond to all requests to review a notice of hospital discharge and won't charge you for their services. If you're admitted to a Medicare-certified hospital or Medicare HMO hospital, you'll receive a notice explaining your rights under Medicare and how to contact the PRO if the need arises.

If you are a Medicare beneficiary, you have the right to:

- Receive all care necessary for the proper treatment of your illness and injury—your discharge should be determined solely by your medical needs and safety, not by the needs of the hospital
- Be fully informed about decisions affecting your Medicare coverage or payment for your stay, *and*
- Request an appeal of any written notice stating that Medicare will no longer pay for your stay

11

TIP

Getting Help

For information about reaching your state's counselors for Medicare, Medigap insurance, benefits for low-income people, and flu shots, call the Medicare hotline at (800) 638-6833.

You can also call this number to report suspected fraud or abuse on the part of Medicare insurers or providers.

At any time, if you have a concern regarding the quality of Medicare-financed care provided to you by a hospital, skilled nursing facility, home-health agency, HMO, or ambulatory surgery center, you or your designated representative can submit a complaint to the PRO. The PRO will help you put your complaint in writing if this would be difficult for you, and it will also provide information and written materials on a variety of health and wellness topics.

In all states, the PRO has a phone number, usually toll-free, for Medicare beneficiaries to call with questions or complaints. For the phone number in your state, call the Medicare hotline and ask for assistance: (800) 638-6833.

Discharge Rights

If a hospital informs you that Medicare will no longer cover your care *and* that you are ready for discharge, but you believe you still need care:

■ First, speak with your physician about your condition and medical care needs.

■ If that doesn't resolve your concern, ask the facility to issue a written notice of noncoverage.

■ Call the PRO. Ask it to review your case. If you choose to appeal a discharge, do so as soon as possible—by noon of the day after you receive the notice.

As long as you ask the PRO for an appeal by noon of the business day after receiving the discharge notice, you can't be discharged against your wishes or be held liable for any charges until noon of the day following the PRO's decision. It should issue its decision within a few days.

State health insurance counseling networks. Every state, plus Puerto Rico, the Virgin Islands, and the District of Columbia, has a health-insurance counseling program for elders. These statewide networks of trained volunteers and staff educate and assist people with health insurance and related issues, including Medicare, long term care insurance, managed care, and Medicare supplements. The advisers are trained and supervised by experts in the program, and their services are *free*. They have no affiliation with any insurance company or product and do not sell, endorse, or recommend any specific insurance.

Counselors are an impartial, confidential source to help you evaluate, choose, and use health insurance. They have up-to-date information on all senior health-insurance concerns. They can answer questions, assist with insurance planning, and offer you free copies of helpful publications.

Area Agencies on Aging. Specialists trained to help elders with insurance and many other matters are available in most communities. The key to finding them, as well as many other services for seniors, is your local *Area Agency on Aging* (AAA). These offices, usually appointed by regional governments to serve elders, provide or coordinate a wide variety of community-based services—from health-insurance information and referrals to meal programs, multiservice and drop-in senior centers, transportation, and other programs.

For more information on AAAs, turn to chapter 15.

Resources

For resources on long term care, turn to chapter 15. For resources on home-health care, turn to chapter 16. For resources on death with dignity, turn to chapter 20. For general issues, turn to chapter 22.

Organizations

American Association of Retired Persons
601 E Street, N.W.
Washington, DC 20049
(202) 434-2277
AARP is the largest organization for Americans age fifty and over. It offers a wide range of benefits, including *Modern Maturity* magazine and the monthly "Bulletin." Call or write for membership information and a catalogue of publications and audiovisual materials. For legal assistance, call AARP's Legal Council for the Elderly at (202) 434-2120. Publications include "When Your Medicare Bill Doesn't Seem Right: How to Appeal Medicare Part B" and "Managed Care: An AARP Guide."

Center for Health Care Rights
520 S. Lafayette Park Plaza
Los Angeles, CA 90057
(213) 383-4519
Send $1 per pamphlet and a self-addressed stamped envelope for fact sheets on Medicare assignment, how Medicare works, Medicare HMOs, Medigap insurance, long term care insurance, and Medicare nursing-home benefits. Send $3 for "Your Rights to Medicare Skilled Nursing Home Care: An Advocate's Guide."

Children of Aging Parents, Inc.
Woodbourne Office Campus
1609 Woodbourne Road
Levittown, PA 19057
(800) 227-7294
Call or write for information, referrals, and publications for caregivers.

Health Insurance Association of America
P.O. Box 41455
Washington, DC 20018
(202) 824-1600
Write for a free copy of their pamphlets: "A Consumer's Guide to Medicare Supplement Insurance," "A Consumer's Guide to Disability Insurance," and "A Consumer's Guide to Long Term Care Insurance."

11

Medicare Rights Center
1460 Broadway
New York, NY 10036-7393
(212) 869-3850
Contact the fund for a copy of its publication, "Medicare Basics: What You Need to Know."

National Academy of Elder Law Attorneys
1604 N. Country Club
Tucson, AZ 85711
(602) 881-4005
Call for referrals to attorneys who serve elders or to order a national directory.

National Association of Area Agencies on Aging
1112 16th Street, N.W.
Washington, DC 20036
(202) 296-8130
The association runs the Eldercare Locator for identifying information and referral services provided by state and local Agencies on Aging. Call (800) 677-1116 to get free referrals to elder services in your area and to order a copy of *The National Directory for Eldercare Information and Referral.*

National Association of Professional Geriatric Care Managers
1604 N. Country Club
Tucson, AZ 85711
(602) 881-8008
Call or write for referrals to geriatric care managers. You can also order a national directory for $35.

National Center on Elder Abuse
810 First Street, N.E., #500
Washington, DC 20002-4267
(202) 682-2470
Call or write for a list of publications and for information on research about elder abuse.

National Council of Senior Citizens
1331 F Street, N.W.
Washington, DC 20004
(202) 347-8800
Call or write for general information and assistance in finding a nursing home and solving Social Security and Medicare problems.

National Council on the Aging
409 Third Street, S.W.
Washington, DC 20024
(202) 479-1200
Call or write for publications and information on elder services, independent living, and other forms of long term care.

National Institute on Aging Information Center
P.O. Box 8057
Gaithersburg, MD 20898-8057
(800) 222-2225
(800) 222-4225
Call or write for free information and publications on health-related issues, including "Age Pages" on menopause, flu and pneumonia vaccines, exercise, incontinence, nutrition, and other topics.

National Senior Citizens Law Center
1815 H Street, N.W.
Washington, DC 20006
(202) 887-5280
Call or write for information about Medigap insurance and referrals to legal services in your area.

Older Women's League
666 11th Street, N.W.
Washington, DC 20001
(202) 783-6686
This membership organization advocates for the rights of midlife and older women. Call or write for low-cost information on caregiving.

United Seniors Health Cooperative
1331 H Street, N.W.
Washington, DC 20005
(202) 393-6222
USHC works to improve the quality and reduce the cost of health and social services for elders. Call or write for membership information and a list of publications and other services. *United Seniors Health Report* ($15 for five issues per year) keeps subscribers informed about health care, financial issues, and USHC activities.

U.S. Department of Health and Human Services
Health Care Financing Administration
6325 Security Boulevard
Baltimore, MD 21207
(410) 966-3000
Write to HCFA or contact any Social Security office for many publications related to Medicare, including "Medicare Q & A: 85 Commonly Asked Questions," "The Medicare Handbook," "Guide to Health Insurance for People with Medicare," "Medicare and Coordinated Care Plans," "Medicare Hospice Benefits," "Medicare Coverage for Second Surgical Opinions," "Medicare and Advance Directives," and "Medicare and Your Physician's Bill."

U.S. Department of Health and Human Services
Social Security Administration
Baltimore, MD 21235
(800) 772-1213, 7 A.M. to 7 P.M. weekdays
Call or write for free copies of many publications in English and Spanish on Social Security benefits, including "Medicare," "Understanding Social Security," "Retirement," "Disability," "Survivors," and other topics. For the most up-to-date figures on deductibles and coinsurance payments, ask for a copy of *Social Security Update*.

Publications

Beyond Medicare: Achieving Long Term Care Security, by Malvin Schechter (Jossey-Bass, 1993), $34.95.

The Caregiver's Guide: Helping Elderly Relatives Cope with Health and Safety Problems, by Caroline Rob (Houghton Mifflin, 1991), $14.45.

Caring and Coping When Your Loved One Is Seriously Ill, by Earl Grollman (Beacon Press, 1995), $10.

Choosing Medical Care in Old Age, by Muriel Gillick (Harvard University Press, 1994), $19.95.

The Columbia University School of Public Health 40+ Guide to Good Health, by Robert Weiss and Gesell Subak-Sharpe (Consumer Reports, 1992), $27.95.

Elders Assert Their Rights: A Guide for Residents, Family Members, and Advocates to the Legal Rights of Elderly People with Mental Disabilities in Nursing Homes. Order from Elders Project of the Bazelon Center, 1101 15th Street, N.W., Washington, DC 20005; tel. (202) 467-5730. $6.95.

50+: People's Pharmacy for Older Adults, by Joe Graedon and Teresa Graedon. Order from The People's Pharmacy, P.O. Box 52027, Durham, NC 27717-2027; tel. (800) 732-2334. $12.

How to Care for Your Parents: A Handbook for Adult Children, by Nora Jean Levin (Storm King Press, 1992), $6.95.

The Johns Hopkins Medical Handbook: The 100 Major Medical Disorders of People Over the Age of 50 (Rebus, 1992), $39.95.

11

Looking Forward: The Complete Medical Guide to Successful Aging, by Isadore Rossman (Dutton, 1989), $22.95.

Medicare Made Easy: Everything You Need to Know to Make Medicare Work for You, by Charles Inlander and Charles Mackay (People's Medical Society, 1989), $13.95 ($12.95 for members).

Medicare/Medigap, by Carl Oshiro and Larry Snyder (Consumer Reports, 1994), $13.95.

Parentcare Survival Guide: Helping Your Folks Through the Not-So-Golden Years, by Enid Pritikin and Trudy Reece (Barron's, 1993), $8.95.

The 36-Hour Day: A Family Guide to Caring for Persons with Alzheimer's, by Nancy Mace and Peter V. Rabins (Johns Hopkins University Press, 1981), $7.95.

When Parents Age: What Children Can Do, by Tom Adams and Kathryn Armstrong (Berkley Books, 1993), $7.95.

On the Job: Health and the Workplace

Nancy Lessin and Laurie Stillman

Laurie Stillman formerly directed the Massachusetts Coalition for Occupational Safety and Health (MassCOSH).

Nancy Lessin is MassCOSH's senior staff member for strategy and policy.

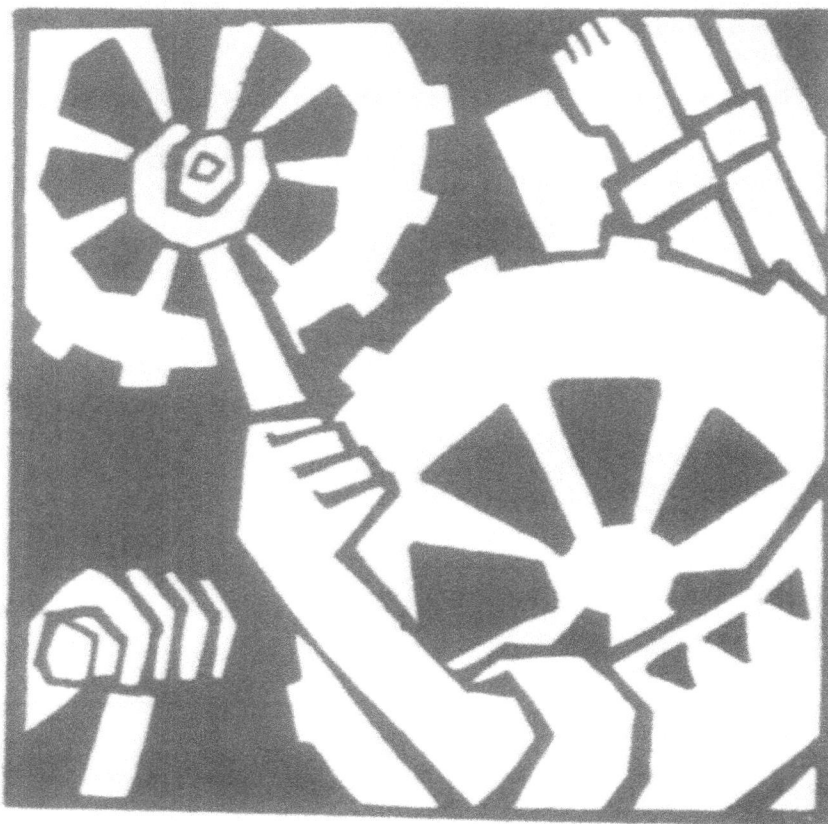

Common Causes of Occupational Illness

■ Workers might inhale dust and fumes that are present in the workplace.

■ Contaminants that get on your hands, food, or cigarettes may be dangerous if you swallow them.

■ Contact with solvents, acids, or dusts can injure eyes, cause skin burns or diseases, or enter the body to cause internal damage.

■ Fumes, dusts, and chemicals can lead to respiratory and lung diseases. About 15 percent of asthma cases may be work-related.

■ Poisoning from metals, gases, sprays, and solvents can lead to liver and kidney ailments, blood disorders, and cancer.

■ Extreme heat or cold can result in heatstroke or frostbite.

■ Radiation can cause cancer.

■ Repetitive work leads to wear and tear on muscles, tendons, ligaments, nerves, and the vascular system.

■ Stressful work is associated with diseases of almost every vital organ. Workers cite too little personal control on the job as the major source of stress.

Work can endanger your health. Nationwide, about 10,000 people are killed on their jobs every year; occupational diseases kill another 50,000 to 100,000 people.

Millions more suffer daily from injuries and illnesses sustained from their employment: Each year, Americans miss about 65 million days of work because of occupational illness and injury, according to the Health Insurance Institute of America. And certain workplace injuries and illnesses are occurring more and more frequently as a result of the rapid pace and repetitive nature of many of today's jobs and the widespread use of toxic chemicals.

You *don't* have to endure unhealthy conditions. Working to support yourself and your family doesn't have to mean compromising your health. Employers are responsible for providing a safe and healthy workplace.

This chapter will help you to learn about some of your options in addressing harmful workplace conditions, to find assistance when you confront risks to your health and safety, and to actively work with your health care providers to get the best treatment.

Occupational Hazards and Your Rights

The causes of many workplace *injuries* are usually obvious—and almost always preventable. For example, proper guards and maintenance for machinery, adequate rest periods, and good training programs go a long way toward preventing calamities.

It's usually much harder to recognize when *illnesses* result from work. In the first place, most occupational illnesses resemble those that result from other causes. A bakery worker with occupational asthma may wheeze and cough the same as another asthma victim. In addition, symptoms can show up long after a person is exposed to hazardous materials. Cancers and other diseases may appear many years later, perhaps well after you have left a job. Even the patient can easily fail to connect an illness to workplace origins.

Nevertheless, job-related illnesses are also preventable. As with injuries, the key is to recognize workplace hazards and control or eliminate them.

Training Shortage

Few health care providers receive enough training in occupational health to recognize possible connections between illness and work. Only half of

U.S. medical schools offer courses on occupational health, and the typical curriculum lasts about four hours. That makes it all the more important for you as a health care consumer to better understand how your work conditions affect your health.

Your Rights to Workplace Hazard Information

Knowledge helps you and your health care providers detect and treat occupational illness. In fact, you have a legal right to obtain a lot of the information—on chemicals and other hazardous conditions—that is crucial to diagnosing work-related disease.

Many rights come via the Occupational Safety and Health Act, which is enforced by OSHA—the Occupational Safety and Health Administration. This federal agency sets workplace health and safety standards and regulations, inspects workplaces, and cites and fines employers who violate the law. OSHA applies to most private employers, as well as to public employers in some states. These employers must provide a workplace "free of recognized hazards" that cause serious physical harm or death.

In the private sector, employers are also required to provide certain health and safety information to unions under the National Labor Relations Act (NLRA). Some states have laws comparable to the NLRA in order to cover public-sector workers. In addition, some states have "right-to-know" laws for state and local government employees not covered by OSHA. Right-to-know laws give workers legal rights to written data on the hazards of chemicals to which they are exposed, plus training and information on necessary precautions.

If OSHA covers your workplace, you have the legal right to:

- Read and keep a copy of your employer's *OSHA 200 Log*, a record of work-related injuries and illnesses in your workplace.
- Learn the results of any hazard tests, such as noise levels or the amounts of chemicals in the workplace air.
- Read and keep a copy of any medical records your employer maintains on you, *and*
- Read and keep a copy of safety and health fact sheets—so-called Material Safety Data Sheet (MSDS)—for the chemicals to which you may be exposed at work.

There is a Material Safety Data Sheet for almost every chemical used in the United States, describing related health effects, physical properties, flammability, emergency procedures, and protective measures to control hazardous or toxic exposure. However, the quality of these documents varies enormously. The "Pocket Guide to Chemical Hazards," pub-

12

- Infectious agents, such as bacteria and viruses, can cause tuberculosis, hepatitis, and many other serious illnesses.

- Many substances and conditions can harm your ability to produce healthy children or have a healthy sex life. Reproductive disorders and damage to reproductive organs are among the ten leading work-related injuries and illnesses. Reproductive hazards can affect fertility, decrease sex drive, promote birth defects or miscarriages, and contribute to childhood cancer. Both men and women need to be concerned about this danger.

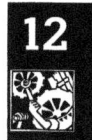

Artists and Hobbyists

Many workplace health and safety issues also apply to hobbyists and artists, especially regarding chemicals, noise, dust, and posture. Artists and craftspeople working in their own studios—perhaps in a garage or attic—should take extra care to learn about proper health and safety procedures regarding the materials they work with. Material Safety Data Sheets are there for private use as well as for industries.

For more information, contact the Center for Safety in the Arts, 5 Beekman Street, #820, New York, NY 10038; tel. (212) 227-6220.

lished by the National Institute for Occupational Safety and Health, and other references can help you check the accuracy of an MSDS.

To obtain a copy of the "Pocket Guide to Chemical Hazards," contact the National Institute for Occupational Safety and Health at (800)35-NIOSH.

OSHA also requires employers to ensure that their workers receive training about such hazards as noise, asbestos, and blood-borne disease-causing agents (specifically, those for HIV and Hepatitis B). Unfortunately, many employer-sponsored training programs are inadequate or nonexistent. OSHA's most frequently violated regulation is its "Hazard Communications Standard," which requires training on dangerous chemicals.

Shock Un-Therapy

Over half of reported occupational illnesses result from repeated physical stresses. Constant loud noises, repetitive lifting and movement, and vibrating machinery or hand tools can lead to deafness, numbness, and other problems.

Rights and Recourses

Some employers resist giving out hazard information, despite the law. If you pursue your right to information under the Occupational Safety and Health Act, it's illegal for your boss to discriminate against you or retaliate in any way. In addition, "whistle-blower" protections in some states offer a recourse for people who face repercussions for speaking out about workplace health or safety hazards. The National Labor Relations Act can also protect workers from unfair employer actions: This protection is strongest when two or more workers act together to obtain health and safety information or engage in other activities related to health and safety.

Be careful, however: All these protections are weak, and they aren't always effective. Unions offer the most protection for workers who request Material Safety Data Sheets, contact government agencies, speak out about health and safety concerns, or refuse unsafe work. If you are a union member, ask your steward to help you get health and safety information.

Getting Care

Ideally, your physician and other health care providers routinely ask you about your exposure to possible workplace hazards. The diagnosis and treatment of many diseases would improve tremendously if every medical history included such simple questions as:

- Where do you work?
- What do you do on your job?
- Have you ever worked with dusts, fumes, or conditions that might be dangerous?

If your health care provider fails to ask these questions, raise the issue yourself. It will also help if you bring your provider the Material Safety Data Sheets for the chemicals to which you are exposed. If you think that asking your employer for these documents may put your job at risk, your health care provider can request the information on your behalf, without divulging your name.

If you suspect your work has injured you or made you sick, it may be best to seek the opinion of a physician or nurse who has special training in occupational health. These physicians and nurses are specifically trained and skilled at diagnosing, treating, and preventing work-related diseases and injuries.

For a table of common occupational illnesses, turn to page 248–49.

To locate a specialist, ask your current health care providers for a referral or call the Association of Occupational and Environmental Clinics at (202) 347-4976. It can refer you to an occupational health clinic in your area.

One advantage of a reputable occupational-medicine specialist or clinic is that they are better equipped than other providers to advance *your* interests effectively. Besides drawing on their own medical training, specialists can refer you to advocates and help you obtain financial assistance through workers' compensation.

Vague Symptoms

Many workplace hazards are linked with vague symptoms—fatigue, depression, and mental confusion are a few examples. Although recognizing the connection with work is particularly difficult in such cases, it isn't impossible.

For example, Janice was getting headaches and her throat and eyes were irritated. She spoke with co-workers in her office, and it turned out that they suffered from similar symptoms. This was the key to identifying and correcting the problem. An investigation showed that the illness was caused by the building's ventilation system.

Reproductive Hazards

In 1977 chemical workers at a plant in California realized that many of the men and their partners couldn't conceive children. Medical tests revealed that many of the men had low sperm counts. Their union, the Oil, Chemical and Atomic Workers, helped the men link this fact with a chemical they manufactured known as DBCP.

In 1978, OSHA responded to the union's petition and issued a very strict exposure limit. Although many of the workers with long-term exposure to DBCP are permanently sterile, the new regulation benefits many current and future workers. It came about because workers talked with one another about their symptoms, and because they had a strong union to pursue the matter medically and with OSHA.

You, the Expert

In the pressroom of a large newspaper, several workers discovered they had blood in their urine. With the help of occupational-health specialists, the press workers linked this symptom with a class of chemicals common in such workplaces—glycol ethers. The workers' union played an important role in getting management to substitute less toxic chemicals for the glycol ethers.

You and your co-workers are the real experts on occupational safety and health. Armed with experience, suspicions, and the specifics of workplace exposures, you can call upon medical, technical, and legal assistance to confirm the links that you suspect. And in the absence of definitive research and strong legal standards, it's often workers who must make the connections and force the corrections.

Work with your union if you are a member, or with co-workers in any case. This can provide both protection and opportunities for safeguarding your health on the job. If necessary, you can pinpoint hazards and collect detailed data on work-related symptoms.

Consumer Alert: Company Docs

If you seek a specialist in occupational health, be cautious about "company doctors." They generally work for your employer, whose interests may differ from yours. Be certain any health care provider you choose is *your* advocate.

More Ways to Get Help

Despite the shortage of trained specialists in occupational health, you're far from alone in your quest for a healthy workplace and for care when your work makes you sick or injures you.

In many states and cities, you'll find a strong advocate in the local committee or coalition on occupational safety and health—a COSH group. These are local organizations of labor unions, other worker advocates, and occupational-health professionals. COSH groups provide training, education, referrals, and medical, technical, and legal assistance.

To find the nearest committee or coalition on occupational safety and health, contact the New York City committee (NYCOSH) at (212) 627-3900.

In addition, many national and international unions have health and safety departments that are excellent sources of information and referrals. Your steward or local union officers can refer you to your union's health and safety department.

At the workplace, many union health and safety committees gather information on specific factories or offices and plan ways to control hazards. Members of these committees may also take part in labor–management health and safety groups that engage in such activities as conducting workplace inspections, investigating accidents and incidents, and recommending hazard controls.

Several government agencies can assist the efforts of workers and unions to improve workplace health and safety and obtain medical care and benefits for people injured or made ill by their jobs. On the federal level:

■ *The Occupational Safety and Health Administration* can inspect workplaces and fine employers who violate health or safety standards.

■ *The National Institute for Occupational Safety and Health* can check your workplace for health hazards, explore links between particular exposures and ill health, and make recommendations on hazard control.

■ *The National Labor Relations Board* can intervene when employers fail to provide unions with certain health and safety information or when employers fire workers for acting collectively to improve health and safety conditions.

On the state level, your sources of help include the Department of Labor (sometimes called the Department of Labor and Industries), Department of Public Health, Workers' Compensation Bureau, Poison Control Center, Rehabilitation Agency, and state OSHA. You can also get help from local public-health graduate schools, work-environment departments at universities, and some other academic departments. To contact any of these, check the phone book, call your local COSH group, or ask your union steward.

And the *OSHA 200 Log* can help you identify unsafe areas that need further attention.

Controlling Hazards

The best response to a hazard is to *eliminate the danger* altogether by substituting safer substances for toxic chemicals or by changing the work. For example, most dry-cleaning processes now use perchloroethylene, a carcinogen. But an alternative wet-cleaning process uses biodegradable soaps and steam heat instead.

Engineering controls are the second most effective way to control a hazard. Engineering controls include attachments to dampen noise or local exhausts to remove toxic fumes. For example, a process to grind hardened steel tips for tools exposed workers to cobalt, chromium, and other toxic chemicals. The factory installed a special grinding-wheel guard that directed air and dust toward a movable local exhaust duct. This cut worker exposure to the dangerous chemicals to under 1 percent of the original level.

Ear plugs, respirators, special clothing, and other *personal protective equipment* are usually the least effective response to hazardous work. In addition to the fact that such equipment is often uncomfortable, it doesn't fully prevent hazardous exposures. However, in certain conditions, such as jobs removing asbestos, personal protective equipment plays a vital role in protecting workers' health.

Money Matters

If a job makes you sick or injures you, you're entitled to *workers' compensation*. You can receive partial payment of the wages you lose and payment for rehabilitation, medical costs associated with the injury or illness, and certain "losses of function."

Repetition Hurts

Musculoskeletal disorders of the back, arms, and legs occur more often than all other types of disabling work-related injuries and illnesses in the United States, accounting for 40 percent of the cases that require time away from work.

Risk factors for these disorders include working in an awkward posture, use of force, repeated motions, and lack of rest. Reducing these disorders requires redesigning workstations and tools so they "fit" workers and redesigning jobs to reduce the pace of work and increase the amount of rest so that one body part isn't overtaxed. Quick fixes—such as the use of back belts—may cause more problems than they solve.

Workers' compensation is insurance for job-related injuries or illnesses. Most employers must buy workers' compensation insurance for their employees.

Without regard to who was at fault, workers' compensation pays your medical bills and part of your lost income while you can't work. It also provides benefits to your family if you are killed on the job.

Workers' compensation is primarily a legal system—not a medical one. That is, a judge, rather than a health care professional, generally decides whether your injury or illness is work-related, the degree of your disability, whether you are entitled to remain off the job, and when you can return to work. However, the opinion of the person who treats you is very important, especially if an employer or its insurance company disputes the work-relatedness of your claim to workers' compensation.

Each state administers its own workers' compensation system, imposes its own rules, and sets maximum weekly wage benefits for people injured severely enough to miss work. In many states, this maximum is 66 percent of the average weekly wage. Rarely do "wage replacement" benefits equal your earnings before an injury or illness. In most cases, the system precludes you from suing your employer to recover full damages or any payments for pain and suffering.

This arrangement compensates injured people more effectively than it does people suffering from occupational diseases. The connection between workplace exposure and ill health can be difficult to prove, with the burden of proof on the worker. Employers and their insurance companies contest over 80 percent of all compensation cases for chronic occupational disease, and less than 5 percent of all workers' comp cases are paid out to workers for occupational disease.

Some workers' compensation laws require you to see doctors your employer designates for treatment. Other states allow you to select your own health care providers. If you have this option, an occupational-medicine specialist can benefit your case significantly.

Filing a Workers' Compensation Claim

You don't necessarily need an attorney to file a workers' compensation claim. In many cases, you can do it on your own, or ask your doctor, union, or other advocates for help. On the other hand, you may need a lawyer to *win* a workers' compensation case if your employer challenges your claim.

Whether and when to obtain legal assistance depends on many factors. COSH groups, unions, and some of the other resource organizations listed in this chapter can help you make that decision.

More Sources of Compensation

Workers who suffer serious long-term injuries or illnesses can apply for Social Security Disability Insurance (SSDI), which provides monthly benefits to people whose injuries or illnesses prevent them from engaging in "substantial gainful employment" for a year or longer. After a five-month waiting period, SSDI benefits, when combined with workers' compensation benefits, equal 80 percent of your average monthly earnings. Social Security denies most SSDI claims initially, but appeals before a Social Security judge often succeed.

At some point, a person injured or made sick by work might feel ready to return to work but not perform all of his or her previous job tasks. According to the Americans with Disabilities Act, employers of fifteen or more workers must provide "reasonable accommodations" that allow disabled workers to perform "essential job functions." Some states have additional protections for disabled workers.

Reasonable accommodations include adjusting the job environment to permit someone with a disability to perform essential job functions. Examples include:

- Physical changes, such as ramps, lower benches, or special equipment
- Training to be able to use special equipment or new systems, *and*
- Job restructuring, such as reassignment of nonessential tasks, job redesign, more rest breaks, or lighter duty

Employers often stop paying your health insurance premiums if you miss work because of a disability. On the other hand, you usually have a right to stay in your employer's group plan if you pay the full premium yourself. If you can't pay the premium, you may be able to obtain medical coverage through state programs or Medicaid.

For more on Medicaid, turn to chapter 4.

An Injury to One . . .

A person may develop carpal tunnel syndrome in his or her wrists from typing on a computer. That worker's situation can raise the awareness of improvements in equipment and job design that would help *all* computer users in the workplace. Making such changes would protect the first worker from a recurrence of this painful, sometimes disabling condition, *and* prevent other people from ever suffering it in the first place.

From a prevention perspective, if an injured worker returns to a job that is modified to prevent reinjury, everyone else doing that job should benefit from the same improvements.

> **TIP**
>
> **Disability and Insurance**
>
> **12**
>
> Check to see if a company or state short-term or long-term disability policy covers your situation. This may supplement your wages while out of work.

Common Occupational Illnesses

Immediate or Short-Term Effects

Symptom	Agent	Type of Work
Dermatoses (allergic or irritant)	metals (chromium, nickel), fibrous glass, epoxy resins, cutting oils, solvents, caustic alkali, soaps	electroplating, metal cleaning, plastics, machining, leather tanning, housekeeping
Headaches	carbon monoxide, solvents	firefighting, automobile exhaust, foundry, wood finishing, dry cleaning
Acute psychoses	lead (especially organic), mercury, carbon disulfate	handling gasoline, seeds, or fungicide, wood preserving, viscose rayon industry
Asthma or dry cough	formaldehyde, toluene diisocyanate, animal dander	textiles, plastics, polyurethane kits, lacquer use, animal handler
Pulmonary edema, pneumonitis	nitrogen oxides, phosgene, halogen gases, cadmium	welding, farming ("silo filler's disease"), chemical operations, smelting
Cardiac arrhythmia	solvents, fluorocarbons	metal cleaning, solvents use, refrigerator maintenance
Angina	carbon monoxide	car repair, traffic exhaust, foundry, wood finishing
Abdominal pain	lead	battery making, enameling, smelting, painting, welding, ceramics, plumbing
Hepatitis (may become a long-term effect)	halogenated hydrocarbons	solvent use, lacquer use, hospital workers

Latent or Long-Term Effects

Symptom	Agent	Type of Work
Chronic dyspnea; pulmonary fibrosis	asbestos, silica, beryllium, coal, aluminum	mining, insulation, pipefitting, sandblasting, quarrying, metal alloy work, aircraft or electrical parts
Chronic bronchitis emphysema	cotton dust, cadmium coal dust, organic solvents, cigarettes	textile industry, battery production, soldering, mining, solvent use
Lung cancer	asbestos, arsenic, uranium, coke oven emissions	insulation, pipefitting, smelting, coke ovens, shipyard workers, nickel refining, uranium mining
Bladder cancer	b-naphthylamine, benzidine dyes	dye industry, leather, rubber-working chemists

Latent or Long-Term Effects		
Symptom	Agent	Type of Work
Peripheral neuropathy	lead, arsenic, n-hexane, methyl butylketone, acrylamide	battery production, plumbing, smelting, painting, shoemaking, solvent use, insecticide
Behavioral changes	lead, carbon disulfide, solvents, mercury, manganese	battery makers, smelting, viscose rayon industry, degreasing, manufacturing and repair of scientific instruments, dental amalgam workers
Extrapyramidal syndrome	carbon disulfide, manganese	viscose rayon industry, steel production, battery production, foundry
Aplastic anemia, leukemia	benzene, ionizing radiation	chemists, furniture refinishing, cleaning, degreasing, radiation workers

Source: "The Occupational and Environmental Health History," *Journal of the American Medical Association (1981).* Copyright 1981, American Medical Association.

Resources
Organizations

AFL-CIO
Department of Occupational Health
    and Safety
815 16th Street, N.W.
Washington, DC 20006
(202) 637-5210
Call or write for information on reaching the health and safety department of any international member union.

Association of Occupational and Environmental Clinics
1010 Vermont Avenue, N.W.
Washington, DC 20005
(202) 347-4976
The AOEC can refer you to an occupational health clinic in your area.

Center for Safety in the Arts
5 Beekman Street, #820
New York, NY 10038
(212) 227-6220
Contact the CSA for information on health and safety in the visual and performing arts. CSA offers newsletters, education and consultation programs, and many books, pamphlets, and other resources.

Coalition of Labor Union Women
1126 16th Street, N.W.
Washington, DC 20036
(202) 296-1200
Call or write for publications and information on job hazards for working women, including a copy of *Is Your Job Making You Sick? A CLUW Handbook on Workplace Hazards* ($4).

National Coalition of Injured Workers
12 Rejane Street
Coventry, RI 02816
(401) 828-6520
This is an association of organizations that help injured and ill workers obtain support, medical care, and benefits. The groups advocate for better workers' compensation systems. Contact the NCIW to find the injured-workers group in your area.

National Institute for Occupational Safety and Health
4676 Columbia Parkway
Cincinnati, OH 45226
(800) 35-NIOSH
NIOSH can check your workplace for health hazards, explore links between particular exposures and ill health, and make recommendations on ways to control hazards. Contact NIOSH to request workplace inspections or to receive information on training programs and a list of publications on various health and safety issues.

National Labor Relations Board
1717 Pennsylvania Avenue, N.W.
Washington, DC 20570
The NLRB can intervene when employers fail to provide unions with certain health or safety information or when employers fire workers for acting collectively to improve health and safety conditions. There are regional offices throughout the country.

Occupational Safety and Health Administration
200 Constitution Avenue, N.W., #N3647

Washington, DC 20210
(202) 219-8148
OSHA can inspect workplaces and fine employers that violate health or safety standards. Call or write for a list of publications and ordering information. There are regional OSHA offices around the country; look in the government listings of the phone book under U.S. Department of Labor.

Publications

Confronting Reproductive Health Hazards on the Job. To order, contact Massachusetts Coalition for Occupational Safety and Health, 555 Amory Street, Jamaica Plain, MA 02130; tel. (617) 524-6686. $9.

Preventing Occupational Disease and Injury, edited by James L. Weeks, Barry S. Levy, and Gregory R. Wagner (American Public Health Association, 1991). To order, contact APHA, 1015 15th Street, N.W., Washington, DC 20005; tel. (301) 893-1894. $28.50 plus $5 shipping and handling.

Part Four

The Complete Package

13 Physician Specialists

June Ellen Mendelson

June Ellen Mendelson is a health policy analyst. She has a doctorate in social welfare from Brandeis University.

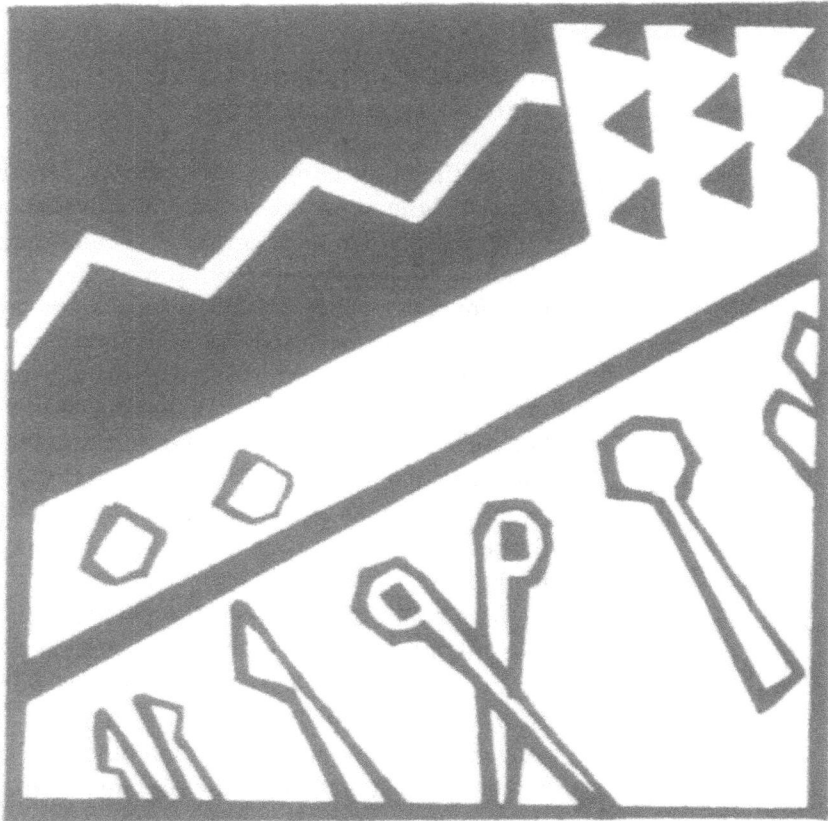

From cardiologists to oncologists, psychiatrists to surgeons, we often turn to specialists when we need complex medical care—and thereby encounter some of our most perplexing medical decisions. When should you see a specialist? What kind of specialist is best for you? What can the specialist do for you? How can you pay for the high cost of specialized medicine?

Fortunately, the person you visit for primary care—the family physician, your child's pediatrician, a gynecologist, a nurse practitioner—will be your key to answering these questions. Most people visit a specialist on the advice of a primary care provider, so this chapter will help you be an informed partner in making the best possible choices.

Indeed, the questions surrounding your use of a specialist highlight the importance of forming a strong partnership with your primary care provider. He or she will be your first—though not exclusive—source of information both about specialists and about other options. And if the two of you decide that you should consult a specialist, your primary care provider can continue to monitor the adequacy of your care.

Choosing a Specialist

The distinctions among the multitude of medical specialties often seem to make little sense from the patient's perspective. For example, three types of physician focus on patients of a particular age—pediatricians for children, adolescent-medicine physicians for teenagers, and gerontologists for older people—while obstetricians and gynecologists treat only women. Many more specialists focus on parts of the body, such as the heart or the lungs. Surgeons constitute a particularly large and broad group; most specialize further, dealing with only one organ or area of the body. Psychiatrists treat behavior but share their domain with nonphysician psychologists, social workers, and others in the field of mental health. Moreover, the list of "official" medical specialties is in flux, and the realms of various specialists overlap, complicating your choice even further.

As a result of this system, a person with a pain of unknown origin faces a challenge. Do you choose a provider appropriate to your age or gender? Or one who specializes in the part of your body where it hurts? How do you find proper treatment? And how do you get the right amount of treatment—neither too much nor too little?

As you face these and other dilemmas, an invaluable asset is your primary care provider. He or she plays a strong role as coordinator of your care from all medical professionals, including specialists, who undertake additional medical training that qualifies them to treat less-common ailments. If you have a debilitating chronic disease or a severe medical condition, your primary care provider will help you find a specialist to consult. And even though the conditions treated by the specialist may affect only one part of your body, you will still benefit from a primary care provider's comprehensive and continuous approach.

For more information on primary care, turn to chapter 5.

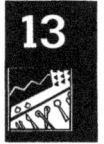

What to Look for in a Specialist

Experience is extremely important. Ask a specialist how many patients with your condition he or she has treated. What have been the results? For certain surgeries, you'll want a specialist who has conducted the procedure hundreds of times.

Good specialists—like good primary care providers—devote the time it takes to respond to your concerns about health care, explaining diagnoses and the choices inherent in different treatment plans.

The Referral

If you agree with your primary care provider on the need to see a specialist, he or she will refer you to an appropriate person. At this point, make sure you understand why you need to see a specialist, why that type of specialist, why that particular person, and what the specialist will do. Ask your primary care provider about dangers, costs, time, and options—and what happens if you disagree with a specialist's recommendation. You might also ask if your primary care provider has ties to this specialist. Such ties may exist if your primary care provider belongs to a group practice of which the specialist is also a member.

Ties certainly exist if you belong to a health maintenance organization or other form of managed care health plan, where the primary care provider acts as a gatekeeper and makes referrals to a selected panel of specialists within the plan. These managed care plans are more likely than traditional health insurers to monitor physicians' recommendations and your choice of procedures and treatments. Rarely will a physician in a managed care plan refer you to a specialist outside the plan's network, although he or she may do so if you require highly specialized care. Certainly, you can expect your primary care provider to be your ally in convincing the plan of your need for specialized care.

For more information on managed care, turn to chapter 4.

TIP

Know Your Insurance

Find out what types of specialty care your insurance covers, including restrictions on who provides it. Glossy brochures advertising the benefits of health insurance seldom include a frank discussion of referrals to out-of-plan specialists. Ask before joining a new plan.

Few people have a problem getting a referral to a specialist when the primary care provider considers it *medically* necessary. But physicians and patients don't always agree on what is necessary. If you disagree with your primary care provider, you can:

■ *Call* your insurance company or a managed care plan's medical director or member-services department. Explain your concern, and perhaps file an appeal or grievance. Explain that you have requested a referral and that your doctor has refused to make one. You'll have to present a strong case.

■ *Persist* with your primary care provider. Evidence from your own library research might convince him or her that a specialist's care is warranted.

■ *Find* a specialist on your own and foot the bill yourself, at least until the specialist provides the evidence you need to convince your primary care provider or insurer of your need for such care.

Consumer Alert: Required Referrals

Some specialists will make an appointment with you only if you have a referral from a primary care provider. And some insurers require such a referral for the specialist's service to be covered.

Getting a Referral for Complex Care

If you need highly complex care, either your primary care provider or a specialist may refer you to a subspecialist who has completed additional training in an even more specific area of medicine. Subspecialists are usually associated with academic health centers or teaching hospitals.

More and more consumers are enrolled in managed care systems that may have few subspecialists in their networks. Some managed care plans also restrict your choice of medical facilities, perhaps excluding teaching hospitals, where more subspecialists and the most advanced technology are usually found. For example, if a specialist recommends cardiac bypass surgery for you, your managed care plan may restrict you to specific surgeons and facilities.

Medicare beneficiaries considering a managed care plan should be especially careful to select one with an adequate number of specialists. Seniors frequently need specialist care.

For more information on Medicare, turn to chapter 11.

Managed care plans occasionally refer patients out-of-plan. An educated consumer can enter into a discussion with plan providers and perhaps convince them to authorize a controversial treatment. Managed care plans do have an interest in your health, and they certainly want to avoid malpractice lawsuits, so consumers have some leverage to obtain the care that they need.

Evaluating a Specialist

The decision you and your primary care provider make about which person is best qualified to perform a proposed diagnostic procedure or treatment will make a significant difference in the care you receive. So express your preferences, regardless of whether you have traditional indemnity insurance, participate in a managed care plan, or lack insurance coverage altogether.

As you decide on a specialist, look for many of the same qualities you seek in anyone from whom you receive health care. First, the specialist must be *competent* to treat your illness. Second, the specialist should inspire *trust* and *respect.* Look for a specialist who treats you as an individual, *listens* to you, and *explains* your problems and options without condescension and in language you can understand.

You can assess personal characteristics by interviewing a specialist. However, judging competency is a challenge. As a start, your state's Board of Registration in Medicine can provide some information about licensing and credentials. These boards keep public records on all physicians in the state, including:

- Medical school and date of graduation
- Board certification, *and*
- Hospital privileges

State medical boards also keep records of formal disciplinary actions against physicians. They also sometimes revoke a physician's license to practice in a state as a result of mental illness, Alzheimer's disease, drug or alcohol abuse, or fraudulent billing. And most state medical boards keep records of medical malpractice cases, but not out-of-court settlements. If your state has a Freedom of Information Act, you can request information from the state board; some state boards release the information as a matter of course. Many boards will mail you copies of letters of complaint against a physician and the physician's response to the complaint, so you can judge for yourself if the physician is one you would want as your doctor.

Complex Questions

If you or a family member has a very rare problem, chances are a hospital affiliated with a medical school is the best place for treatment. These tend to be the most up-to-date and best-equipped institutions, with relevant specialists and subspecialists on staff.

13

If a specialist refers you to a hospital for complex care, ask him or her many probing questions, such as:

- How often does this hospital treat patients with a problem like mine?

- What are the most common complications resulting from treating this condition? What are they in this hospital?

- Who is on call at night? Is a senior physician available?

- Will a case manager coordinate all aspects of my care? Is this person available by phone? What kind of training does the case manager have?

- What type of care can the hospital deliver to my home?

For more information about hospitals, turn to chapter 6.

TIP

Disciplinary Record

To order a copy of *Questionable Doctors*, contact the Public Citizen's Health Research Group, 2000 P Street, N.W., Washington, DC 20036; tel. (202) 588-1000. $200 for complete U.S. listing; $15 for a single state.

Physician disciplinary actions hit an all-time high in 1994, with 3,685 doctors disciplined by state medical boards. In 1,498 cases, the board revoked or suspended the doctor's license, imposing milder sanctions on the others.

The National Practitioner Databank identifies doctors who have been involved in incidents of medical incompetence. Because the licensing system is organized by state, this computer database helps prevent doctors who have trouble in one place from moving to another location to practice. It includes malpractice payment reports, losses of license or clinical privileges, and disciplinary actions by a professional society. Hospitals and medical boards may use this information to evaluate physician credentials. Unfortunately, the data isn't available to you, although Congress may change this soon.

You can also consult *Questionable Doctors,* available from Public Citizen's Health Research Group. It names over ten thousand doctors that have been disciplined by the states and the federal government in the past decade. More than twenty-five thousand disciplinary actions were taken against doctors named in the report. Nonetheless, only one-fourth of the physicians lost their licenses to practice, even temporarily. The offenses ranged from overprescribing drugs or prescribing the wrong ones to criminal convictions for alcohol or drug abuse to sexual misconduct with a patient.

Certification Boards

Specialist practice differs from primary care by focusing on one aspect of medical care. Any licensed physician can limit his or her practice to any specialized field without receiving additional training or certification. That doctor can even list the practice in the Yellow Pages under that specialty. However, this physician wouldn't necessarily be a *board-certified specialist.* (Maryland and a few other states require physicians to have the proper training and credentials before claiming to be a specialist.)

Although the licensing of physicians is regulated by the state, the medical profession itself controls certification. The American Medical Association regulates specialty boards that set requirements for specialty training. This certification assures you that a physician has completed additional hospital training, passed oral and written exams, and kept up with the continuing medical educational requirements in a particular specialty.

Board certification offers some confirmation of a physician's competence in a field. Conversely, physicians practicing outside their specialty may be less experienced and thus more prone to error. And it's increasingly important for physicians to become board certified in a particular specialty to get a job at a hospital and health plan, maintain a private practice and get referrals, and obtain insurance compensation for the care they deliver.

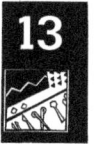

Checking Up on a Specialist

Most physicians display their certifications and diplomas on the office wall. If you don't see these credentials, you can ask:

- What specialty training have you completed?
- Are you board certified? If so, by what boards?
- With what hospitals are you affiliated?

To check if a doctor is certified, call the American Board of Medical Specialties Certification Line at (800) 776-2378, or contact your state medical board. Before you call, know the doctor's first and last name, and, if possible, the middle initial.

Note, however, that over one hundred self-styled medical boards offer membership with few or no requirements, according to *Money* magazine. Make sure the certifying agency is affiliated the American Board of Medical Specialties.

Osteopathic Specialists

Although osteopathic medicine is most often associated with primary care, osteopathic physicians can also specialize and in essentially the same fields as conventional doctors. These specialists are board certified by the American Osteopathic Association.

For more information on osteopathic medicine, turn to chapter 5.

Getting Good Specialist Care

Specialists, like primary care providers, deal with three general facets of medical care: diagnosis, prognosis, and treatment. To find the right specialist, seek satisfactory answers to questions about all three areas of care. If the specialist doesn't have time to answer all your questions on the first visit, or you think of new questions, set up another appointment or ask for a telephone conference.

Insist that the specialist take all the time you require to understand what's going on with your body. A frank discussion and probing ques-

Video Assist

♥ Some specialists use interactive video programs to educate patients about treatment options and involve them more deeply in making decisions. Developed by the Foundation for Informed Medical Decision Making, these videos provide the patient—and the doctor—with the information and options needed to make smart decisions about treatment.

The video on breast cancer, for example, includes interviews with several women regarding their surgical experiences. It provides clear and simple explanations of the risks and benefits of the various options that arise after surgery, such as chemotherapy and hormone treatment.

The foundation's programs present information about the potential harms and benefits of surgical and nonsurgical treatments. In one study, conducted at Group Health Cooperative, an HMO in Washington State, surgery rates were cut in half among men who watched the video on prostate disease, with many viewers opting instead for watchful waiting. Yet the video contains no apparent bias against surgery. No wonder both patients *and* insurers have

tions will aid you in making the best decisions in collaboration with your doctors. Also, feel free to seek the help of your primary care provider in evaluating what the specialist recommends.

If a specialist proposes a particular test, ask:

- Will this test tell you if you are all right?
- What are the chances the test will be wrong?
- How will I find out about the results?
- How often will I need another test?
- What additional tests will I need?

If the specialist says you have a serious medical problem and recommends a particular treatment, ask:

- What is wrong? What is my illness or condition?
- What are the immediate and long term risks and side effects of the recommended treatment?
- What are the benefits of the recommended treatment?
- Will I be better in one year due to the treatment? In five years?
- What is your experience with cases like mine?
- What complications might arise?
- Can I see my medical record and keep a copy?

Before Agreeing to Surgery

Because any surgery or invasive procedure involves risks, it makes sense to check the credentials of your provider before proceeding. If you are contemplating major surgery, the hospital may tell you if your physician is in good standing at that hospital and is approved to perform the contemplated procedure. Hospitals keep information on the credentials of their physicians, which may include licensing, performance, and quality-assurance records. The trend today is to make some of this information available to the consumer.

To minimize the risks involved—and because you only want to receive surgery that is absolutely necessary—talk to your surgeon. Ask:

- What will happen during the surgery?

- What will happen if I refuse surgery?

- Who will perform the surgery? How often has he or she done it in the past? What's his or her success rate? How often has he or she seen a condition like mine?

- Who will choose the anesthesiologist? What is his or her experience?

■ Will the anesthesiologist be present during the entire operation? Will the anesthesiologist monitor the recovery room afterward?

■ What is the general success rate for this kind of procedure?

■ What alternative treatments are available? What are the risks and benefits of each?

■ How much will the surgery cost?

■ What are the most common complications?

■ Will I be able to resume my former activities?

■ When will I be able to return to work?

■ What's the best I can expect?

■ What's most likely to occur?

■ What if I wait until next year—or until I have insurance coverage?

Surgery Advice

The American College of Surgeons publishes a series of free pamphlets, "When You Need an Operation." For copies, write to the ACS, Office of Public Information, 55 E. Erie Street, Chicago, IL 60611; tel. (312) 664-4050.

The American Society of Anesthesiologists and the American Association of Nurse Anesthetists both have free booklets on what you should know about anesthesia. For copies, contact ASA, 520 Northwest Highway, Park Ridge, IL 60068, tel. (708) 825-5586; or AANA, 222 S. Prospect Avenue, Park Ridge, IL 60068, tel. (708) 692-7050.

Second Opinions

If you disagree with a specialist on what constitutes the best care for you, try again to work things out. That physician already knows a great deal about you and your problem. Moreover, your care is essentially under way, and it's possible that you misunderstood the initial explanations. If you can't resolve the problem this way, consult your primary care provider for advice about your options.

One of those options is getting a "second opinion" from another specialist. Remember, medicine is an inexact science. Uncertainties about treatments and diagnoses arise because doctors differ in their practice styles, education, and training—sometimes in controversial ways.

positive comments about this tool for strengthening the partnership between you and your health care providers.

For more information, contact the Foundation for Informed Medical Decision Making, P.O. Box 5457, Hanover, NH 03755-5457.

13

Outpatient Surgery

More and more surgeries that don't require an overnight stay take place in ambulatory care centers as well as hospital operating rooms. In such cases, take special care to insist that the physician explains what you can expect during recovery and where to go for emergency care if complications arise.

Surgery performed in a doctor's office may present even greater risks. Ask the doctor what emergency procedures are in place in the office. If an emergency arises, what hospitals are available for backup? What precautions are in place for the use of anesthesia? Some physicians who do office surgery regularly have their office inspected by the Accreditation Association of National Health Care.

For more information on ambulatory care, turn to chapter 6.

TIP

Shopping Around

Second opinions can be invaluable, but don't seek one just to shop for the diagnosis you'd like to hear.

TIP

Copy Your Records

Your insurance company might pay for a second opinion but not for a repeat test. Get copies of your test records or X rays and bring them to the person providing the second opinion.

Indeed, the list of conditions for which the treatment plans are disputed is long, and it changes constantly as evidence accumulates in favor of or against long-accepted practices. A few examples of maladies and procedures about which doctors differ significantly are breast cancer, prostate cancer, back pain, recurrent colds in children, tonsillectomies, high blood pressure, and cardiac bypass surgery.

This list is far from comprehensive; rather, it illustrates what physicians and patients confront in the absence of one definitive solution. This is a major reason patients seek—with the support of insurance companies—second opinions before accepting a specialist's diagnosis or recommended treatment.

Two doctors rarely offer greatly divergent diagnoses. More likely, they'll differ on the alternatives they propose and your chances of getting better. If the outcome is especially uncertain, you might find almost as many opinions as there are doctors; you must then pay special attention to working with health care professionals to make a wise decision.

A second opinion is especially critical for surgery and other invasive procedures. In fact, many insurers, and even some states, require second opinions before many types of surgery. A second opinion helps you and the doctor decide if such a drastic step is really needed. It can also help you discover alternatives that could be safer, cheaper, less painful, and even more effective.

Usually, you'll want a board-certified doctor for the second opinion. And try to get the second opinion from someone independent of the person who gave the first opinion. Don't let your specialist refer you to a friend of his or hers or to someone with essentially the same training. Of course, finding a truly independent physician can be more difficult in an HMO, where you normally consult only doctors within the plan. Check with the HMO's member-services department about going outside the plan for a second opinion.

Fortunately, it's not as hard as you might expect to tell a specialist you want a second opinion. Because it's such a common practice, even an insurance requirement in many instances, few doctors will treat you as uppity for suggesting it. To find a good person to give you a second opinion, you can ask your primary care provider or check with local medical societies.

Money Matters

Specialists cost more. How much that fact matters to you is a very personal issue that rests in part on one point: Do you have medical insurance?

If you have insurance, find out what your policy covers. Will the insurance pay for the kind, quality, and quantity of specialized care you and your physician decide is warranted? After all, that's one purpose of insurance: to ensure that your personal finances don't force you to go without care you need. Remember, your insurance status doesn't affect your need for a particular procedure, only your ability to pay for it.

The insurance company may encourage you to use less-expensive providers or seek less-expensive forms of care—*both of which may make sense for you as well.* If you have insurance through your employer, he or she may share the interest of the insurer in limiting the medical bill, perhaps leading him or her to pay less attention to quality than you would yourself.

If you don't have insurance, or your insurance doesn't cover the recommended care, you'll have to add a strong concern for cost-effectiveness to your demand for quality. Seek out the same data that cost-conscious insurers use, comparing the specialist's fees to standard rates for the procedures he or she is recommending. To get this data, you can look in major libraries for *Medical Economics* magazine, which regularly publishes price information. You can also ask in the library's business section for insurance publications that include the data you need. Alternatively, private companies sell information on fees.

Bargaining

"While most of us might feel uncomfortable haggling with our doctors, and while most doctors would rather not have to justify their fees, there are times when medical bills could and should be discussed." That's the advice of *Boston Globe* health care writer Madeline Drexler.

Most health insurers bargain with providers in some way, and you can too—if you lack insurance or if you decide to get care that your insurance doesn't cover.

"If you can't pay up," notes Drexler, "your physician or hospital billing department might offer to discount the charge, arrange payment over time, or in rare cases, throw out the bill."

Primary Means First

If at all possible, see a primary care provider before consulting a specialist. This saves money, plus you benefit from the doctor's more general knowledge.

Primary care providers can handle about 70 percent of physician office visits effectively. However, specialists provide most medical care

Third Opinions

A third opinion may be in order if two specialists differ significantly in their reports. Also consider a third voice if you feel you have good cause to be dissatisfied with the first two opinions. Check with your primary care provider or insurer to find out if you are covered for a third opinion.

Convincing insurers to pay for a third opinion is usually simple if two specialists disagree. It will be harder to convince insurers you need a third opinion if the first two say treatment isn't warranted. You may have to become a sleuth and conduct research in medical libraries. And you may decide to consult a lawyer.

If you are a member of an HMO, you might choose to pay for a visit to an out-of-plan physician. It may be worth it, both in terms of your financial health and your medical care.

in the United States, and most practicing physicians limit their practice to a specialty. In fact, one-third of all primary care is delivered by specialists, often at higher specialist rates. This contrasts with the situation in Western Europe and Canada and is yet one more reason why U.S. medical bills are sky-high.

The predominance of specialists in the United States contributes to rising costs and compromises quality by contributing to a patchwork, procedure-oriented medical system. Specialists tend to use more health care resources than primary care providers because they depend more on technology, tests, and procedures. One indicator of the impact this has on cost and quality comes from studies by Dr. John Wennberg revealing the incidence of back surgery "epidemics" upon the arrival of a neurosurgeon to an area.

Consumer Alert: Two-Way Rules

Medicare, almost all managed care plans, and most insurers pay for second opinions. But beware of the reverse. If you *don't* get a second opinion for surgery and other procedures, you may be stuck with the whole hospital bill, no matter how critical the care.

Check your insurance policy carefully. Does it cover a second opinion? Does it *require* one? Does it dictate whom to see?

Judgment Calls

For certain types of specialty care, you may have to fight to get your insurer to foot the bill, especially if the treatment could be considered experimental or optional. For example, according to a study published in the *New England Journal of Medicine,* insurers are "arbitrary and capricious" about paying for experimental bone-marrow transplants and high-dose chemotherapy for breast cancer.

Conducted by Duke University physicians William Peters and Mark Rogers, the study found that insurers refused to pay for the procedures for 121 out of a group of 533 patients. The major reason given for the denial: The treatments are experimental. Of course, insurers also resist paying for these procedures because of the price tag: $100,000 or more for a bone-marrow transplant.

On the other hand, the study illustrates the payoff for consumer persistence. Of the 121 people the insurers initially told No deal, 62 ultimately received payment after hiring attorneys.

Managed Specialties

The Council on Graduate Medical Education recommends that 85 to 105 specialists are needed for every 100,000 people. In the interest of quality care, managed care organizations should not fall below this number. You have a right to insist that your primary care provider refer you to a qualified specialist, trained and experienced to treat your particular problem.

Physician Self-Referral and Unnecessary Tests

If you have insurance, your health plan will scrutinize a specialist's bill for unwarranted tests and other procedures and may even insist that you get authorization for tests in advance. If you are paying the bills yourself, it's up to you to watch out for unnecessary tests and padded bills.

Consider the results of a 1994 investigation by the federal General Accounting Office. The study analyzed 2.4 million records involving seven types of diagnostic tests and found strong patterns of abuse. Physicians who belonged to a practice owning the equipment for special imaging tests, such as MRIs and X rays, were far more likely to recommend such tests than were physicians who sent patients to unaffiliated providers. "The in-practice rates were about 3 times higher for MRI scans, about 2 times higher for CT scans, 4.5 to 5 times higher for ultrasound, echocardiology, and diagnostic nuclear medicine imaging, and about 2 times higher for complex and simple X rays." An MRI costs $400 to $1,000.

This problem goes by the name of *self-referral,* where physicians benefit financially from sending you to certain providers for care. About 10 percent of physicians have ownership interests that raise issues of self-referral. Only New York, Florida, Illinois, and New Jersey restrict self-referral in any way, and these restrictions don't apply to many situations.

AMA on Physician Self-Referrals

The Council on Ethical and Judicial Affairs of the American Medical Association suggests that physicians not refer patients to an outside health care facility in which they have an investment, unless they also directly provide care or services at the facility.

The council also says that physicians should disclose their investment interest to patients when making a referral. Patients should get a list of alternative facilities.

TIP

Don't Pay for Unnecessary Tests

Some lab tests are simple and inexpensive, but others are costly. Before agreeing to any test, have the doctor explain how, or if, the test results will affect your choice of treatment.

13

Who Does What

No introduction to physician specialists would be complete without some explanation of the many types of specialists you might encounter. The American Board of Medical Specialties recognizes twenty-four medical specialty boards and seventy-three subspecialties. Subspecialists must be certified in one of the specialties before completing their subspecialty training.

The categories of specialists and subspecialists have steadily grown in number over the past decade, as have the requirements for training. The ABMS publishes a book listing board-certified physicians. You can find it in many libraries.

Primary care providers can help you choose among the many specialties. As you can see from the list of specialties, the areas of expertise overlap significantly from the point of view of patients. For example, a cardiologist and thoracic surgeon both treat heart disease, but their approaches to treatment reflect their different training. Similarly, for back pain, you might consult a neurologist, orthopedic surgeon, neurosurgeon, or a sports-medicine doctor.

For information on alternative specialists and specialties, turn to chapter 19.

Medical or Surgical

Specialists and subspecialists fall into two major categories: medical and surgical. Among the surgical specialists and subspecialists are *colon and rectal surgeons, neurosurgeons, ophthalmologists, orthopedic surgeons, plastic surgeons, thoracic surgeons,* and *urologists.* Medical specialists and subspecialists include *cardiologists, endocrinologists, gastroenterologists, hematologists, pediatricians,* and *rheumatologists.*

The Medical and Surgical Specialties

For each of the following specialties, a member board of the American Board of Medical Specialties certifies physicians in that field. For example, there is an American Board of Allergy/Immunology, an American Board of Anesthesiology, and an American Board of Colon and Rectal Surgery.

Allergists and immunologists diagnose and manage disorders of the immune system, such as asthma, eczema and other adverse allergic reactions.

Anesthesiologists administer medications during or after surgery. They work with surgeons in operations, and some work independently to treat chronic pain and relax patients.

Colon and rectal surgeons deal with disorders affecting the lower digestive tract.

Dermatologists deal with diseases of the skin, mouth, external genitalia, hair, and nails, and with related sexually transmitted diseases.

Emergency medicine deals with care in a hospital emergency ward, including recognizing and treating a wide spectrum of physical and mental conditions.

Family practice deals with preventing, diagnosing, and treating a wide variety of ailments in patients of all ages.

Internists focus on managing common and acute illnesses, including long term follow-up. They provide primary care, but over half of all internists also train in a subspecialty. For example, a growing subspecialty in gerontology focuses on aging.

For more information on primary care, turn to chapter 5.

Medical geneticists diagnose and advise patients with diseases that are inherited.

Nephrologists treat diseases of the kidney.

Neurological surgeons perform surgery on the nervous system. This includes the diagnosis and surgical treatment of disease or impaired function of the brain, spinal cord, peripheral nerves, muscles, and autonomic nervous system.

Neurologists deal with the diagnosis and treatment of diseases and impaired functions of the brain, spinal cord, and autonomic nervous system.

Nuclear medicine makes use of radioactive isotopes for diagnosis, therapy, and research.

Obstetricians and gynecologists specialize in the female reproductive system and associated disorders.

For more information on health care providers for women, turn to chapter 9.

Ophthalmologists provide comprehensive vision and eye care, including surgery.

For more information on eye care, turn to chapter 18.

Orthopedic surgeons use surgery to restore function to damaged joints, backs, feet, and other extremities.

Otolaryngologists are surgeons who diagnose and treat disorders of the head and neck. The specialty focuses on hearing and speech pathology and disorders of the esophagus, nose, throat, face, and jaw.

Pathologists examine clinical samples for the purpose of diagnosing and understanding disease. Pathology has many subspecialties, including forensic pathology, which contributes to criminal investigations.

Pediatricians care for children. The many subspecialties of pediatrics include adolescent medicine, pediatric emergency medicine, and pediatric infectious disease.

For more information on care for children, turn to chapter 8.

Physical medicine focuses on diagnosing and treating patients with disabilities that impair their ability to complete the activities of daily living.

Plastic surgeons repair and reconstruct all areas of the body. They reduce scars, reconstruct breasts for cancer patients, and correct undesirable structures.

Preventive medicine aims to promote and maintain the health of selected groups of people. Screening programs for tuberculosis, cholesterol, and AIDS are the province of this specialty.

Psychiatrists diagnose and treat disorders of the mind and brain, including mental, emotional, and addictive disorders.

Pulmonary specialists treat diseases of the lung and respiratory system.

Radiologists use X rays to diagnose and treat diseases, especially malignant tumors.

General surgeons receive training to manage a broad range of surgical conditions affecting almost any area of the body. Most continue their training with education in a subspecialty.

Thoracic surgeons operate on the chest.

Urologists manage medical and surgical problems of the genitourinary system. Their expertise encompasses disorders of the kidney, bladder, adrenal gland, and the male reproductive system.

Sports Medicine

Sports medicine is a rapidly growing focus for physicians who specialize in enhancing health and fitness and preventing injury and illness. Many are trained in orthopedic surgery and add training in such diverse areas as exercise physiology, training regimens, and the psychological aspects of competition.

Specialists in sports medicine can be certified as subspecialists by the boards for emergency medicine, family practice, or internal medicine.

Generalist Specialists

Several recently established medical specialties and subspecialties each cover a broad range of diseases, reflecting a trend toward more generalized care:

■ *Family medicine* resembles general medical practice as a field. Family medicine practitioners fulfill an obvious need, and consumers seek them out.

■ *Occupational medicine* focuses on the myriad diseases associated with the workplace.
For more on occupational illnesses and hazards, turn to chapter 12.

■ *Preventive medicine* focuses on ways to prevent disease. These physicians study internal medicine and public health.

Resources

For more resources on primary care, turn to the resources section in chapter 5 and for general resources, turn to chapter 22.

Organizations

American Board of Medical Specialties
1007 Church Street
Evanston, IL 60201
(708) 491-9091
Send $1.50 for a copy of the ABMS's thirty-page pamphlet, "Which Medical Specialist for You?" The ABMS can also provide you with the names and addresses of the various boards of specialization it recognizes. *The Directory of Medical Specialists,* published by the ABMS, lists all board-certified specialists throughout the United States; copies are available in major libraries.

American Osteopathic Association
142 E. Ontario Street
Chicago, IL 60611
(800) 621-1773
Contact the AOA for information about osteopathic medicine. For referrals to osteopathic physicians, call ext. 7401.

Publications

Good Operations, Bad Operations, by Charles Inlander and the staff of the People's Medical Society. Order from People's Medical Society, 462 Walnut Street, Allentown, PA 18102; tel. (800) 624-8773. $27.50 ($22.50 for members).

"Medicare Coverage for Second Surgical Opinions: Your Choice Facing Elective Surgery." Write to the Health Care Financing Administration, Office of Public Affairs, Room 403B, 200 Independence Avenue, S.W., Washington, DC 20201. Ask for Publication No. HCFA 02173. Free.

The Patient's Guide to Surgery, by Edward L. Bradley (Consumer Reports, 1994), $24.95.

Surgery Electives: What to Know Before the Doctor Operates, by John McCabe (Carmania Books, 1994), $14.95.

14 Mental Health

Cindy Brach and Gail K. Robinson

Cindy Brach works for the Agency for Health Care Policy and Research. She was associate director for research and analysis at the Mental Health Policy Resource Center in Washington, D.C., and has been a human services consultant, a state-level administrator, and a municipal policy analyst.

Gail K. Robinson works for The Lewin Group. She was deputy director of the Mental Health Policy Resource Center. She also has been director for the Bureau of Demonstration Projects and associate director of strategic planning and project development for the New York State Office of Mental Health, as well as having directed Maryland's Office of Planning and Analysis for Mental Health, Addictions and Developmental Disabilities.

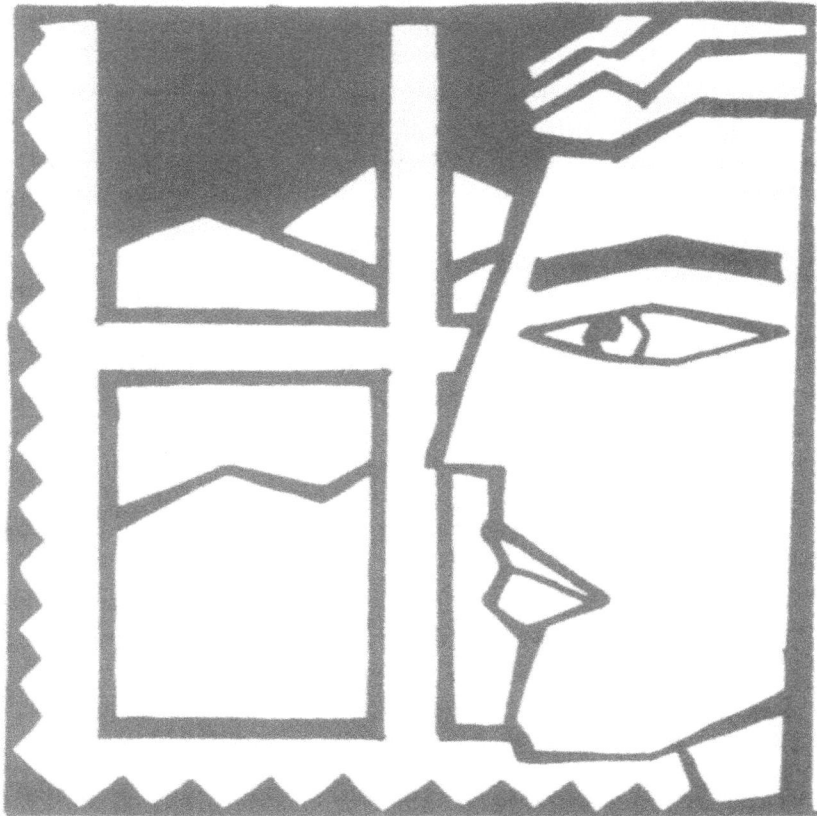

Some Common Mental Disorders

Phobias: Obsessive, unrealistic, and persistent fears of particular objects or situations. For example, people with claustrophobia fear enclosed spaces.

Panic: Discrete periods of sudden, overwhelming anxiety that produce terror and actual physical effects on your body, such as hyperventilation.

Obsessive-compulsive behavior: Persistent intrusion of unwanted and uncontrollable thoughts or actions. Repeated hand washing is an example.

Eating disorders: Severe disturbances in eating behavior, such as anorexia nervosa (refusal to maintain a minimally normal body weight) and bulimia nervosa (repeated binge eating followed by self-induced vomiting, misuse of laxatives, fasting, or excessive exercise).

Depression: Feeling sad or desperate for no apparent reason.

Manic-depression: Depressed feelings alternating with manic periods characterized by euphoria, an expansive or irritable mood, hyperactivity, less need for sleep, distractibility, and impaired judgment.

In any given year, mental disorders affect 22 percent of the adults in the United States. From 5 percent to 22 percent of children and adolescents suffer from mental disorders. Suicide is the third leading cause of death among teenagers.

Mental illness encompasses a variety of disorders, from minor to serious and complex conditions. Furthermore, some people experience severe problems for a brief time; others may have long term illnesses but with symptoms that occur only once in a while.

Today, you can get effective treatment for many mental health problems—whether your condition is mild or severe, short term or long-lasting. You should seek professional help if you are distressed and your efforts—such as exercising, meditating, or talking to friends—haven't helped you overcome your problem.

Step One: Educate yourself. The start of any treatment is learning where your distress comes from and studying the options for getting help. Education is the key to consumer empowerment. Read this chapter, contact the organizations listed at the end, and then move on to the library and the self-help aisle of your local bookstore.

Step Two: Create a partnership with a provider. As you travel the road to better mental health, a wide variety of professionals can provide you with many forms of assistance and treatment.

Responsible mental health providers actively contribute to their patients' knowledge and insight about distress. Good relationships with providers are characterized by trust and equality. Join with your provider to figure out what is wrong, why it's wrong—and what to do about it.

Recognize, however, that providers take many different perspectives on mental health and therapy. Don't assume that the first person you consult makes a good match for you and your needs. Take time to discover the right provider with the right approach for you.

Step Three: Continually assess and reassess your treatment. Caregivers, friends, and family may offer valuable advice, but you are ultimately responsible for yourself. You say when to continue or stop a treatment. Can you manage your distress without professional support? If the answer is yes, you can stop treatment for the time being.

You can measure the mental health care you receive by how well it helps you meet four primary goals:

■ Does it reduce or eliminate the symptoms of your disorder?

- Does it restore or improve your ability to socialize and work?
- Does it maximize your sense of well-being and that of your family?
- Does it prevent injury to yourself and to others?

If you now receive mental health care yet feel unable to manage on a day-to-day basis, consider two possible explanations: One, you need to allow yourself more time, working with your current providers. Two, the services don't fit you. It's probably time to investigate new providers.

Hotlines

The National Alliance for the Mentally Ill provides mutual support and education for people with severe mental illnesses and their families. Call NAMI's toll-free help-line at (800) 950-6264. The National Depressive and Manic Depressive Association also runs a mental health hotline: (800) 82-NDMDA.

Substance Abuse

One out of six adults abuses alcohol or drugs at some point in his or her lifetime. Although mental health and substance abuse services overlap to some extent, the two systems are largely distinct.

For more information on substance abuse, contact:

- The National Clearinghouse for Alcohol and Drug Information: (800) SAY-NO-TO
- Alcoholics Anonymous: (212) 870-3400, *or*
- Narcotics Anonymous: (818) 780-3951

Choosing a Provider

Psychiatrists, psychologists, clinical social workers, psychiatric nurses, marriage and family therapists, and professional counselors all provide mental health services. These practitioners vary in their level of education, their orientation, the amount of regulation to which they are subject, and whether insurance will cover their bills.

Your selection of the right professional is critical. As in so many other areas of health care, research mental health providers carefully. For recommendations, you can look to a variety of sources:

- Your physical health care provider
- Your former mental health provider, if you've moved since being treated

Dysthymia: A mild but chronic despondency lasting for months, often years. The person can work and maintain relationships, but everything is flat and colorless. Brief breaks in mood don't last.

Schizophrenia: A group of psychotic disorders characterized by a disintegrated personality. People with schizophrenia can misinterpret reality; for example, they may suffer delusions and hallucinations, mood changes, and withdrawn, regressive, and bizarre behavior.

For in-depth information about specific mental disorders, you can contact a host of organizations, such as the Anxiety Disorders Association of America. For information on some of these organizations, turn to pages 288–90.

14

- Family and friends—ask them to ask their health care providers
- Your health plan—a managed care plan may have a list of providers in its network
- Professional societies of mental health providers
- University psychiatric or psychology departments
- Government mental health, health, or social services agencies
- Religious organizations and your priest, rabbi, or minister
- Community-based agencies, such as neighborhood service centers
- Local hospitals and mental health and health clinics.

Ask every contact to recommend two or three individuals, institutions, or organizations. Interview potential providers. And don't be afraid to "comparison shop"—to make appointments with more than one provider and choose among them. You can also get a diagnostic assessment, which may take several sessions, before you commit yourself to treatment, but expect to be billed for each session.

Consider the kinds of services you want. If you think you may need medication, seek a provider with the authority to write a prescription—for example, a psychologist who works in collaboration with a physician.

For more information on the types of mental health care, see page 278.

Can Your Regular Doctor Do the Job?

Primary care providers deliver a significant proportion of mental health treatment, especially for depression and anxiety. Consider the pros and cons of receiving mental health care from the same person who is responsible for your regular health care.

Pros:

- You know and trust the provider.
- If it's a doctor, he or she can write prescriptions.
- You have ready access to the person.
- Your insurance is more likely to cover all or part of the bills.

Cons:

- The provider may be too close to you or other family members.
- Medical doctors are more likely to medicate.
- Short appointments, which are not appropriate for psychotherapy, are more likely.
- The provider probably lacks in-depth mental health training, making it more likely that he or she will misdiagnose or even fail to recognize depression or other mental conditions.

Your Choice of Provider

Choosing a mental health provider can be even more difficult than choosing a primary care provider, in part because you can select from among a variety of types and specialties. The decision-making process can resemble picking out a new car: Your choice depends on your needs, the extra features you value, and what you can afford.

Cost is almost always a factor. Some health insurance (including Medicaid and Medicare) covers only certain care from certain types of providers; other plans may restrict you to providers who are on the plans' staff or are part of their network. Some policies may limit the number of covered visits. Find out how much your insurer will pay. And check for copayments and for gaps between the reimbursement level and what providers charge.

For more information on insurance, turn to page 283.

The specialties presented here are listed roughly in order of cost, beginning with the most expensive.

Psychiatrists are physicians who specialize in diagnosing and treating mental and emotional disorders. As medical doctors, they may be more likely than other mental health practitioners to see physical roots to mental illness, although they also practice psychotherapy and may have psychoanalytic training. As medical doctors, psychiatrists can write prescriptions. The American Board of Psychiatry and Neurology certifies psychiatrists.

Of all mental health providers, psychiatrists charge the most. On the other hand, all insurance policies that cover mental health treatment accept psychiatrists as providers.

Clinical psychologists have master's or doctoral degrees in psychology and training in psychotherapy. Like psychiatrists, some psychologists receive psychoanalytic training. However, psychologists can't prescribe drugs unless they also have a medical degree. The American Psychological Association and the American Board of Professional Psychology both credential clinical psychologists. Many states license only psychologists with a doctorate and two years of clinical experience. Virtually all insurance policies that cover mental health accept Ph.D. psychologists as providers.

Clinical social workers have a degree in social work—usually a master's degree—and special training in counseling. Clinical social work is an increasingly popular credential for providers and clients. For the providers, the training doesn't require getting a doctoral degree. For

Depression

Genette is 68 years old, married, and retired. Recently, she has found herself inexplicably fatigued. She has lost energy, stopped eating, and wakes at night feeling down. Although she'd like to organize the house, she has difficulty concentrating and can't seem to accomplish anything. Even the art classes she loves have fallen by the wayside. She feels worthless.

Like Genette, one in four women and one in ten men will suffer from depression in their lifetime. Two out of three depressed people don't get appropriate treatment because their symptoms are not recognized, blamed on personal weakness, so disabling that the person can't reach out for help, or misdiagnosed and wrongly treated.

Some people experience a few symptoms; others experience many. The severity of the symptoms varies as well. Seek professional advice if you experience several of the following symptoms for more than two weeks or if they interfere with work or family life:

■ Persistent sad or "empty" mood

clients, social workers are usually cheaper, easier to find, and they are frequently oriented toward problem solving and advocacy. All but three states certify or license social workers. Health insurance covers social workers more now than in the past but still less frequently than psychiatrists and psychologists. Thirty-two states require insurers to reimburse clinical social workers treating people who have mental health coverage.

Professional counselors have completed a master's degree, received clinical training, and passed an exam. Some counselors specialize, such as in treating seniors. Forty-two states credential professional counselors. In the past, insurers didn't pay for professional counseling, but a growing number of states (currently fifteen) require reimbursement of professional counselors treating people who have mental health coverage.

Marriage and family therapists consider the family as a whole, whether the problem relates to marital and family relationships or to a specific mental or emotional disorder. Most marriage and family therapists have a graduate degree in the field. The remainder are psychiatrists, psychologists, psychiatric nurses, clinical social workers, and pastoral counselors. Most states license or certify marriage and family therapists. Most insurance policies exclude marriage and family therapy from coverage, although this is changing. Six states require insurers to reimburse marriage and family therapists treating people who have mental health coverage.

Psychiatric nurse specialists are registered nurses who specialize in treating mental disorders. They often assist with drug therapy and electroconvulsive therapy and act as psychotherapists under the direction of a psychiatrist. Psychiatric nursing services are often dispensed in conjunction with physician services or to patients who stay overnight in a hospital or other institution. As a result, they usually aren't billed separately.

Pastoral Counselors

In pastoral counseling, the counselor represents a religious tradition or community and uses the insights and principles of religion, theology, and modern behavioral sciences to help individuals, couples, families, groups, and institutions work toward wholeness and health. Many pastoral counselors also receive training and mental health credentials in other fields, such as social work.

Interviewing the Candidates

It's very important to select a mental health provider you trust. Of course, you'll probably have to spend some time with a provider before deciding whether you feel comfortable, but you may be able to look for some characteristics at the outset. To shorten your search process, think about which criteria are most important to you. For example, if you are gay you might feel strongly that your provider have experience with gay clients.

Ask a potential provider the following questions to help you decide if he or she is the right person for you:

What is your education and what are your certifications and licenses? Make sure the provider has the minimum qualifications to practice. Some certifications signal advanced achievement but aren't prerequisites for a mental health provider.

With which hospitals are you affiliated? You may prefer a particular facility should you need hospital services.

What teaching or staff appointments do you have? Associations with universities or treatment facilities can yield insight into a provider's orientation.

How many years of clinical experience do you have? If a provider is relatively inexperienced, ask if he or she is receiving supervision.

In what settings have you practiced? Some clinicians have primarily private practices, and others see clients at a clinic or a hospital.

What type of clientele do you generally serve? You may want a provider who has experience with clients who are culturally similar to you or have similar mental health problems.

How long is an average appointment and how frequently do you usually see clients? You may want more or less intensive services.

What is your therapeutic style and what techniques do you use? For example, do you tend to recommend drugs for treatment? Are you active in your questioning? Do you use behavioral techniques like assigning homework or teaching relaxation exercises? Finding out about

- Loss of interest or pleasure in activities you used to enjoy, including sex

- Decreased energy, constant fatigue, feeling "slowed down"

- Feelings of hopelessness, guilt, worthlessness, or helplessness

- Trouble sleeping or sleeping too much

- Increased or decreased appetite or weight

- Difficulty concentrating, thinking, remembering, or making decisions

- Thoughts of death or suicide

- Excessive crying or irritability

- Chronic aches and pains that don't respond to treatment

Treatment can help about four out of five severely depressed people, often in a few weeks. However, severely depressed people may need encouragement from family and friends to seek treatment. For information, contact your family physician, your employee assistance program, the local health department or mental health center, or one of the national groups listed at the end

(continues)

of this chapter. Also, many university medical centers have special programs for treating depression.

While you are waiting for treatment to take effect:

- Don't set difficult goals or take on a great deal of responsibility.

- Break large tasks into small ones, set some priorities, and do as much as feels comfortable at your own pace.

- Try to be with other people—it's usually better than being alone.

- Do activities that may make you feel better, such as mild exercising, going to a movie, or participating in religious activities.

- Don't expect to snap out of your depression. People rarely do.

- Postpone important decisions, such as changing jobs or getting a divorce, until your depression has lifted or you can at least consult others who know you well.

- Remember that your symptoms are part of the depression and will disappear as your depression responds to treatment.

the style and techniques can help you determine if there's a good match between you and the provider.

Do you have any specialties? Some providers concentrate in particular areas, such as treating eating disorders.

Drugs and Mental Health

Medications have gained widespread acceptance in treating people with either severe or mild mental illnesses. Proven agents combat some psychoses, depression, and anxiety. Frequently, several classes of drugs can be used for any given disorder.

No hard-and-fast rules determine which drugs and what dosages will be most successful with a particular patient. Moreover, some patients try more than one drug before finding one or a combination of drugs that is satisfactory. If you have an unusually hard time finding an appropriate medication, enlist the services of a psychiatrist who specializes in the use of drugs for treating mental disorders.

Drugs aren't necessarily an alternative to psychotherapy—and some people believe that combining both treatments is superior to either one alone. This is especially true for people who don't respond to either psychotherapy or drugs alone. Furthermore, psychotherapy plays a role during the weeks it takes patients receiving drugs to respond to medication, helps patients deal with emotional turmoil and reluctance to take long-term medication, and addresses social functioning and interpersonal relationships, not just reducing symptoms.

All drugs have side effects, some more serious than others. In fact, some drugs—Prozac (fluoxetine) is an example—are popular because they have fewer bad side effects rather than because they succeed more often. Make sure your mental health provider explains the most common side effects before you start any medication. If you experience side effects, discuss them with your provider immediately and before you stop taking your medication—some drugs have to be stopped gradually to give your body time to adjust.

Many drugs used to treat mental disorders present a risk to fetuses. If you are pregnant or are trying to become pregnant, consider discontinuing medication, at least for the first trimester if not for the whole pregnancy. Also talk to your health care providers about switching to medications that are less harmful to fetuses.

For more information on medications, turn to chapter 7.

Reviewing the Options for Mental Health Services

Most people receiving mental health care live at home and visit their providers for care. In seeking quality outpatient mental health services, people can turn to private practitioners and public outpatient mental health clinics and organizations. For example, large university hospitals with mental health outpatient facilities and community mental health centers can be prime places to receive care. Also, some psychiatric clinics operate under the auspices of general hospitals, mental hospitals, and family-service agencies. General hospitals often provide psychiatric treatment in emergency rooms.

If you decide to seek professional help for yourself, you'll encounter not only diverse providers but also a broad—perhaps bewildering—array of services. Indeed, your choice of a mental health provider can depend on the service you feel is right for you.

The first step in mental health treatment is a psychiatric examination—a systematic look at your emotional state and mental functions. Based on this exam and your history, the examiner will make a provisional diagnosis and recommend certain services and treatments. You might receive the following services as an outpatient or as part of an inpatient or residential program:

Individual psychotherapy. Treatment of mental and emotional disorders based primarily on communication between a client and a provider.

Group psychotherapy. Application of psychotherapy to a group, usually six to eight people. The interactions in the group provide some of the material for the therapy.

Family therapy. Treatment of two or more family members in the same session. This approach assumes that a mental disorder in one person may relate to a disorder in other members of the family and affect how they all interact and function.

Self-help and peer groups. Troubled people with a common problem helping one another through personal and group support. Self-help groups exist for many common mental disorders and in many communities.
For more information on self-help groups, turn to chapter 22.

Psychoeducation. Education to promote behavioral changes, such as educational counseling to prevent AIDS.

TIP
Check It Out

If you want to know if a provider is a member in good standing, contact the relevant professional association. Associations will not tell you if there have been complaints against a provider, but they will usually tell you if a practitioner has been expelled or suspended. For example, call or write the American Psychological Association for information about psychologists. Also check with the state board that examines and certifies your provider. Psychiatrists, clinical psychologists, and clinical social workers may all have different licensing bodies.

14

TIP
Putting It Together

Your options for mental health services aren't necessarily mutually exclusive. Many people combine two or more, either concurrently or sequentially, to create a personalized treatment package.

TIP
Workplace Help

Employee assistance programs (EAPs) can help with personal concerns of employees—such as health, marriage, family, stress, financial matters, alcohol or drug abuse, or emotional issues. Many employers sponsor work-based EAPs that provide confidential assessment and referral services, including follow-up services in many cases. Frequently, employees can reach EAPs by phone twenty-four hours a day. Ask your personnel department for information.

Psychoanalysis

Based on the theory that repressing memories of painful or undesirable events influences mental health, psychoanalysis attempts to elicit past emotional experiences. Psychoanalysis is an intensive treatment that strives to resolve patients' conflicts. Even patients who don't suffer from mental illness often use it to gain insight into their personality and behavior.

Psychoanalysis differs from psychoanalytic psychotherapy, which uses some of the same principles to reduce symptoms and improve functioning. Psychoanalytic psychotherapy undertakes less profound personality changes and emphasizes the person's life situation rather than the relation between the analyst and patient.

Services for People with Severe Mental Illnesses

Many mental health services focus on severely ill people. Some services are offered on a short-term basis, while others last indefinitely to help the person continue to live in the community rather than in an institution. These services are generally available through the state or local department of mental health, as part of follow-up care after a person leaves a hospital, or from a local mental health organization.

In-home mental health services. Assistance in such areas as activities of daily life, budgeting, managing behavior, respite services, and responding to a crisis.

Drop-in programs. Members discuss mutual concerns without feeling stigmatized. They also socialize and enjoy refreshments. At some drop-in centers, professional staff offer counseling, provide information and referrals, and conduct educational and recreational activities on a scheduled or ad hoc basis.

Crisis stabilization. Nonresidential professionals are on call in the event of a crisis. Programs may offer hotlines—to prevent suicide, for example—and staff who provide in-home services.

Adult protective services. Government-sponsored services available to people with mental health or physical conditions that keep them from managing their own affairs or protecting themselves from exploitation. Protective services clients have no guardian, relative, or other person available to assist them.

Case management. An assessment of a person's need for services, plus coordination, planning, and follow-through on the provision of those services.

Many programs for people with severe mental illnesses help them learn critical skills. These programs focus on such topics as:

Independent living. One-on-one or group instruction in cooking, the use of leisure time, money management, meal planning, housecleaning, obtaining needed services from the community, and so on.

Health and hygiene. Instruction in nutrition, relaxation, physical fitness, grooming, clothing, sexuality, self-care, and use of medication.

Problem solving and alternative coping. Instruction on how to identify a problem, devise a set of options, and then decide what to do.

Job-related skills. Instruction to help trainees understand the meaning, value, and demands of work; training in identifying sources of job leads, writing a resume, and interviewing; and actual job placement using leads provided by counselors who identify the best options and help clients develop realistic expectations and deal with stress.

Transitional employment. Entry-level, part-time, or full-time jobs, with clients and program staff cooperating until both feel the client can handle the job successfully.

Supported employment. Part-time or full-time jobs in the community that receive less staff backup than transitional employment.

Family Aids

Some services for people with severe mental illness target families and other caregivers:

■ *Respite care:* Temporary relief for the caregiver from some tasks. For a short time, the person with mental illness gets assistance at home or in a residential facility.

■ *Behavioral family management:* Education for the families of people with mental illness about mental disorders, treatments, communication skills, and problem solving. The goals are to meet the needs of families and involve them in treatment and rehabilitation.

Hospitalization and Residential Alternatives

People with more severe mental illnesses and those who need intensive, long-term treatment might receive inpatient care—twenty-four-hour care in an institution. Sites for such care include state or county mental hospitals, private psychiatric hospitals, and psychiatric wards or scattered beds in general hospitals or Veterans Affairs medical centers.

Hospital care is generally a last resort, used on a short-term basis to stabilize a person's condition so that he or she can return to a less restrictive environment. Nursing homes provide long-term residential care for those who either have a physical condition requiring twenty-four-hour nursing care or whose mental condition (as specified by law for such conditions as Alzheimer's and dementia) requires a specialized setting and services, while not requiring continuous active mental health treatment.

For more information on nursing homes, turn to chapter 15.

The following types of residential care represent differing levels of patient independence and professional oversight:

Community residences, including halfway houses, group homes, and boarding houses all are nonmedical facilities with three or more beds and overnight or round-the-clock staffing. Clients receive room, board, supervision, and some supportive or rehabilitative services. The most common forms of in-house mental health care are individual therapy, group counseling, group meetings, and recreational services. Other services may include remedial and basic education, training in the skills of daily living, prevocational and vocational training, social services, medication monitoring, nursing services, and case management.

Fairweather lodges are long term, unstaffed living arrangements that are affiliated with a business that provides jobs and job training for residents.

Supportive community living ranges from supervised apartments with twenty-four-hour live-in staff and semisupervised apartments with part-time live-in staff to cluster apartments in which clients live close to one another and cooperatives in which clients share an apartment with staff available on-call. The supports can range from service planning and intervening when a person behaves inappropriately to providing meals and transportation.

Foster care families provide room, board, and minimal services to one or more individuals in the family's home. Sometimes mental health professionals supervise and back up the foster-care family. Family foster care is also known as, or available as part of, substitute family care, alternate homes, home care, family care, alternate families, community living, community residential care, supportive living, and cooperative living.

Partial Hospitalization

Partial-hospitalization programs provide a set of coordinated clinical services for people with a significant psychiatric, emotional, or behavioral disorder. Partial hospitalization offers three or more hours of programming daily.

Treatment includes such services as individual and group psychotherapy, medication evaluation, family and expressive therapies, and psychoeducational therapy groups as well as other therapeutic activities, including cooking, budgeting, personal hygiene, and recreation.

Emergencies and Hospitals

In case of a crisis—when a person is violent or suicidal, for example—a hospital emergency room can be the appropriate place to seek help.

Some hospitals are better equipped to deal with mental health emergencies than others. If you help care for someone who might require such services in the future, investigate now which hospitals can best handle the person's problem. And keep handy the phone numbers of whoever has been providing mental health treatment so you can call in case of an emergency.

Money Matters

As with other forms of medical care, there are a variety of ways to pay the bills, control expenses, and get financial assistance. And even if you don't have private insurance or qualify for public assistance, you can often obtain public mental health services at little or no cost. Many of the organizations listed in this chapter can provide information about such options. Private practitioners may offer a sliding-scale fee that takes into consideration your ability to pay.

Insurance and Mental Health

If you are shopping for health insurance or choosing among plans offered by your employer, check the mental health coverage of the

Children and Adolescents

Children and adolescents receive many of the same mental health services as adults, and their systems of care are largely parallel. For example, specialized psychiatric hospitals treat children and adolescents, community residences for children and adolescents provide therapeutic residential care for small groups, and therapeutic foster care places children with emotional disturbances with trained foster parents.

Some services focus on children and adolescents:

■ *Family-based treatment:* Surrogate families ("professional parents") maintain and treat severely emotionally disturbed youths in their homes.

■ *Family support:* Parent education, support groups, advocacy training, respite care, and after-school care help families care for their own emotionally disturbed child.

■ *Home care:* Families of children and adolescents with emotional disturbances get support in the home, such as help supervising the child and education in parenting and administering medications.

available policies. Some plans don't cover mental health, and those that do may deny some or even most benefits or make them prohibitively expensive to actually use.

When assessing the mental health coverage of any insurance policy, ask:

What does the plan cover? Does it include a broad range of treatments, such as partial hospitalization and residential services? Does it cover family counseling, substance abuse counseling, children's mental health? Inpatient care? Outpatient care?

What criteria does the plan use to exclude people from mental health benefits? Some policies don't cover conditions you have before you join the plan; other policies won't provide mental health benefits to anyone who has *ever* used mental health services. Still other policies restrict or exclude benefits for specific disorders, such as attention deficit disorder for children or chronic schizophrenia for adults.

Is there an extra premium for mental health coverage? Whether or not it's assessed separately, insurance plans with mental health coverage generally cost more.

What are the annual or lifetime limits on mental health benefits? For example, a plan may allow twenty outpatient psychotherapy visits each year, or it may cover 120 days lifetime maximum of inpatient treatment. Are your needs likely to exceed such limits? Treatment for difficult life events, such as divorce or work stress, tends to be short. But severe mental disorders, such as depression, can require prolonged and expensive care. Effective in 1998, federal law prohibits insurance plans from imposing a different limit for mental health than for other medical conditions.

What types of providers does the plan cover? For example, would it cover a visit to a clinical social worker? Are there different limits for different providers?

How do you get care? Does a physician or other "gatekeeper" need to give you authorization *before* you receive mental health treatment? Will care be subject to review during treatment to obtain approval to continue it?

If you belong to an HMO, PPO, or other managed care plan, find out how you'll get mental health care. For example, you may receive care from a primary care physician or have to see a primary care physician first for a referral to a mental health specialist.

Learn about the quality of mental health services a managed care plan offers:

How quickly can you get mental health care? Does the health plan offer a toll-free access number twenty-four hours a day? Does it require providers to offer acute care for a crisis, such as a paralyzing depression, within six hours? Less immediate care, such as for a major marital dispute, within twenty-four hours? Routine care within seventy-two hours? And theory may differ from reality: How long is the *actual* wait for a mental health appointment?

How large is the provider network? Can you receive care within thirty minutes of home or work? Are enough providers in the network to allow you a real choice?

How specialized is the provider network? Do you have access to enough specialists to ensure high-quality care for special needs, from schizophrenia to anorexia nervosa?

Is there any coverage for providers who aren't part of the network?

Does the plan have providers who meet your language and cultural needs?

Does the plan regularly monitor and strengthen its mental health services using:

■ *Consumer satisfaction surveys:* A sample of patients should receive a survey after they receive treatment. Check whether the plan pays its providers partially based on consumer satisfaction ratings.

■ *Questionnaires to determine what treatment is provided for specific conditions:* This practice helps members know that the treatment they receive is accepted and valid.

■ *Measures of the outcome of care:* Investigate whether the health plan tells consumers its record on the results of treatment.

■ *Educational tools:* Ask if the health plan continually educates its staff. Plans that participate in the Consortium for Clinical Excellence have access to a national program to help clinicians stay abreast of treatments for specific conditions.

■ *Risk-factor-specific programs:* These programs help youths cope with a specific risk, such as parental divorce, school transition, or gang violence.

In addition, schools often have counselors and health clinics that address mental health problems. Some before-school and after-school programs are also connected to school systems. The child welfare system and the juvenile justice system may provide services—such as respite care and psychiatric evaluations—for children and adolescents with mental or emotional problems. And some suicide-prevention programs are based in schools.

For more information on health care for children, turn to chapter 8.

TIP

Reimbursement

If you qualify for Medicaid or Medicare, ask your provider if she or he accepts Medicaid and Medicare reimbursement as payment in full.

Insurance Copayments

Check the copayments on policies you consider. Policies may subject mental health treatment to a different copayment than other health services, and copayments typically increase with the length of treatment. And check whether copayments for mental health services are applied to your overall annual deductible. Is there a ceiling on out-of-pocket payments?

If Your Insurance Doesn't Cover Mental Health

Federal and state programs can pay for some mental health treatment for some people. If you are receiving cash assistance from the government, such as Aid to Families with Dependent Children or Supplemental Security Income, you are automatically eligible for Medicaid if you have no health insurance, and most states offer some Medicaid coverage to low-income, medically needy persons.

Medicaid covers outpatient and inpatient general hospital services, physician services, and Early and Periodic Screening, Diagnosis, and Treatment (EPSDT). In many states, it also includes rehabilitative and clinic services, prescriptions, services by practitioners other than physicians, inpatient psychiatric hospital services for children, and services in institutions for mental diseases for children and the elderly.

Most people over sixty-five receive Medicare, which is available to those eligible for Social Security and others with specified conditions. Medicare Part A provides coverage for hospital inpatient care, with lifetime limits, deductibles, and copayments. Part B covers some outpatient mental health services, although you pay half the bill.

For more information on Medicare and Medicaid, turn to chapters 4 and 11.

Medical schools often operate large outpatient clinics that provide mental health services and may be part of a local, county, or state mental health system. These clinics may base their bills partly on your income or accept reimbursement by Medicare or Medicaid. Community mental health centers and community health centers also base their bills partly on your income or accept reimbursement from Medicare or Medicaid.

Consumer Alert: Insurance Un-Coverage

Not every insurance policy covers mental health care. And even if your policy includes more than the minimum coverage for mental health, it may limit benefits in other ways. For example, your insurance may cover only a few visits to a mental health provider, or you may have to pay a higher proportion of the bill yourself than for other health care.

More and more policies that ostensibly allow you a relatively large number of visits may apply very stringent review procedures. In other words, your providers may need to justify your need for services after just a few visits.

What Can You Pay?

If you don't have insurance coverage, ask yourself how much you're prepared to pay. Bear in mind that you can get some mental health care in many communities at little or no cost from public or nonprofit agencies.

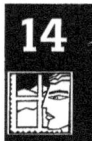

The Rights of Mental Patients

If you have a mental illness, you don't give up your rights. Some legal rights apply specifically to people receiving mental health care, while most belong to every patient—and every citizen. Remember, however, that laws vary among the states, and the courts are constantly refining the interpretation and breadth of your rights.

For more information on patient rights, turn to chapter 3.

Your rights include:

The right to refuse treatment. Except in limited circumstances, adults can refuse any mental health treatment. This includes the right to refuse medication or painful techniques to change behavior, such as electroshock therapy. This is based on the principle that your informed consent is necessary before any medical treatment can begin.

There are two exceptions to bars on forced medication: to prevent serious harm to the patient or to others in an emergency situation in an institution and to treat a patient who has been declared legally incompetent by a court.

Inpatient psychiatric treatment can be required for a person who is dangerous to himself or herself or to others. However, procedural due process is required *before* an adult can be hospitalized without his or her consent. A person can be detained in an emergency, but most states require a commitment hearing within two to four days. As at any civil hearing, a person is entitled to an attorney and must be allowed to cross-examine witnesses, get an independent evaluation, and see relevant information such as medical records.

If you are receiving mental health services, you also have:

The right to treatment. Institutionalized mental patients have a right to treatment. In many states, this includes the right to an individualized treatment plan and treatment that meets professionally accepted standards in the least restrictive setting possible.

The right to protection from intrusive and hazardous procedures, such as forced sterilization, and from harm, such as corporal punishment or unsanitary conditions.

The right to communicate with relatives, friends, and counsel.

The right to confidentiality and access to records. Just like other medical records, psychiatric records are confidential. Without a court order, they can't be disclosed to people not involved in your treatment without the informed consent of you or your guardian. Conversely, you are entitled to know the content of your records.

The right to control your own assets. Mental patients are presumed to be capable of handling their own funds.

Leaving Can Be Difficult

Legally, people who voluntarily enter inpatient facilities can discharge themselves at any time. However, getting out is often hard. Inpatients who express an intention to leave can be threatened with civil commitment as a way of deterring them from exercising this right.

If Someone Is Mistreated in the Mental Health System . . .

In every state the federal government funds Protection and Advocacy programs for individuals with mental illness. Contact your state's P&A agency for assistance or to complain about abuse, neglect, or rights violations.

To locate your state P&A agency, call the National Association of Protection and Advocacy Systems at (202) 408-9514.

Discrimination

The Americans with Disabilities Act (ADA) prohibits discrimination against disabled people, including those with mental disabilities. The act also requires employers to make reasonable accommodations for people with disabilities.

A number of organizations can help you learn about, and protect, your rights under the ADA:

■ *The Job Accommodation Network* specializes in responding to employment discrimination. Call (800) 526-7234.

■ *The Disability Rights Education and Defense Fund* specializes in combating discrimination in public accommodations and by state and local governments. It operates an ADA Hotline: (800) 466-4232.

■ *The ADA Information Center* of the Disability and Business Technical Assistance Centers provides general information about rights under the ADA. Call (800) 949-4232.

Resources
Organizations

American Association for Marriage and Family Therapy
1100 17th Street, N.W.
Washington, DC 20036
(202) 452-0109
For referrals: (800) 374-2638
Call or write for a list of marriage and family counselors in your area and a copy of their consumer pamphlet.

American Group Psychotherapy Association
25 E. 21st Street
New York, NY 10010
(212) 477-2677
Contact AGPA to locate a state association that can provide local referrals.

American Psychiatric Association
Division of Public Affairs
1400 K Street, N.W.
Washington, DC 20005
(202) 682-6220
Call or write for information and referrals to local societies. Write for a list of publications.

American Psychological Association
Public Affairs
750 First Street, N.E.

Washington, DC 20002
(202) 336-5700
Call or write for referrals to local associations and a list of brochures.

Anxiety Disorders Association of America
6000 Executive Boulevard, #513
Rockville, MD 20852
(301) 231-9350
Call or write for information, literature recommendations, and referrals to professional treatment providers.

Center for Mental Health Services
Knowledge Exchange Network
(800) 789-2647
Call this federally sponsored toll-free service to ask about mental health and to order CMHS publications.

National Alliance for the Mentally Ill
P.O. Box 923
Arlington, VA 22201
Toll-free help-line: (800) 950-6264
This family support and advocacy organization for people with severe mental illnesses has a thousand affiliate groups in all fifty states and operates networks that focus on children and adolescents, forensics, religious outreach, and veterans. Write or call for a list of publications.

National Association of Social Workers
750 First Street, N.E.
Washington, DC 20002
(800) 638-8799
Call or write for referrals. Chapters in every state can also provide referrals, and the national registry is available in major libraries.

National Depressive and Manic Depressive Association
730 N. Franklin Street, #501
Chicago, IL 60610
(800) 82-NDMDA (826-3632)
Call or write for information, a catalogue of books, videos, and pamphlets, and referrals to their network of 275 local chapters and support groups.

National Empowerment Center
20 Ballard Road
Lawrence, MA 01843-1018
(800)POWER-2-ALL
(800) TTY-POWER (TTY)
Call or write to locate consumer-controlled alternatives to professional treatment.

National Federation for Societies of Clinical Social Work
P.O. Box 3740
Arlington, VA 22203
(800) 270-9739
Call or write for help with managed care, general information on clinical social work, or referrals to a state chapter.

National Foundation for Depressive Illness
P.O. Box 2257
New York, NY 10116
(800) 248-4344
Call for a recorded message about depression. Write for referrals and information.

National Institute of Mental Health
Information Resources and Inquiries Branch

5600 Fishers Lane, #7C-02
Rockville, MD 20857
(301) 443-4513
This federal agency supports research on mental illness and mental health. Call or write for a list of publications.

National Mental Health Association
1021 Prince Street
Alexandria, VA 22314
(800) 969-NMHA
This national organization performs education and advocacy through state and local affiliates. Write or call for free pamphlets, fact sheets, and referrals.

National Mental Health Consumers' Self-Help Clearinghouse
311 South Juniper Street, #902
Philadelphia, PA 19107
(800) 553-4539
Write or call for referrals to self-help organizations.

Publications

Consumer's Guide to Psychotherapy, by Jack Engler and Daniel Goleman (Simon & Schuster, 1992), $17.

"Depression Is a Treatable Illness: A Patient's Guide," free pamphlet available from the Agency for Health Care Policy and Research. Call (800) 358-9295.

The Essential Guide to Psychiatric Drugs, by Jack M. Gorman (St. Martin's Press, 1995), $6.99.

"Mental Health: Does Therapy Help?" in *Consumer Reports*, November 1995.

"Principles of Good Mental Health," pamphlet available free from United Seniors Health Cooperative, 1334 G Street, N.W., Washington, DC 20005.

15 Long Term Care

Peggy Denker

Peggy Denker researches and writes on long term care and other issues for Families USA. She directs *a.s.a.p.*, Families USA's grassroots advocacy network.

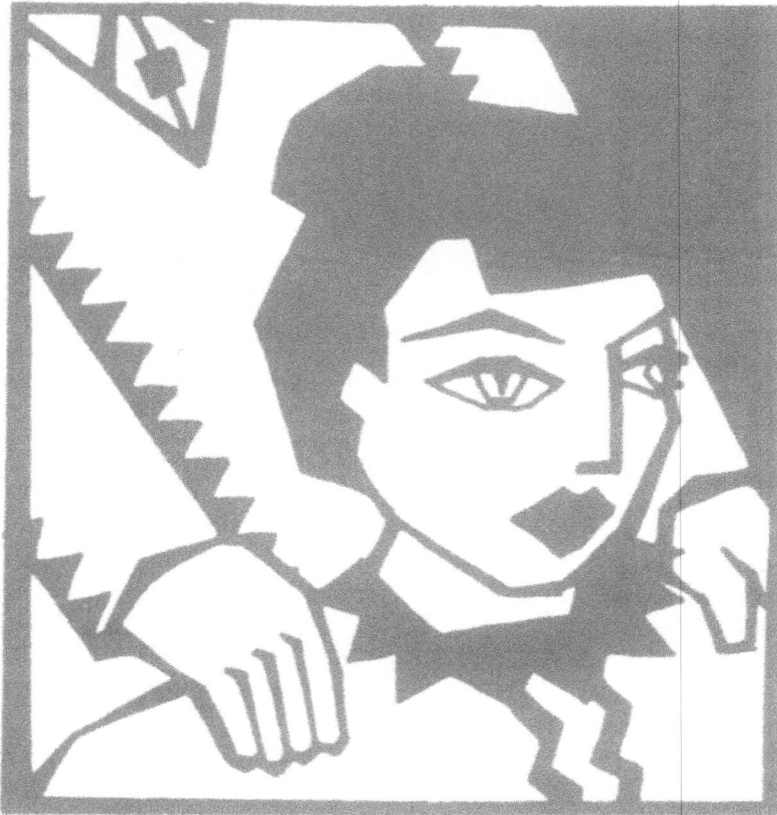

How Severe Is the Disability?

Professionals measure the need for long term care by looking at how well a person can manage certain tasks. Bathing, dressing, eating, going to the toilet, or getting in or out of a bed are called "activities of daily living," or ADLs. Other important functions necessary to independence—cooking, cleaning, shopping, taking medicine, paying bills—are "instrumental activities of daily living," or IADLs. The severity of a person's disability—and often his or her eligibility for assistance—is generally expressed in terms of the number of ADL or IADL limitations.

Over 10 million Americans can't perform one or more of these activities. Although people of all ages are affected, two-thirds of those with ADL or IADL limitations are sixty-five and over, and the likelihood of limitation increases dramatically with age. Fewer than one in ten people age sixty-five to sixty-nine have difficulty with even one ADL or IADL, but nearly six in ten people over age eighty-five do.

While ADL and IADL limitations are common measures of dependency, these aren't always appropriate yardsticks.

*J*oan Evans has had a stroke, and her prospects for full recovery are uncertain. Until the stroke, Joan had enjoyed a full and independent life in the town where she and her late husband had raised their children. Her children no longer live nearby.

Saul Miller was recently diagnosed with Alzheimer's disease. He had been living with his daughter's family—partly to save money but mostly to be a part of his grandchildren's lives. In fact, Saul often cared for the grandchildren while his daughter worked. Physically, Saul is robust, and his other children support their sister's determination to care for their father. But the mystery and tragedy of Alzheimer's confuses and frightens them.

Claudia Taylor takes care of her husband, Oscar, who has Parkinson's, but her heart condition has worsened, and she requires surgery. Claudia will need to recuperate in a skilled nursing facility after leaving the hospital, so she confronts two decisions. What kind of care can she arrange for her husband during her hospitalization and recovery? What arrangements can she make for both of them in the longer term?

What options do these families have as their lives change? How much control can they keep?

Because every family's situation is different, this chapter can't cover all issues in depth. Instead, the needs of these three families introduce you to issues and services to help you develop your own plan for long term care, a challenge most of us will face, whether for ourselves or someone in our family. Their situations can help you understand long term care *before* you or someone you love needs it. Or, if you have an immediate need for information, this chapter can help you find assistance now. In either case, it will guide your way through a complicated and emotionally challenging landscape.

Long Term Care: A Family Concern

Families caring for a loved one indefinitely are both consumers and providers of care. They struggle to assemble an assortment of services, often despite limited resources and funds. They care for loved ones, sometimes to the detriment of their own physical and financial well-being. And they turn to "respite programs," where available, to give themselves a breather from caregiving responsibilities.

What Is Long Term Care and Who Might Need It?

Long term care is just that: care provided over a long period of time to people who can't take care of themselves without assistance. The kind and amount of care depend on the nature and severity of the disability. Care can be as simple as providing occasional help with meals and running errands for an older person. Or it can be as complex as around-the-clock medical attention for someone with a serious illness.

Nursing homes provide long term care, but they are neither the only source nor even the major one. In fact, most long term care takes place at home, provided free of charge by family members who run errands, prepare meals, help with medications, and otherwise attend to the needs of a relative who has difficulty functioning independently.

Getting Started

Whether looking ahead or dealing with a crisis, you'll answer five basic questions as you develop a plan of action:

1. What kind of care is needed?
2. Who will provide care?
3. Where will care be provided?
4. What will care cost?
5. Who will pay for care?

For example, people with Alzheimer's disease may be *able* to eat or go to the toilet but forget to do so.

People are usually considered "severely disabled" if they need help with three ADLs. Many people who need help with two also require some form of long term care.

15

Plan Ahead

Arranging long term care, whether for yourself or a relative, is much easier if you plan ahead. If possible, start looking into facilities before you need them. The more time you take to thoroughly research and think through the issues you will confront, the more confident you will be about the decisions you make.

As you conduct your research, you'll find that some facilities and services aren't immediately available. Ask about placing a name on waiting lists, particularly if you anticipate a need for a nursing home. If your circumstances change or you decide on other arrangements, you can always withdraw the name.

The available services for long term care vary tremendously across the country, as do their costs and insurance coverage. By learning now what is available—and what kinds of help you or your family might need—you can make yourself a wiser consumer of long term care.

Question 1: What Kind of Care Is Needed?

The first step is to get a clear idea of what help is needed. Very ill people may require around-the-clock, highly skilled nursing care. But many

TIP

Be Organized

Keep track of the information you gather by putting it all in one place—a notebook, for example. Note the date and the name of the people with whom you speak, and take a moment to write down the most important points of each conversation. Use these notes to keep track of information and refresh your memory as you go along.

older people are basically in good health and can get by with someone who looks in on them occasionally and perhaps runs errands from time to time. To address this range of needs, begin by arranging for a comprehensive assessment of the physical and mental health and self-sufficiency of the person who will use long term care.

A person disabled by a serious illness or injury may need *medical care* or *skilled nursing care*. Make an appointment with the attending or family physician. He or she can tell you what kind of medical care is needed and how often.

Consumer Alert: Simpler Solutions

Keep in mind that medical professionals don't always consider non-medical issues and options when proposing a plan of care. And many of the medical services your doctor may propose can be provided in your home, a hospital outpatient wing, a health care center, or other facility.

Medical needs are important, but address them as part of an overall plan of care, taking into account your family's needs and resources. In fact, most long term care doesn't require special medical training. Assistance in getting to the toilet and preparing meals are typical aspects of caring. This kind of help is often called *custodial care*.

The plan you develop won't be static—you'll modify it as circumstances change. For example, rehabilitation can improve functioning, and that could lessen or eliminate the need for care. Or the caregiver may become ill and need to make alternative arrangements. It may be possible to manage Alzheimer's or Parkinson's at home in the early stages, but a different living situation may become necessary as the condition worsens.

Self-Determination

If you're planning care for another person, consider his or her wishes and feelings. And leave him or her free to make choices you might not like. Everyone dreads losing independence, and we're all entitled to as much control over our lives as is reasonable. If possible, consult your loved ones as you plan.

Question 2: Who Will Provide the Care?

Once you thoroughly assess needs, match them to the resources available. Start by deciding how much care your family can realistically provide: 70 percent of the severely disabled not in nursing homes receive all their care from family and friends, without the assistance of any paid services.

However, when care is needed at unpredictable times of the day—such as help going to the toilet—someone must be available. In those cases, the primary caregiver would have to work at home.

Both the cost and availability of services affect decisions about the family's role in caregiving. As you search for affordable, high-quality care, research alternatives thoroughly. This will give you the tools to construct the best possible plan, one that meets the needs of both the person getting care and the family. Careful research can also save you money.

Be Realistic: What Care Can You Give?

For the sake of the person needing care, as well as for the rest of your family, be honest about how much each person can do. Don't underestimate the difficulties of caregiving. It may be physically taxing and will certainly make substantial emotional demands.

Respite Care

If family members provide most of the care, investigate *respite care*. Family members may take a temporary break from caregiving with assistance from government or private programs.

Question 3: Where Will Care Be Provided?

Many people automatically assume that only nursing homes provide long term care, but that isn't the case. Long term care can also be provided in the home, in the community at facilities that people visit during the day, or in other family-like housing arrangements. Most people who are chronically ill, disabled, or infirm live at home. Most seniors in need of long term care—5.6 million people—live outside nursing homes.

Sometimes a family supplements the care they can handle themselves by hiring a person to come into the home and help out or by taking advantage of services in the community—senior centers or adult day care centers, for example. Many communities have volunteer and nonprofit long term care programs, and for-profit businesses have identified long term care as a market niche to fill.

In any case, the time may come when care in your home no longer makes sense. You'll need to make alternative arrangements if the dis-

Stay Involved

Family members often hesitate to place a parent or spouse in a nursing home. You fear that the nursing home won't ensure high-quality care. You may also feel guilty, believing you'll no longer play a role in your loved one's life.

In fact, families do stay involved, managing the selection of a home, dealing with the admissions process, and monitoring the care continually. You also consult with nursing-home staff and often retain financial responsibility. In fact, you're needed now as much as before: You provide the personal contact that helps transform a facility into your relative's new home.

The members of your family might arrange their schedules to visit on different days to bring news of the family and listen to your relative talk. Whenever possible, take your relative home for holidays and weekend visits or even for a few hours. Remind other family members to telephone regularly, especially on birthdays, anniversaries, and other important dates.

Some facilities suggest that family members not call or visit for the first

ability is no longer manageable at home, if no family members can realistically provide the care, or if the family can no longer cope, even with help from community services.

You may find a solution from the growing array of housing alternatives: retirement communities, congregate housing, assisted-living units, adult foster care. These facilities often provide some limited assistance to residents, such as meals or cleaning. But at times, a nursing home is the most responsible choice.

Who Are the Caregivers?

Thousands of Americans work all day, then go home to feed and bathe and otherwise care for their aging parents. Three-quarters of these family caregivers are women. Many wives, daughters, and daughters-in-law tend disabled husbands or parents around the clock.

Younger members of a family also may help out. Children may help look after a grandparent with Alzheimer's disease, for instance.

Most family caregivers spend at least four hours a day, seven days a week, providing care, despite the fact that one in three caregivers is also in relatively poor health.

Question 4: What Will Care Cost?

Even unpaid family care involves costs. When family members make a commitment to care for someone, they may give up some income or even jeopardize their careers. Other costs can result from remodeling a home to compensate for a disability; for example, your disabled parent might be able to stay in your home if you add a handrail in the bathroom and augment stairs with ramps.

Still, family care, even if supplemented with paid services, usually costs less than a nursing home. On the other hand, if someone is severely disabled and requires around-the-clock medical care, a nursing home may actually cost less. With these considerations in mind, you can begin to estimate the cost for a plan of care.

The total cost for paid services provided in the home or the community ranges from just a few dollars a week for someone to come in occasionally to lend a hand, to $200 a week for an adult day care center, to $5 to $20 an hour for a paid aide, to $50,000 or $60,000 a year for intensive home care. For a nursing home, the cost may be less than $20,000 a year in rural areas—or more than $60,000 in major cities. The average is around $38,000 a year.

Question 5: Who Will Pay for Care?

As you flesh out a plan of care, considerations of cost and reimbursement will influence your choices. What financial contribution, if any, can the family make toward buying needed services? Even if care is desirable, you may not be able to afford it unless you are reimbursed by private insurance or covered by a program such as Medicaid.

Medicaid is a federal-state program for the very poor. It is reserved for people meeting very strict income and asset levels, but the high cost of health care could consume an individual's income and assets so that he or she might become eligible for Medicaid.

Medicare, also a federal program, covers skilled nursing care and rehabilitation therapy in the home if it is provided by a Medicare-certified agency and a physician stipulates that the patient's condition is expected to improve. Medicare is the largest payer for home health, despite severe limitations on what it covers.

For more information on paying for care, turn to page 304 and chapters 4 and 11.

few weeks, to give the residents time to adjust. *This is bad advice.* Do just the opposite: Visit as often as possible. Residents are happier when family and friends visit regularly.

Nurses and aides may pay more attention to residents whose families visit regularly. And an occasional word of thanks and encouragement to the staff helps, too.

15

Consumer Alert: Check the License

If you locate a suitable program or agency, find out if it has the licenses and certifications to qualify for reimbursement from the relevant sources—Medicare, Medicaid, the Department of Veterans Affairs, or your private insurance.

High-Cost Care

Overall, nursing-home care is the costliest long term care, and sources of financial help are woefully inadequate. In 1992 the total cost of nursing-home care amounted to nearly $65 billion, and families paid nearly half that amount out of their own pockets. The Department of Veterans Affairs, Medicare, and private insurance paid only about 8 percent of the total, around $5 billion.

Medicaid paid the balance. In part, Medicaid's large share results from a sad irony: Nursing homes cost so much that the bills impoverish people who then qualify for Medicaid.

Finding Services

The array of long term care services is neither well coordinated nor fully funded, and not all services are available everywhere. Finding a full set of services is particularly challenging in rural communities.

TIP

Eldercare Locator

Call the Eldercare Locator at (800) 677-1116 for free information on services in your community. When you call, you'll be asked for the name and address of the older person for whom you seek information and a brief description of the problem.

In many cases, you can start with the Eldercare Locator. Operated by the National Association of Area Agencies on Aging, it can direct you to information and referral services in your community. The Locator can also direct you to your local Area Agency on Aging. Established under the Older Americans Act, these agencies provide information and referral services either directly or by subcontracting with another local group.

The Department of Veterans Affairs is a good source of information for veterans who need long term services. For your local VA office, look in the federal government section of the telephone directory.

Senior centers can also help you locate services. Religious service organizations, visiting nurses associations, and other volunteer service groups may have suggestions. And many associations (the Alzheimer's Association, for example) operate information and referral services for families that have a member with the disease. If an illness had led to hospitalization, you might consult the hospital's social worker or discharge planner.

Finally, ask everyone you know about services for long term care. In all likelihood, many of your neighbors and co-workers have been through a similar experience. Clergy may also be able to help. Any of these people may know of unique local services—grocery stores or pharmacies that provide home delivery, for example. What is more, they may give you information about the quality and affordability of various options.

Assessment Services

Assessment or *care-management* services can help you develop a plan of care, find services to carry it out, and monitor the care provided. The Eldercare Locator, your local Area Agency on Aging, and the National Association of Professional Geriatric Care Managers can direct you to care-management services in your community.

Your local department or office on aging, as well as nonprofit or charitable agencies, may also offer free or low-cost assessment services. Look under Social Services in the phone book. The local chapter of the National Association of Social Workers may be able to refer you to social workers who can manage and coordinate care. Hospitals run geriatric screening programs that can be especially helpful if the diagnosis is Alzheimer's disease. Independent social workers or *care managers* employed by local home-health agencies are also skilled in conducting assessments.

If there are no free or low-cost care-assessment services near you, or you don't qualify for them, expect to pay from $50 to $150 an hour or a flat fee of $75 to $300. The cost will depend on where you live as well as the scope and depth of the assessment. Be sure to ask for a fee schedule and for written information detailing what the fee includes.

Home-Care Services

Volunteers and paid professionals offer a wide scope of services that can be provided in your home.

Skilled medical care, such as that offered by a nurse or a physical therapist, can be arranged in consultation with your doctor or hospital. It is referred to as *home-health care.* However, many people who don't need medical care still need some assistance with daily activities. These services are referred to as *home care* or *custodial care.*

For more information on home care and home-health services, turn to chapter 16.

Personal-care services, such as help with grooming or dressing, may be available through volunteer programs or home-care agencies.

Homemaker or *chore services,* including household repairs, cleaning, laundry, cooking, yard work, and shopping, are available from many volunteer and paid sources.

Friendly visitor services provide volunteers from churches, synagogues, service groups, and other organizations to look in on and lend a hand to people who live alone.

Home-delivered meals—"Meals on Wheels"—can help homebound elders get nutritious meals even if they can't cook for themselves.

Loan closets are free, informal "lending libraries" of equipment such as walkers, bedside toilets, bath seats, and even wheelchairs.

Telephone-reassurance services are volunteer programs that periodically phone those who live alone to make sure they are doing well.

Respite care gives family members a breather from caregiving responsibilities while ensuring them that their loved one remains in good hands.

Support groups give families a chance to share their caregiving concerns and express their feelings.

Emergency-response systems link seniors to hospitals, other health facilities, the fire department, or social-service agencies through buzzers installed in the home or through a small push-button control worn around the neck like jewelry.

Home improvements, such as ramps in place of stairs, can help those who use wheelchairs or walkers to get around.

TIP

Care Managers

If possible, consult a care manager who is independent of the services he or she recommends. Care managers who work for agencies have an incentive to recommend the services their employers offer.

15

Younger People and Long Term Care

Not all people receiving long term care are seniors. About 40 percent of nursing home residents are between the ages of eighteen and sixty-four, while 3 percent are under eighteen.

Some younger people requiring long term care are disabled from birth; others are victims of accidents or disease. If you seek a nursing home for someone under fifty-five, ask facilities about their special programs for young adults.

Too often, younger residents have no one their own age with whom to talk. Traditional programs do little to meet the emotional needs of young adults, who must struggle in an environment designed for the elderly. Try to choose a facility geared to young adults or one that has young adult residents already.

For more information, call the Brain Injury Association at (800) 444-6443. Many young adults in need of long term care are head injury victims. Local chapters of the Arc may also be able to assist you. To find a chapter near you, call (817) 261-6003.

Community-Based Care Services

Most cities and towns, even small ones, provide a variety of community-based programs to serve people with disabilities and senior citizens and help them live in their own homes. Many programs offer services to people in need of care and to their families—services such as meals, counseling, and referrals.

Adult day care covers a variety of health, social, and related support services for adults who have functional impairments and need supervision. Adult day care can provide a chance for a person to interact with others, lessening the sense of isolation, and it can also offer a useful respite for caregivers. Adult day care centers often employ staff skilled in responding to the special needs of people with Alzheimer's disease. Be sure to inquire. These centers may provide transportation to and from the facility. In cities, the usual fee for adult day care is about $30 or $40 a day.

Adult day health centers offer skilled health services, generally rehabilitation therapy or other services specifically related to health care. These centers may also help with specific tasks that are especially hard for a family to manage, such as bathing. Medicaid may cover adult day health care. Your Area Agency on Aging can direct you to local services.

Congregate meal programs provide nutritious hot meals to older people in senior centers, schools, churches, and other community settings. A meal program may request a modest donation for each meal served. Congregate meal programs provide at least one-third of the recommended daily diet, as do Meals on Wheels programs. Contact your local Area Agency on Aging.

Senior centers, sometimes called multipurpose senior centers, are community or neighborhood facilities offering older people social and recreational opportunities and a broad spectrum of supportive services. Senior centers may provide health, educational, counseling, and legal services along with congregate meals. Many senior centers offer transportation to and from the facility. Senior centers may ask for a modest donation for some of their services.

Transportation and escort services take people to and from medical appointments, senior centers, shopping, and other local services. Some of these services, funded by the Older Americans Act, charge no fee (although they may suggest a contribution). Many local and state governments operate van or dial-a-ride programs for seniors or offer other forms of transportation assistance. For example, some counties sell vouchers that seniors can use toward taxi fare. Associations such as the Multiple Sclerosis Society provide transportation or offer financial assistance for transportation services.

Hospice programs assist people with terminal illnesses by offering comfort and controlling pain. Often sponsored by religious organizations, services may be provided in your home, in a hospital, or in a nursing home. To be accepted for hospice care, a person generally expects to live less than six months. Medicare pays for hospice care, and a few private insurance policies cover it as well.

For more information on hospices, turn to chapter 20.

Legal-assistance programs have attorneys who specialize in elder law, including reverse mortgages, Medicaid planning, and nursing-home insurance, as well as complaints about rights abuses. In addition, the local bar association can direct you to estate-planning attorneys who specialize in drawing up wills and trusts, planning for inheritance taxes, and dealing with guardianship for mentally incapacitated people.

For more information on legal services for seniors, turn to chapter 11.

Housing Options in the Community

A person needing long term care has many more options than staying in the family home, selling it and moving in with a relative, or entering a nursing home.

Senior housing or retirement communities feature apartments or town houses that are suitable for people who can care for themselves with little assistance. Some are rental units, and some are condominiums. Many of these communities include such features as bathroom handrails and electrical outlets at a convenient height. They may also offer meals, transportation, planned social activities, and other supportive services.

Assisted-living units offer private apartments. This option emphasizes privacy, independence, and personal choice and serves those who need daily assistance but not constant nursing care. These are also called *board-*

TIP

Senior Center Search

There are more than twelve thousand senior centers across the United States. To locate those in your community, call your local Area Agency on Aging or the Eldercare Locator.

TIP

Transportation Help

To find out what assistance is available in your community, call the National Transit Hotline, operated by Community Transportation Association of America, at (800) 527-8279.

15

TIP

Assisted-Living Resource

Consult the Assisted Living Facilities Association of America, 10300 Eaton Plaza, Fairfax, VA 22031; tel. (703) 691-8100. The association can send you a checklist of questions to ask providers.

TIP

How Old?

When looking into alternative housing, consider the ages of the residents. Some older people may be happy in a home with a wide age range; others may feel more comfortable with their peers.

and-care homes, sheltered housing, domiciliary care, or *adult foster care.* Assisted-living accommodations vary from single or double rooms to suites or apartments and are staffed twenty-four hours a day. Typical services include reminders about or physical assistance with meals, bathing, dressing, eating, medication, transportation, shopping, housekeeping, laundry, and other activities. Some assisted-living arrangements are strictly regulated; others aren't. Be sure to ask questions and get references because the appropriateness of facilities varies. Make sure that a home that claims to offer personal care or supervision actually does so.

A continuing-care retirement community is an attractive option for those who can afford it. These communities are unique because they provide a continuum of care, offering residents a long term contract covering housing, nursing care, and other services. Typical offerings include nursing and other health services, meals and special diets, housekeeping, transportation, emergency help, personal assistance, and recreational activities. Whether operated as for-profit or nonprofit enterprises, continuing-care communities have substantial entrance fees and monthly fees.

Congregate Housing

For many seniors who don't require constant supervision, congregate housing offers a long term alternative to "institutional" life in a nursing home. These residences integrate a cooperative living environment with supportive services on-site or nearby. In part because people share certain facilities—kitchens, for example—congregate housing encourages residents to socialize and support one another.

Nursing-Home Services

Contrary to popular belief, not all stays in a nursing home are long. Nursing homes are often used for short periods to recuperate from an illness or injury: 45 percent of people who enter nursing homes leave within three months. A long term stay in a nursing home is more often appropriate for a person with a degenerative disease such as Alzheimer's or Parkinson's.

Public programs and private insurance often classify nursing homes according to the kinds of care offered—skilled care or custodial care.

Skilled nursing care is twenty-four-hour specialized medical care for people convalescing from serious illness or injury. A registered nurse or other medical specialist provides the care. Medicare, Medicaid, and private insurance all cover skilled care under certain conditions:

- The patient needs *daily* skilled care
- The facility is certified for reimbursement by Medicare, *and*
- The care is provided under the orders of a doctor who stipulates that improvement is expected

Custodial care refers to assistance with nonmedical activities: bathing, grooming, getting in and out of bed, going to the toilet. Most long term care is custodial and requires no medical training.

To find a suitable nursing home, begin with a list of the facilities in your area—you may have to compile it yourself. Your doctor or care manager will have suggestions. And seek recommendations from the local Area Agency on Aging. Friends and neighbors may also have ideas.

Once you have a list of nursing homes, telephone to get basic information about location, costs, and services. Follow up with a visit to each facility that sounds promising.

As you tour a nursing home, ask questions. Speak to the appropriate staff person for specific information. For example, speak to the director of nursing to find out how the facility would manage requirements for specific care. Talk with the activities director for information on the activities program. Keep in mind that quality is the most important issue in choosing a facility.

Federal law requires states to inspect nursing homes periodically as part of the certification process for Medicare and Medicaid. The inspection results are on file at the facility, and you are entitled to see them. Ask a staff member to show you the survey report. You can also get a copy from your state's nursing-home inspection office for a small charge.

If you want to find out about health-and-safety violations at a particular nursing home, you can read the deficiency lists. These provide a detailed history of a nursing home's problems and the state's efforts to correct them. Keep in mind that some of the lists contain hundreds of pages. It takes patience and determination to fully understand these materials.

Some deficiencies are more serious than others. A facility with a lot of deficiencies may actually provide better care than one with fewer but more serious violations. When touring a nursing home, see if you notice any of the same problems that appear on the deficiency lists.

Inquire about the nursing home's policy on physical and chemical (drug) restraints. Who decides when restraints are appropriate? How closely monitored are residents who are restrained? Federal law prohibits nursing homes from using physical and chemical restraints on residents for discipline or for the convenience of nursing-home personnel. Restraints are only in order when necessary to treat medical symptoms or to ensure the safety of the person being restrained or other residents. Except in emergencies, physical and chemical restraints require written orders of physicians.

If you see residents with restraints, carefully question the staff about the nursing home's philosophy on the use of restraints. Ask what kind of activities and rehabilitation are used to keep residents restraint-free.

The Transition

A person's transition to a nursing or rest home can be eased by:

■ Frequent visits by family and friends
■ Family outings as often as possible
■ Providing comfortable, washable clothing with name tags sewn in
■ Providing a supply of writing paper and stamps
■ Arranging for subscriptions to newspapers and magazines
■ Encouraging the resident to participate in activities, *and*
■ Providing personal items to make the room as homelike as possible

Money Matters

Americans spend some $65 billion a year on nursing-home care and additional amounts for supplemental care in the home or the community. In most states, public programs (Medicaid, Medicare, the Department of Veterans Affairs, etc.) or private insurance pay a small portion of this bill—leaving the disabled and their families to pay the major part themselves.

While no one knows the full out-of-pocket costs for long term care, the overwhelming bulk of the money goes to nursing homes. With annual costs for a nursing home averaging over $38,000 a year, many older people face bills upward of $150,000. Unless you plan ahead, you could find your life savings wiped out. Nearly one-half of the total cost of nursing homes comes directly from the pockets of American families, a burden that is increasing steadily.

And the remaining half of the bill?

The Supplemental Security Income program covers six weeks of care in a skilled nursing facility for the elderly poor. This program, plus small ones operated by the states and private long term care insurance, account for a few percent of the total payments for nursing-home care.

Medicare, the government health-insurance program for elders, pays about 4 percent of the total. Aimed chiefly at insuring against major illnesses, Medicare only pays for nursing-home care under very narrow circumstances. Medicare only covers nursing-home care when needed to recuperate from an acute illness or injury. It *doesn't* cover nonmedical, or custodial, care.

Medicare pays for up to one hundred days in a skilled nursing facility for those who require daily skilled nursing care or rehabilitation services. The facility must be Medicare-certified. Medicare pays the full cost of the first twenty days in a skilled nursing facility and, in 1996, all but $92 a day for the next eighty days. After one hundred days, the patient or his or her insurance policy must pick up the whole tab.

For more information on Medicare, turn to chapter 11.

If your doctor discharges you from a hospital to a skilled nursing facility, be sure to find out which services Medicare will cover. Ask your doctor and your hospital discharge planner. If you have questions, contact the insurer that administers Medicare in your area. (The discharge planner can give you the phone number.)

The Department of Veterans Affairs operates 133 nursing homes; they served nearly 31,000 veterans in 1994. In addition, the VA paid for care in private nursing homes or state homes for another 47,000 veterans.

Veterans suffering from service-connected disabilities, former prisoners of war, and World War II veterans eligible for Medicaid are all eligible for VA care. For most other veterans, a complicated "eligibility assessment" determines if you qualify for care. If the assessment finds that your income is above a specified level, you must pay part of the bills for your care. Nursing-home care may be provided to any qualifying veterans *if space and resources are available.*

If you think you may qualify for VA nursing-home care, contact the nearest VA office or medical facility. They are listed in the federal government section of the telephone directory under "Department of Veterans Affairs."

The primary government program covering long term care is Medicaid, which pays nearly half the total cost. The Medicaid program, established in 1965 to provide health care to the nation's poor, covers care for those with limited income and assets.

The federal government and the states administer and finance Medicaid jointly. The federal government pays half or more of the states' costs and sets guidelines on who must be covered and what services must be provided. Within those broad guidelines, states have great leeway in determining eligibility and coverage, and specific features of the Medicaid program vary substantially from state to state. All states *must*

■ Telltale signs of good care in facilities

There is no charge for ombudsman services. To locate the long term care ombudsman in your community, call the Eldercare Locator or your Area Agency on Aging.

TIP

Shop Around

15

If you can, visit more than one nursing home and visit each one that looks promising. And also pay several visits at different times of the day to the ones that appear best.

Nursing-Home Residents Have Rights

♥ If you live in a nursing home, you have many rights under federal and state law. The facility must provide you with a written statement of these rights when you sign a contract.

■ *Services and Fees.* The nursing home must inform you about its services and fees in writing before you enter the home and periodically during your stay.

■ *Managing Your Money.* You have the right to manage your money or to designate someone you trust to do so. If you allow a nursing home to manage your funds, you must sign a written agreement and receive regular account statements.

■ *Privacy.* You have the right to privacy in all aspects of your medical care, as well as privacy in your room. The home must provide safe and secure storage for your possessions.

■ *Respect.* You have the right to be treated with consideration, respect, and courtesy.

■ *Visitors.* You have the right to associate privately with anyone you choose at any reasonable hour. You have the right

cover care in a skilled nursing facility for those who qualify for Medicaid under the "categorically needy" definition. These services, for people who need daily skilled nursing or rehabilitation services, must be ordered by a doctor and be directly under her or his supervision.

For those who don't need daily skilled nursing care, all states cover care in a state-licensed intermediate care facility or nursing home, either through the categorically needy or the "medically needy" programs. Medicaid will cover room and board, nursing care, and custodial care. Although the amount Medicaid pays for these services is less than the going rate for the facility, the nursing home *can't* charge the patient or family extra for these items. The nursing home may charge patients for materials and services not covered by Medicaid, such as a visit by a hairdresser or a dental hygienist.

Medicaid is a mixed blessing. For many seniors, it provides much-needed financial support for the staggering burden of nursing-home costs. Unlike Medicare, Medicaid pays for the less-specialized care most often needed—and does so indefinitely. Unlike private insurance, Medicaid doesn't require you to pay very high premiums for many years before you can collect limited benefits.

It has been estimated that about one-third of those going into nursing homes are already enrolled in Medicaid. Sixty-five percent of all nursing-home residents receive Medicaid at some time while they are in an institution. Medicaid is the only major safety net against the catastrophe of nursing-home bills.

And now the bad news. Medicaid is, in essence, a welfare program: You must use up your income and assets—impoverish yourself—before you receive benefits. If your spouse is not institutionalized, he or she is left with very little in assets or income.

Planning Ahead for Medicaid

$ If you think that you or someone in your family might qualify for Medicaid assistance to help pay for nursing-home care, get specific information on your state's Medicaid program. Do your homework early. What are the eligibility criteria? What is counted as income? As assets?

If you are not eligible now, are there steps you can take to receive Medicaid benefits later? Call the Eldercare Locator for a referral to help in your state.

Consumer Alert: Medicaid and the "Snapshot Date"

❗ Under the Spousal Impoverishment Law, Medicaid must permit the at-home spouse to retain a share of the couple's combined assets.

Unless you plan ahead, Medicaid will determine how much the at-home spouse can keep based on an accounting of total assets at the time of application.

Protect against this unnecessary loss of assets by asking the state to establish the total value of your assets *on the first day of institutionalization.* This is sometimes called the "snapshot date." Medicaid will use this higher amount as the basis for determining how much the community spouse can keep.

Consumer Alert: Medicaid Discrimination

Medicaid pays nursing homes less than do individuals who aren't on Medicaid. As a result, some nursing homes accept only "private-pay" patients. But even Medicaid-certified nursing homes often try to limit the number of lower-paying Medicaid patients by limiting the number of beds available for Medicaid patients.

When you apply to a nursing home, the staff will ask about your financial resources and your plans for paying for care. Some homes will demand that you prove you have the resources to pay for your own care at the private-pay rate for one or even two years, delaying the time when they might have to accept the lower Medicaid rate for you. This is illegal in many states and of questionable legality under federal law. Contact your long term care ombudsman to find out your state's laws.

In addition, some nursing homes insist that Medicaid recipients or their families "supplement" the Medicaid payment with contributions, gifts, or donations. Whether required as a condition of admission or continued stay, *this is expressly prohibited under federal law.*

If you enter a nursing home as a private-pay patient but then deplete your resources and qualify for Medicaid, a private-pay facility can transfer you to another nursing home if one is available. Medicaid-certified nursing homes must continue to serve patients, but many people encounter discrimination once their status changes. They may be transferred to less desirable rooms or denied services they once received. In some instances, Medicaid patients sit in separate areas of the dining room, receive different food selections, or aren't allowed to participate in the same activities. *Federal law prohibits discrimination in the services provided on the basis of the source of payment.*

If you or a family member encounter Medicaid discrimination, voice your concerns to the administrator of the nursing home. Make it clear that you are monitoring the care provided and that you know your legal rights. State your concerns clearly and forcefully, without unnecessary rancor.

to send and receive mail without having it opened and to use a telephone for private conversations at reasonable hours. The home must give you immediate access to family, friends, and any agency or individual who provides you with health, social, or legal services.

■ *Moving Out.* Living in a nursing home is voluntary. You are free to move to another nursing home—or to any other place. You can call a taxi or your family or friends to take you home. If a court has declared you to be incompetent, your guardian can authorize your leaving.

■ *Medical Care.* The nursing home's doctor or your private physician must keep you informed about your medical treatments and your physical condition. You have the right to see all your medical records, to participate in planning your medical care, and to refuse any medications or treatments. You also have the right to use your own doctor.

■ *Going to the Hospital.* If you must go to the hospital and you are paying for the nursing home, the facility must hold your place as long as you continue to pay for it. If you are on Medicaid, the law

(continues)

requires the facility to hold your bed for up to fifteen days.

■ *Durable Power of Attorney.* You have the same rights in a nursing home that you have elsewhere. You can make all your own decisions, or you can choose someone you trust to make them for you by signing a Durable Power of Attorney.

For more information on rights, turn to chapter 3.

If you don't get satisfactory answers, contact your state's long term care ombudsman. In addition, the Office of the Inspector General at the U.S. Department of Health and Human Services maintains a toll-free hotline for complaints about Medicaid discrimination: (800) 447-8477. Or write to HHS, Office of the Inspector General, Hotline, P.O. Box 23489, Washington, DC 20026. Or contact the National Senior Citizens Law Center, 1815 H Street, N.W., Washington, DC 20006; tel. (202) 887-5280.

Insurance for Long Term Care: Buyer Beware!

The insurance industry has developed special types of policies in response to public alarm over skyrocketing costs for long term care. Private insurance today pays less than 2 percent of the total national bill for nursing homes.

A strong word of caution is necessary regarding long term care insurance. Most financial experts advise against purchasing these policies unless you have substantial assets. The United Seniors Health Cooperative, a consumer group, advises seniors to skip long term care insurance unless they have at least $30,000 annual income and $75,000 in savings for individuals or $60,000 in income and $150,000 in savings for couples.

Many policies offer very little coverage for the services described in this chapter. Policies may also have exceptions for preexisting conditions or stringent medical requirements. Before *considering* a purchase of any long term care policy, examine it carefully and get a second opinion—including the advice of a lawyer familiar with the needs of seniors.

Criticism of these policies revolves primarily around high costs and stingy benefits. What's worse, so many insurance agents have been guilty of outright fraud and abuse in the sale of these policies that Congress has taken up legislation to clean up the long term care market.

If you are interested in a long term care insurance policy, look for:

■ Guaranteed renewability for life
■ A "waiver of premiums" provision that continues your coverage at no further cost while you're collecting benefits
■ Coverage of any level of care, from custodial care to skilled care without any requirement that hospitalization or skilled care precede the care
■ Coverage of Alzheimer's and other mental impairments
■ A deductible (also called a "waiting period" or "elimination period") of no less than twenty days, no more than one hundred
■ A grace period for late payments to guard against cancellations
■ No limitations on preexisting conditions, *and*

■ "Nonforfeiture provisions" that give you a partial refund if you cancel your policy.

What Now? Assembling a Plan

Now that you've read about the possibilities, let's revisit the three families who introduced this chapter and see how they meet their needs for long term care.

Joan Evans had a stroke. She probably won't fully recover, but a needs assessment determined that, with physical therapy, she'll be able to move on her own from her wheelchair to a chair or bed. Since Joan's doctor diagnosed that therapy will improve her condition, Medicare covers part of those costs. Her Medigap insurance covers a significant portion of the remainder.

For more on Medigap insurance, turn to chapter 11.

Although her speech is slow, Joan can make herself understood, and she retains all her mental faculties. Joan has begun therapy and regained considerable stability and strength. She'll receive home-delivered meals until she feels more competent in her own kitchen. Through personal-care services, Joan gets help with bathing every other day.

A borrowed walker from a loan closet lessens the expense of equipment. Through her local Area Agency on Aging, Joan learned about a volunteer group that provides some housekeeping. At present she relies on neighbors to pick up her groceries, but she is exploring alternatives, being reluctant to become a burden on their good will.

In short, Joan faces much uncertainty, but her stroke hasn't devastated her life. Although she doesn't expect to remain in her home permanently, the changes she faces are far less frightening now.

Checklist: Choosing a Nursing Home

The first question to ask is "Do you have an opening?" Many nursing homes have waiting lists. If you are not facing a crisis, get on the waiting list.

■ Is the facility clean, friendly, and attractive? Be wary of unpleasant odors.
■ Check the food service. Visit at mealtime.
■ Are the nursing home and its administrator licensed by the state?
■ If you seek coverage under Medicare or Medicaid, is the facility certified by Medicare and/or Medicaid?
■ Is the location convenient for family visits and visits by the family doctor? If your doctor won't travel to nursing homes—and many won't—what doctors visit patients in the facility?

- How many registered nurses, licensed practical nurses, and nurse's aides does the facility have? What are their qualifications? What is the ratio of these staff to residents? How does staffing change from the day shift to the night shift? There are no "right" answers to these questions, but they will help you compare one facility to another.
- How long have staff members worked at the facility? Rapid turnover often signals problems.
- What are the visiting hours? Is the family welcome at all times?
- What activities are provided for residents? Are activities challenging and tailored to the interests of the residents? Does the nursing home have special activities that engage residents with a particular disease such as Alzheimer's?
- Does the nursing home allow residents to keep some of their own furniture and to decorate their rooms?
- Does the nursing home require residents to sign over personal property or real estate in exchange for care?
- Is care coordinated with a health plan or an HMO?
- What is the "typical profile" of residents? For example, if you require temporary rehabilitation services and the home specializes in caring for people with Alzheimer's, it's probably not a good match.

Saul Miller, diagnosed with Alzheimer's disease, is fine physically, but he wanders from home at all hours and can be alternately combative and withdrawn. His behavior threatens his own well-being, and his family can't supervise him twenty-four-hours a day indefinitely.

An adult day care center with a special component for people with Alzheimer's offers Saul a program well suited for his needs. The center costs $200 a week, and Saul's children split the bill. His daughter's family can carry on with their daily lives. Saul returns to his daughter's home each evening, and family members share responsibility for ensuring his safety during the night.

Recognizing the progressive deterioration of Saul's condition, his family is exploring nursing homes, reserving a decision while they investigate more intensive home care. The family is reluctant to place Saul in a nursing home, but they have put his name on a waiting list in case this option becomes necessary in the future.

Claudia Taylor had to cope with the impact of her own heart surgery *and* the effect of her absence and poor health on her husband, Oscar, who had Parkinson's. Because Oscar's health was failing and she herself would have to convalesce for two months after surgery, Claudia placed her husband in a nursing home, knowing that his placement was permanent. After her surgery, Claudia recuperated in the same nursing home. After thirty days, she returned home. Medicare paid in full for her nursing-home care, but Claudia uses savings to pay for Oscar's care.

As the savings have been drawn down, Claudia has sought the advice of an elder-law attorney about getting Medicaid coverage for Oscar. The attorney has reviewed Claudia's financial situation, explained how Medicaid coverage of her husband would affect *her,* and advised her of her options.

Checklist: Before You Sign a Nursing-Home Contract

Obtain a copy of the contract and review it ahead of time in the privacy of your own home. If the home won't give you a copy, ask why not. And get a lawyer's advice.

Ask the nursing facility about any part of the contract you find confusing or unfair. If you make changes in the contract, both you and the institution's representative must initial them. If the nursing home is uncooperative, take an advocate with you to help negotiate.

Make sure the contract has no blank spaces and that it's fully completed and correct at the time you sign it.

A comprehensive contract:

- States your rights and obligations as a resident, including safeguards and grievance procedures
- Specifies how much you must pay each day or month to live in the nursing home
- Details the prices for items not included in the basic monthly or daily charge
- States the facility's policy on holding a bed if you temporarily leave the home for hospitalization, vacation, or other reasons, *and*
- States whether the facility is Medicaid- or Medicare-certified

The Special Needs of Alzheimer's Patients in Nursing Facilities

If you plan on placing a family member in a nursing home, keep in mind that most homes integrate Alzheimer's patients onto existing, nonspecialized floors. As many as 40 percent to 60 percent of patients in most nursing homes have Alzheimer's disease.

Only a few specialized units for people with Alzheimer's are available. Because these facilities are in very short supply and have admissions priorities, don't apply *only* to special-care units.

In examining a nursing home without a special-care unit for a person with Alzheimer's, interview admissions personnel about the facility and its programs. Trust your instincts as you seek answers to the following questions:

✓ *Does the facility acknowledge that it has other Alzheimer's patients?* Ask to speak with family members who have Alzheimer's patients there.

✓ *Is the environment simple?* Simple design and lower levels of auditory and visual stimulation are more appropriate for patients with cognitive impairments.

✓ *Is the environment safe?* Doors and windows should be secure, especially if the patient is a wanderer. Is there a security system to prevent wandering outside? An uncluttered space for the patient to walk?

✓ *What is the staff-to-patient ratio on all shifts, including weekends?* The generally accepted optimal ratio is one to six; the minimum is one to nine.

✓ *Do activities include the Alzheimer's patient?* Talk to the activities director and look at the weekly schedule of activities. Do activities meet the needs of cognitively impaired patients? Some facilities conduct parallel activities that benefit patients for whom standard activities are difficult. Is a staff person available to supervise activities on at least two shifts?

✓ *Does the staff address patients with respect or with condescension and scolding?*

✓ *Is there assistance at meals, and are special diets available to patients?*

✓ *How does the facility deal with unruly or inappropriate behavior?*

✓ *Do staff members talk with the family and let the family's experience help guide the care of the patient?*

✓ *As a patient's condition declines, is he or she moved to another area of the facility?* Moves should be kept to a minimum and are most appropriate when the patient reaches a severe stage of the disease.

✓ *What is the policy on the use of physical and chemical restraints?*

✓ *What is the procedure for care of a terminal patient?* For example, will the facility allow families to refuse feeding tubes or extraordinary measures for later-stage patients?

✓ *How and by whom has the staff been trained in the care of Alzheimer's patients?*

✓ *Who provides primary medical care for the facility?* You may want to interview these providers.

✓ *Who provides psychiatric services for Alzheimer's patients?*

✓ *What is the policy on visiting?*

✓ *Does the facility sponsor an Alzheimer's family-support group?*

✓ *Does the facility or its staff belong to the Alzheimer's Association?*

✓ *Does the facility have a written waiting list?* Will you receive notice when your turn comes?

✓ *Does the facility accept Medicaid after the patient's private funds are exhausted?*

✓ *Are there any additional costs (now or later) because the patient has Alzheimer's disease?*

—Adapted from *Guide to Nursing and Rest Homes in Massachusetts,* edited by Diane K. Goldman (Women's Education and Industrial Union, 1994)

Resources

For additional resources on long term care, turn to chapter 3 on consumer rights, chapter 11 on elders, chapter 16 on home care, and chapter 22 for general resources and organizations dealing with specific diseases.

Organizations

Alzheimer's Association
919 Michigan Avenue
Chicago, IL 60611
National Help-Line: (800) 272-3900
Caregiver Help-Line: (708) 933-1000
Call or write for a free brochure.

American Association of Homes for
    the Aging
901 E Street, N.W.
Washington, DC 20004
(202) 783-2242
Call or write for publications for caregivers and elders.

American Association of Retired Persons
601 E Street, N.W.
Washington, DC 20049
Consumer Affairs: (202) 434-6030
Social Outreach and Support: (202) 432-2290
Call or write for a free catalogue of AARP publications, many of which are free. Among the titles are "Care Management: Arranging for Long Term Care," "A Checklist of Concern: Resources for Caregivers," "Coping and Caring: Living with Alzheimer's Disease," "Making Wise Decisions for Long Term Care," "Nursing Home Life: A Guide for Residents and Their Families," and "Selecting Retirement Housing." AARP also maintains a database of retirement communities, with information on fees, services, amenities, sponsorship, and other factors. To obtain a list of communities in one or two metropolitan areas, write the Retirement Communities Database, Correspondence Unit at AARP.

Assisted Living Facilities Association
    of America
10300 Eaton Place, Suite 400
Fairfax, VA 22030
(703) 691-8100
Call or write for brochures, including a consumer checklist of services and information on assisted living.

B'nai B'rith International
1640 Rhode Island Avenue, N.W.
Washington, DC 20036
(202) 857-6600
For a small fee, the Caring Network Program will give you referrals to organizations that provide assistance and information.

National Association of Meal Programs
101 N. Alfred, #202
Alexandria, VA 22314
(703) 548-5558
Call for information on meal programs in your area.

National Association of Professional
    Geriatric Care Managers
1604 N. Country Club
Tucson, AZ 85711
(520) 881-8008
An association of private professionals who help caregivers identify needs and resources in the community. Call for referrals to local providers.

National Citizens' Coalition for Nursing Home Reform
1424 16th Street, N.W., #202
Washington, DC 20036-2211
(202) 332-2275
Call or write for a catalogue of publications on nursing homes, physical and

15

chemical restraints, and other long term care topics.

National Senior Citizens Law Center
1815 H Street, N.W., #700
Washington, DC 20006
(202) 887-5280
Contact the center for assistance if you encounter discrimination in connection with the Medicaid program.

Publications

Beating the Nursing Home Trap: A Consumer's Guide to Choosing/Financing Long Term Care, by Joseph Matthews (Nolo Press, 1993), $19.95.

The Complete Nursing Home Guide: Finding Quality Care for Your Loved Ones, by Mary B. Forrest, Christopher B. Forrest, and Richard Forrest (Taylor Publishing, 1993), $18.95.

"A Consumer Guide to Home Health Care," $4. and "A Consumer Guide to Life Care Communities," $3. Both are published by the National Consumer's League, 815 15th Street, N.W., Washington, DC 20005.

Consumer Reports, August, September, and October 1995. For information on ordering a three-part report on nursing homes, write CU/Reprints, 101 Truman Avenue, Yonkers, NY 10703-1057.

A Family's Guide to Selecting, Financing, and Asserting Rights in a Nursing Home. Published by the Center for Public Representation, 520 University Avenue, Madison, WI 53703. 1986. $15.

"Guide to Choosing a Nursing Home." Published by the U.S. Department of Health and Human Services, Health Care Financing Agency. Pub. No. HCFA-02174. Free.

How to Evaluate and Select a Nursing Home, by R. Barker Bausell, Michael A. Rooney, and Charles B. Inlander (People's Medical Society, 1988), $7.95.

"How to Pay for Nursing Home Care: Here's Help." For a free copy, contact the American Health Care Association, 1201 L Street, N.W., Washington, DC 20005-4014; tel. (202) 842-4444.

Long-Term Living: How to Live Independently as Long as You Can and Plan for the Time When You Can't, by Susan Polniaszek (Acropolis Books, 1990), $7.95.

National Directory for Eldercare Information and Referral. Published by the National Association of Area Agencies on Aging, 1112 16th Street, N.W., Washington, DC 20036. $40 ($30 for members).

"Nursing Home Insurance: Who Can Afford It?" (Families USA, 1993), $5.

"Nursing Home Patients Bill of Rights: An Illustrated Guide for Consumers and Providers." Published by the National Senior Citizens Education and Research Center, Nursing Home Information Service, 925 15th Street, N.W., Washington, DC 20005. Free.

"Nursing Homes: What You Need to Know." Published by the Maryland Attorney General's Office, Consumer Protection Division, 200 Saint Paul Place, Baltimore, MD 21202. Free.

The 36-Hour Day: A Family Guide to Caring for Persons with Alzheimer's, by Nancy Mace and Peter V. Rabins, M.D. (Johns Hopkins University Press, 1991), $11.95.

You, Your Parent, and the Nursing Home, by Nancy Fox. 1986. Available from Prometheus Books, 700 E. Amherst, Buffalo, NY 14215. $17.95.

Home Care*

Anne P. Werner and James P. Firman

Anne P. Werner is director of member and community services for the United Seniors Health Cooperative.

James P. Firman is president of the National Council on the Aging and the former president of USHC.

This chapter is excerpted and adapted from *Home Care for Older People: A Consumer's Guide*, published by USHC.

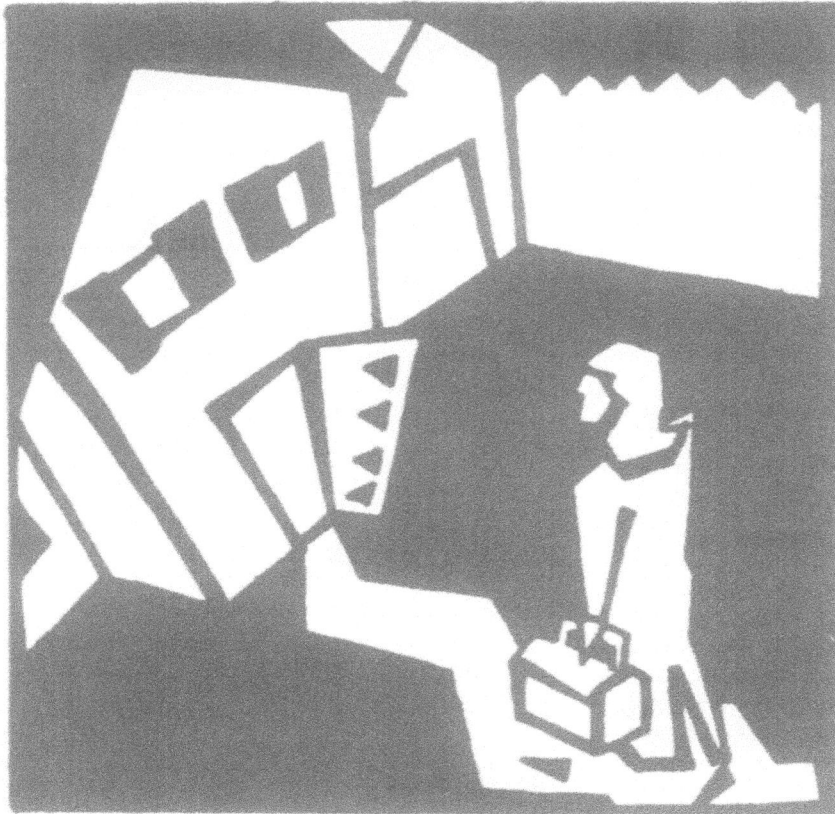

"Home Services" Outside the Home

In many communities, a wealth of services enrich the lives of people needing home care, as well as those of the family caregivers. Here are a few:

■ *Adult day care or day health centers* offer a safe, pleasant environment for people who can't safely remain at home alone or who can benefit from spending more time with others of similar age and interests. Day health centers also offer preventive care, health screenings, and therapy programs. Adult day care programs are a real health care bargain.

■ *Respite care*, either at home or in a nursing home, provides a temporary "vacation" for the family members providing care. This refreshes caregivers and can greatly reduce burnout. Respite care may be given by someone who comes into the home or by staff in a nursing home or assisted-living facility during a short admission.

■ *Home-delivered meals*, often called Meals on Wheels, are available in many communities at a modest cost. Hot and cold meals are delivered to a person's home, three to five days a week.

"**H**ome care." These two simple words encompass a wide and complex range of services. Home care can mean anything from help with the everyday tasks of living to advanced medical care. But the many kinds of home care all share one thing in common: They take place where most people prefer to be—in their own homes.

Whether you live in an apartment, a house, a room in your child's house, or a retirement residence, home care can benefit you when you are frail, ill, or disabled. The goal is to maintain or restore your ability to function well enough to continue living at home.

You *do* have choices. If you need care at home, you don't need to surrender control over your life and let others tell you what you must do.

Getting Started

As many as 7 million elders, plus millions of disabled people of all ages, need help with at least one of the five "activities of daily living"—bathing, dressing, walking, eating, or using the toilet. Even more people need occasional assistance with other routine tasks, such as grocery shopping, getting to the doctor, managing chores, and paying bills.

Home care varies to fit these and other situations. For example, after surgery, a physical therapist may visit you at home for a few weeks. As you recover, you may progress to much simpler needs that a home-health aide might provide.

Supplemental Care

Home care often supplements care that a spouse or other family member provides. A woman may not be strong enough to help her husband bathe, even though she can manage most of his care. Or the many tasks of caring for his disabled wife may be too much for a husband who has arthritis. In both cases, an aide can preserve the mental and physical health of the caregiver.

Who Provides Home Care?

Family members—mainly women—provide nearly 80 percent of home care. When your family can't handle the amount of assistance you need, or lacks the required technical training, you can choose from two types of outside home care: *home-health care* and *home-support services*. Sometimes these categories are distinct; on other occasions, they can blend into each other.

Home-health care is administered by professional practitioners. A doctor orders the care, and a registered nurse, licensed practical nurse, or trained rehabilitation therapist provides it. Sometimes, a medical social worker or nutritionist joins a home-health-care team.

Home-health aides, trained professionals or semiprofessionals, are also members of home-care teams. Sometimes called home-care aides, they assist nurses or therapists with such tasks as taking your temperature, helping you with prescribed exercises, and doing household tasks—shopping, cooking, and laundry.

Homemaker's duties overlap with those of home-health aides when it comes to managing a household. The homemaker normally does more extensive housecleaning, including dusting, vacuuming, and cleaning the kitchen and bathroom. However, homemakers aren't trained to check a pulse or assist with exercise routines.

Home-support services include all the other nontechnical services a person may need to continue living at home. You can get these from an agency or from an individual working independently. Sometimes volunteers help with certain tasks, such as transportation to a medical appointment or the grocery store. The various people providing home-support services include:

- Homemakers and home-health aides
- The person who comes to do heavy chores and yard work
- The aide or volunteer who handles paperwork, such as filing Medicare claims or balancing checkbooks

■ *Personal emergency-response systems* are often called Medical Alert Programs. A person wears an electronic device around the neck or wrist. When activated, the device signals a hospital or central dispatcher to summon assistance.

■ *Adult protective services* protect older and disabled adults from physical or mental abuse, neglect, and exploitation. Your Area Agency on Aging can tell you how to contact the local protective service. All health care workers must report suspected abuse, neglect, or exploitation. Whether you file a report yourself or on behalf of someone else, your identity will be confidential.

16

Living Alone

Women usually outlive men, so they are more likely to need home care at some time during their lives. Regardless of gender, people who live alone and lack a network of friends, neighbors, and other helpers most often take advantage of home-care services.

Assessing Your Needs

If you have been in a hospital, your doctor and hospital personnel will help you plan for home care. If you haven't been hospitalized, a variety of local organizations can help you assess your needs and figure out how to meet them. And if your requirements are relatively simple, this chapter may be all you need to get started.

As you prepare to leave the hospital and get skilled home care, your doctor should write a *plan of care* for you. Even if the doctor doesn't give you a formal plan, ask for written information about what you'll need—and need to do—at home. You'll have too much on your mind to remember everything, and written instructions will also help others who assist you.

Ask the doctor or nursing supervisor to arrange for a *discharge planner* to talk with you about arranging your home care. All hospitals have a social-services department to help you plan your discharge. In addition, about one-third of the nation's hospitals offer home-health services, either through their own staff or through an affiliated agency.

Alternatively, the discharge planner may call on an outside agency to provide services for you at home. In many cases, the agency will write your plan of care and present it to your doctor to sign. When your home-health care requires a doctor's oversight and a nurse's supervision, the plan will describe exactly what care you'll need, who'll provide it, and how often. It will also specify treatments, medical equipment and supplies, medications, and any special diet.

If the plan is complex, involving providers outside the agency, it should include a clear, written statement of who is in charge and who will do what, how often, and at what cost to you. One key question your plan should answer: Who assumes responsibility for coordinating all the care providers? Find out who to call if there are any problems with an outside provider.

If you don't have access to discharge services through a hospital, you can determine your home-care needs with a *geriatric assessment*. In addition to identifying your medical, nursing, and rehabilitation needs, this assessment will consider your family circumstances and lifestyle. How much care can you or your family provide? How safe is your home? How well does it suit your current needs?

A home-health agency can conduct this assessment. Normally agencies don't charge for the service if you are likely to become a client. If your case is complicated and your budget permits, consider hiring a private geriatric-care manager. Some long term care insurance will pay for or provide an assessment. As a less-expensive alternative, ask a nurse or social worker to advise you. The local Area Agency on Aging may direct you to these professionals.

For more information on the health care needs of elders, turn to chapter 11.

The Family Plan

Discharge planners and other home-care advisers can do a lot, but they can't do their job alone. Your input is vital to devising a plan that meets your needs and considers your preferences on timing, frequency, and manner of care. A good plan gives you, the client, the responsibility you wish to assume. And family members should take part in the discussion with the discharge planner or adviser, if possible.

When Home Care Is Not Enough

Family unity, health, and finances are all part of an equation that must be measured against the desires and needs of the person receiving care at home. While older people may fear going into a nursing home, they usually don't want to burden others either.

One way to deal with this issue is by convening a family council. It may also help to consult a member of the clergy, a trusted friend, or an attorney. And learn about the growing number of alternatives to nursing homes, such as assisted-living facilities. You may be pleasantly surprised when you investigate the variety of living arrangements offered in your community.

For more on long term care, turn to chapter 15.

Choosing the Right Providers

After surgery, you may need skilled nursing care. In this case, you'll look for a Medicare-certified home-health agency. On the other hand, if you are living at home and simply finding daily tasks difficult to manage, you'll probably look for a homemaker or a companion. If your requirements fall somewhere between skilled and basic care, three main sources of help are available: a home-health agency, a registry of nurses or aides, and independent workers.

Should you decide to use an agency, you'll receive more support than you will if you decide to hire help on your own. The care provided through home-health agencies often qualifies as *skilled care,* the type of home care that health insurance is most likely to cover. However, if you don't need skilled services, *homemaker* or *home-health-aide agencies* may fulfill your needs. These frequently aren't Medicare-certified but tend to cost less because they don't have to satisfy many regulations or hire highly trained personnel.

If you decide to use a registry or a private source instead of an agency, you'll be the direct employer, which gives you more control over the situation as well as lower costs.

Assembling Information

As you address the following considerations, suggested by the National Association for Home Care, seek answers from the home-care agencies themselves as well as from other sources, such as local organizations that advocate for elders. Base your ultimate decision on the balance of factors that suits your situation.

- How long has the agency served the community?
- Is the agency accredited?
- Is the plan of care written out?
- Does the plan make clear the purpose and amount of care deemed practical for the conditions being treated or served?
- What are the arrangements for emergencies?
- How does the agency protect the confidentiality of its clients?
- Does the agency describe its services, eligibility requirements, fees, and funding sources in writing?
- What are the financial arrangements?
- What arrangements will the agency make for you if you exhaust your reimbursement sources?

Selecting a Home-Care Provider—Who and What to Ask

What to find out	Home-Health Agency	Homemaker/ Aide Service	Registry	Independent Worker
Is the agency Medicare-certified?	✓	✓		
Is it state-licensed?	✓	✓		
What is its reputation?	✓	✓	✓	✓
Is home assessment available?	✓	✓		
How are workers supervised?	✓	✓	✓	
How are workers trained?	✓	✓	✓	
Is there an established complaint process?	✓	✓	✓	
Is there client input in the plan of care?	✓	✓		
Who handles paperwork?	✓	✓	✓	
Will the agency refer you to another source if necessary?	✓	✓		

The Job Offer

Whether you hire an aide directly or through a registry, prepare yourself to become a "home-care manager."

The job description. As the first step in hiring your own aide, write down exactly what you want the person to do for you. List all the steps that each task entails. If the aide will help you bathe, you'll want the tub cleaned afterward. Make the job description specific. How often will each task be done? How long should it take to do the tasks right? Outline a typical daily routine. Include the salary or hourly rate in the job description. If you don't know how much to pay, ask your Area Agency on Aging to suggest a fair wage.

The interview. Ask a prospective homemaker or aide:

■ *Where have you worked before?* Get the names and phone numbers of three previous employers and contact them.

■ *What were your duties?* Look for an aide who has had direct experience with the duties and conditions your situation entails.

■ *How long were you employed in previous jobs?*

■ *How long can you work on this job?*

■ *Do you smoke?* If you don't smoke, a nonsmoker is your obvious choice. If your best candidate smokes, consider how you might work this out.

■ *Are there any duties in this job that you feel you can't do?* A caring person may be willing to learn new tasks; an inflexible attitude indicates possible problems ahead.

■ *Would anything in your situation keep you from arriving on time?* You might prepare a backup plan if the aide cannot come due to illness or a family problem.

Making the decision. If you have several good candidates, you may base your final decision largely on personality: how do you feel about inviting this person into your home? Trust your instincts. After all, you must feel comfortable with the person who will spend time with you in your home.

Writing an Employment Agreement

This is a sample agreement between a person needing home care and a provider. It's based on a form developed by IONA Senior Services of Washington, D.C.

EMPLOYMENT CONTRACT BETWEEN

Employer_____   and Employee _____

Salary $_____per hour   Fringe benefits_____

Terms of payment: when_____   how _____

Hours of work: from_____to_____on_____

Changes in scheduled hours are negotiable.

Employee's Social Security Number _____

HOUSEHOLD TASKS:

☐ light housekeeping   ☐ bedmaking   ☐ cooking
☐ laundry   ☐ escort on short trips   ☐ taking out garbage
☐ errands & shopping   ☐ washing dishes   ☐ companionship & support

PERSONAL-CARE TASKS:

☐ bathing & grooming   ☐ dressing   ☐ getting out of bed
☐ getting around   ☐ feeding   ☐ diet planning & cooking
☐ exercise   ☐ medication reminders

SCHEDULE FOR DUTIES TO BE PERFORMED:

Household tasks: dust and vacuum once a week, mop kitchen once a week, change sheets once a week, wash laundry once a week, shop for food once a week, wash dishes after each meal

Personal-care tasks: assist with bath and shampoo once a week, transport to doctor's appointment once a month, provide some conversation, cook lunch

Nonacceptable behavior: smoking at work, using foul language, evidence of intoxication, coming to work late

TERMINATION

Each party will give two weeks' notice before terminating this contract.

Reasons for termination without notice include theft, failure to carry out duties, evidence of nonacceptable behavior, and endangering employer's health or safety.

For unsatisfactory work, the employer will give two warnings. If the work continues to be unsatisfactory, a termination date will be set.

Signed: _____   _____
                    (employer)   (employee)

Date: _____   _____

The contract. After an applicant accepts your job offer, prepare an employment agreement that you both sign. If you hire the worker through an agency, sign the contract with the agency rather than the individual. This document should spell out what the agency will—and won't—do. It should specify the duties of the worker, and how often he or she will perform them.

In some situations, you and an agency may share responsibility for selecting and supervising a worker. For example, a registry may do some screening and provide an orientation. As the employer, you may choose to use either a formal contract or a simpler agreement clarifying the expectations and responsibilities of both parties.

Managing Your Home Care

A home-care worker who comes to you through an agency will be trained by that agency and instructed to contact his or her supervisor about any health-related concerns or changes to the plan of care. Even so, this person works in your home, where you are the daily supervisor. And "employer" may be a difficult role for you when you are not feeling your best, especially if you have never employed anyone in your home before.

To understand the challenge of care management, picture a symphony orchestra. The conductor leads the orchestra through a piece of music, cueing in the strings, woodwinds, brass, and perhaps a soloist in a precise, synchronized fashion. Like the orchestra, a person recovering from a serious illness or accident may need a "conductor" with training to synchronize and coordinate a large array of home-care providers. Fortunately, specialists are available to help in this situation.

Home Care as a Vocation

Some people choose to work in home care because they like helping people. Part of their reward is knowing they are helping you live independently, recover from an illness or accident, or simply find some comfort each day. Others like the flexibility of working only a few days a week or a few hours a day.

That said, most home-care aides take jobs in this field because it is the best work available given their education, training, or language skills. The typical home-care worker earns less than $6 an hour and comes from a family whose total income averages about $20,000 a year. Home care offers low pay, few fringe benefits, irregular hours, and limited opportunities for advancement.

> **TIP**
> ### Care Manager Source
> Your local Area Agency or Office on Aging is the place to start gathering information on care managers. If the agency doesn't manage care, the staff can direct you to an appropriate source. If you can afford to pay for a care manager, the agency may ask you to do so.

16

Empowerment and Dependency

In an earnest effort to do everything possible for a spouse, parent, or other relative, families can do too much, robbing the patient of independence.

If the patient's mental faculties are not impaired, families should present alternatives, discuss the advantages and disadvantages of each, and let the patient decide. Because so many natural losses can come with aging, it's important to preserve the patient's decision making to the fullest degree possible. And take time to listen as well as to talk to the person for whom you are caring.

Even patients with the most debilitating physical problems can give something of themselves to others. A man who worked as an accountant may be able to keep his own books and help someone else as well.

You and Your Home-Care Workers

Managing home-care workers requires sensitivity. Tell aides what you like about their work. Let them know that you appreciate the small, extra things they do. Aides often make efforts above and beyond their assigned duties; recognize and appreciate this.

Be equally clear about problems. For example, if a worker arrives late often, ask if a particular situation is causing the tardiness. Would it be better for the aide to come later in the morning and stay later in the afternoon? Many people have a tendency to slide a bit in their work if they feel it won't be noticed, so speak up *in a constructive way* to deal with such issues early in the relationship.

If your aide comes from an agency, a supervisor should call periodically to ask you about the aide's performance. If this doesn't happen after a few weeks, call the supervisor yourself and volunteer your objective appraisal of the person's work. Use this time to work out any problems *and* to register praise.

Home Rules

Attach a list of "home rules" to the contract you sign with an individual or an agency. Give the rules to each person who comes to work in your home and post them where they can be easily read.

One man listed these rules:

- No smoking in my house, please. It hurts my eyes.
- Be kind to my dog and he will be your friend for life.
- Foul language offends me. Please spare my feelings.
- Please respect my belongings. They may not seem like much to you, but they are very precious to me.

Paperwork, Paperwork, Paperwork

For some people, the prospect of filing reports, keeping records, and handling tax payments is reason enough to use an agency for home-care workers. Others find the paperwork required of employers manageable once the initial forms are filed, and they appreciate the flexibility and control associated with doing their own hiring and supervision. In fact, people who are actively involved in their own care may recover more quickly and completely.

As an employer, you are responsible for making certain payments on behalf of each person you hire directly to work in your home, be it a nurse, an aide, or a person to help with chores. For example, you must report the wages and deduct Social Security taxes if you pay a worker more than $1,000 during a quarter. Also, you and your workers must agree on whether you will withhold federal and state income taxes from their wages. And your state may require you to pay into its unemployment fund.

How to Complain About Quality

If home-care workers or health care personnel come to you through an agency, you have several options should you need to register a complaint:

■ Large agencies generally have a grievance process. Ask for the chief operating officer or the person who handles "quality of care."

■ Call the Better Business Bureau if the agency's practices are unethical or if you think some type of fraud may be taking place.

■ If you receive care under Medicare Part A and feel that the care is inferior, you may ask the state "Peer Review Organization" to investigate. PROs monitor the appropriateness and quality of care. To locate your state's PRO, call the Social Security Administration at (800) 638-6833.

■ Contact your state's long term care ombudsman.

For more information on ombudsmen, turn to chapter 15.

Money Matters

For most people, the biggest challenge of home care is paying the bills. An aide for four hours a day, five days a week can cost from $8,000 to $14,000 annually. And you'll confront a hodgepodge of government programs that, even when pieced together, often leave big gaps in coverage.

Medicare

Most Americans over the age of sixty-five qualify for Medicare. In addition, some 3 million Americans under age sixty-five qualify because they have severe long term disabilities.

If you are enrolled in Medicare and require skilled care, this is the preferred way to finance your home care. Medicare will pay all of the

TIP

Applying for Medicaid

To find out if you qualify for Medicaid or to apply for benefits, contact your local welfare office. In some states, you can also apply at senior citizen centers and other locations.

Medicare-approved amount for skilled health services delivered at home under certain circumstances. You must be homebound, under the care of a physician who signs a plan of care, *and* in need of only part-time or intermittent home-health services. You must also receive the care from a Medicare-certified agency. Consult your local Area Agency on Aging.

For more information on Medicare, turn to chapter 11.

Consumers, Medicare, and Home Care

■ Medicare reimbursement doesn't depend on hospitalization. Your need for skilled services is the key.

■ Get your doctor to document your need for skilled services.

■ If you think your care is being terminated too soon, contact the local Medicare fiscal intermediary. Call (800) 638-6833 to find the appropriate organization.

■ Don't be afraid to appeal decisions made by the certified home-health agency.

Medicaid

Medicaid, a federal/state insurance program for low-income people, can be a viable option to help pay for home care. However, people must meet strict income and asset requirements to qualify for coverage. These amounts vary from state to state.

In many states, people with higher incomes can qualify for Medicaid if they have high medical expenses. Under these "spend down" provisions, your medical expenses are deducted from your income. This is how most people qualify for Medicaid's benefits for long term care.

Medicaid potentially covers five types of home care:

1. *Home-health services covered by Medicare.* If a person qualifies for both Medicaid and Medicare, Medicaid will pay the 20 percent copayment required for some Medicare home-health services, such as durable medical equipment.

2. *Home-health services covered by Medicaid only.* All states offer home-health services to people eligible for Medicaid. These services include skilled nursing, home-health-aide services, and medical equipment and supplies.

3. *Private nursing.* In twenty-eight states, Medicaid pays for extended hours of home nursing care.

4. *Personal-care services.* In about thirty states, Medicaid also pays for personal-care services under certain circumstances.

5. *Home- and community-based waiver services.* States can apply to the federal government for permission to offer additional nonmedical services. Some forty-nine states offer services under this program but often make it difficult to qualify.

For more information on Medicaid, turn to chapter 4.

The Older Americans Act

Your local Area Agency on Aging receives funds under the Older Americans Act to enable older people with frailties or disabilities to remain independent. Anyone sixty or over can receive services, which are directed particularly to people with the greatest social and financial need who could otherwise not remain in their homes.

Each area agency has a degree of flexibility in how it will meet the needs of its community's residents. Services fall into three major categories: home, community, and access.

1. *Services in the home* include homemakers, chore service, and meal delivery. You apply to the Area Agency on Aging, which may provide the service directly or through another agency.

2. *Services in the community* include senior centers, day health care programs, protective services, and legal counseling.

3. *Access services* include transportation to help older people travel to senior centers, medical appointments, Social Security offices, and shopping areas.

Veterans Home Care

Veteran Affairs Hospital-Based Home Care is available in a few communities. Veterans who are at least 50 percent disabled due to a condition connected with their military service are eligible. A team consisting of a doctor, nurse, dietitian, social worker, and physical therapist teaches a veteran's relatives or friends to care for him or her.

Private Payment Options for Home Care

If government programs don't suit your situation, you have several potential private options for paying for home care. Two important options are Medigap insurance and insurance for long term care.

■ While you receive Medicare-covered home-health care, you may be eligible for additional payments if you've bought a Medicare Supplemental Insurance Policy (*Medigap insurance*). If you purchase plans D, G, I, or J of the ten standard Medigap polices, an At-Home Recovery Benefit will include some payment for personal-care services. This benefit could allow you more time for healing or rehabilitation. *For more information, turn to chapter 11.*

■ *Private long term care insurance,* a relatively new type of policy, is intended to protect people from the catastrophic expense of a lengthy stay in a nursing home. However, until recently the home-care coverage of most policies was relatively weak, and the policies themselves are the subject of intense criticism. *For more information, turn to chapter 15.*

An excellent source of information on home care for veterans is the Veterans' Benefits Department of the Paralyzed Veterans of America. *For more information, call (800) 424-8200.*

Resources
Organizations

American Association of Retired Persons
601 E Street, N.W.
Washington, DC 20049
(202) 434-6030
Call or write for a catalogue of publications, including the free pamphlets "A Handbook About Care in the Home," "A Consumer's Guide to Homesharing," "The Doable Renewable Home: Making Your Home Fit Your Needs," and "Your Home, Your Choice."

National Association for Home Care
228 Seventh Street, S.E.
Washington, DC 20003
(202) 547-7424
Call or write for a list of publications.

National Association of Area Agencies
        on Aging
1112 16th Street, N.W.
Washington, DC 20036
(202) 296-8130
Eldercare Locator: (800) 677-1116
Call the Eldercare Locator for assistance in finding the most appropriate information source for home care anywhere in the country.

National Association of Professional
        Geriatric Care Managers
1604 N. Country Club
Tucson, AZ 85711
(602) 881-8008
An association of private professionals who help caregivers identify needs and resources in the community. Call for referrals to local providers.

United Seniors Health Cooperative
1331 H Street, N.W. #500
Washington, DC 20005-4706
(202) 393-6222
USHC is a nonprofit independent consumer organization. For the past decade it has been helping older adults achieve health independence and financial security. Call or write for a list of publications and services. Also call or write to order a copy of *Home Care for Older People: A Consumer's Guide,* $14.50; *Long Term Care Planning: A Dollar & Sense Guide* (1997 edition), $15.00; *Managing Your Health Care Finances: Getting the Most Out of Medicare & Medigap Insurance,* $14.00.

Publications

The Caregiver's Guide: Helping Older Friends and Relatives with Health and Safety Concerns (Houghton Mifflin, 1992), $14.45.

"A Consumers Guide to Home Health Care." Thirty-six–page discussion of home-health care, including a consumer checklist. Order from National Consumers League, 815 15th Street, N.W., Washington, DC 20005. $4.

Golden Opportunities: Hundreds of Money-Making, Money-Saving Gems for Anyone Over Fifty, by Amy Budish and Armond Budish, $27.50; *Home Safety Guide for Older People: Check It Out/Fix It Up,* by John Pynoos and Evelyn Cohen, $13.95; and *Retirement Income on the House: Cashing In on Your Mortgage with a Reverse Mortgage,* by Ken Scholen, $29.95. Order any of these books from Serif Press, 1331 H Street, N.W. Washington, DC 20005; tel. (800) 221-4272.

Home Health Care, by Jo-Ann Friedman (W.W. Norton, 1986), $25.

"The Medicare Handbook." Available free from U.S. Department of Health and Human Services, Health Care Financing Administration. Call (800) 638-6833.

"Safety for Older Consumers: Home Safety Checklist." Available from Consumer Product Safety Commission, Washington, DC 20207.

16

17 Caring for Your Teeth

Robert Krughoff

Robert Krughoff directs the Center for the Study of Services, based in Washington, D.C., and San Francisco. The center publishes *Checkbook* magazine, from which this chapter is adapted.

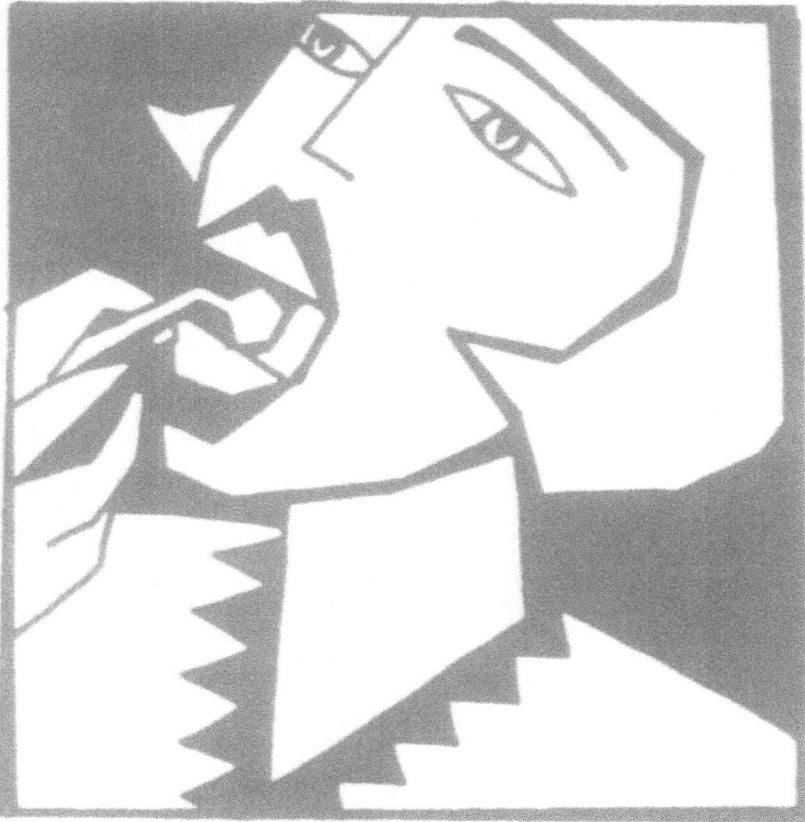

Fluoride: The Magic Ingredient

Throughout recorded history, tooth decay has probably caused more pain than any other infectious disease. It still leads to the loss of more teeth, at all ages, than any other cause.

Fluoride is the magic ingredient in preventing caries. Even for people who benefit from a fluoridated water supply, fluoride toothpastes and mouth rinses, used daily or weekly, reduce caries. Also, a topical fluoride treatment—in which a dentist applies fluoride to teeth—performed twice annually can reduce

Smile. Flash the good news. Teeth and gums are healthier. Decay is down. About half the schoolchildren in the United States have no decay in their permanent teeth, almost twice as good a record as two decades ago. There's a little less gum disease also, and far fewer toothless working adults.

Mouths look better as well. Advanced techniques and materials make it possible to model attractive, natural-looking teeth on top of stained, chipped, or irregular ones. And more and more adults are having their teeth straightened, encouraged by new, barely visible orthodontic appliances.

Improved dental health, particularly in the area of preventing tooth decay, has held back demand for dental care. At the same time, the supply of dentists is up, from 47 dentists per 100,000 Americans in 1970 to more than 60 in 1990. This supply-demand relationship may have slightly restrained prices for dental care.

On the other hand, the ratio of dentists to consumers could return to 1970 levels in ten years because of the recent closure of several dental schools. In any case, the high price of establishing a dental practice will push consumer costs up. The average dentist now starts out with a school debt of over $50,000 and invests about $100,000 to open an office.

Just as important, despite rapid progress in prevention, most Americans' mouths still bear witness to the ravages of dental caries (cavities) and gum disease. In fact, the continuing prevalence of oral diseases in the United States has been called a "neglected epidemic." About thirty thousand oral cancers are diagnosed each year—about 4 percent of all cancers in this country—killing about eight thousand people. The average child has one cavity by age nine, four by age fourteen, and eight by age seventeen. Over half of working adults and 95 percent of people over sixty-five are missing more than one tooth; 10 percent of Americans wear full dentures. Over half of homebound elders haven't seen a dentist in ten years, and 41 percent of people over sixty-five have no teeth.

Keep all this in mind as you begin your search for a dentist or talk to your current dentist about your routine and specialized care.

Prevention $$

Preventive dental care saved close to $100 billion during the 1980s.

What a Good Dentist Does

More important than anything a dentist can do for you is what you do for yourself. That's why you want a dentist or dental hygienist who thoroughly explains proper brushing and flossing and advises you on selecting the best type of brush, floss, fluoride toothpaste, and other supplies. Equally important, the dentist or hygienist should have you demonstrate your technique periodically so he or she can suggest improvements. If your dentist doesn't do this automatically, ask him or her to do so.

The Qualities to Seek

Because many aspects of prevention require regular office visits, you want a dentist who notifies you when it's time for regular checkups and care. For example, one key to prevention is regular "scaling" by a dentist or hygienist to remove the calculus (hardened plaque) that accumulates on your teeth. Another is diagnosis and treatment of decay and gum disease at an early stage.

In addition, a good dentist:

- Takes a thorough medical history at the first exam and updates the history at each subsequent visit
- Gives you complete, up-to-date instructions on how to care for your teeth
- Asks you questions and carefully inspects your mouth during each exam
- Explains your options and provides a written treatment plan before any major procedure
- Shows concern for your safety and comfort by wearing gloves to prevent the spread of infection and uses lead aprons to protect you during X rays
- Works efficiently and gently
- Leaves you with a comfortable bite and nicely finished tooth surfaces, *and*
- Tailors care to each individual—for example, by scheduling different intervals between visits depending on each patient's risk for dental disease

Dentists often vary on these and other items of concern to patients, although this variation doesn't necessarily translate directly into important differences in quality. Most consumers consider their dentists adequate or better. In all cases, the relationship between you and your dentist is very personal, and a dentist others don't like might be just right for you. Nonetheless, asking questions may prove a useful aid as you begin your search.

caries significantly, particularly for people without a fluoridated water supply. It will likely benefit those who drink fluoridated water as well.

Your best defense against dental decay is to live in a community with fluoridated water. However, more than 100 million people in the United States don't enjoy this benefit. Eight of the fifty largest cities lack community water fluoridation. The 3.5 million residents of Los Angeles, the 1 million residents of San Diego, and almost 1 million people in San Antonio don't get fluoridated water from the city. Other major cities lacking community water fluoridation include San Jose; Sacramento; Portland, Oregon; Tucson (which voted for fluoridation in 1992); and Honolulu. Also, many communities have marginally safe water supplies or provide water that tastes bad; so some consumers purchase bottled drinking water that is clean and good-tasting but unfluoridated.

To find out if your community has fluoridated water, ask a dentist or call the local or state board of health.

Finding a Dentist

Start looking for a dentist by consulting friends, especially those with needs similar to yours. When you identify a few possible dentists, ask your friends for more details and talk to the dentists yourself. Call your county dental society for referrals to dentists in your area, or ones that meet your specific requirements, such as speaking your language, familiarity with a disability you may have, or charging based on ability to pay.

Seek a dentist who:

- Discusses symptoms you have, such as loose teeth, bleeding gums, pain when eating, or a continual bad taste in your mouth

- Instructs you on prevention

- Checks your technique in flossing and brushing

- Is gentle

- Explains diagnoses, treatment plans, and costs

- Offers alternatives

- If a treatment fails, volunteers to redo it at no charge

- Encourages second opinions in complex cases

How Often?

Not everyone needs to visit the dentist with equal frequency. If you have healthy gums and accumulate plaque and calculus slowly, once a year might be enough. Six months is common, and a few people need a checkup and cleaning every three months. Ask your dentist to recommend the best interval for you and to explain why. Ask what notices you will receive when it's time for your next appointment.

A Thorough Diagnosis

Good diagnosis is essential to good treatment. A flawless technician is of little use if he or she misses the problem requiring treatment.

As a central aspect of diagnosis, your dentist should keep a written record of your dental history, beginning with a complete history taken at the first exam. Knowledge of your past toothaches, swelling, bleeding gums, and other problems will help alert the dentist to possible trouble. In addition, knowledge of drug allergies and other medical factors may affect your treatment. A new dentist should request copies of recent X rays and possibly other records from your previous dentist.

At each visit, a thorough dentist inspects the soft tissues of your mouth, tongue, lips, cheeks, and salivary glands. This can reveal oral cancers and other problems. Next, the dentist checks for cavities and has you close your mouth and move your jaw from side to side to check your bite. Finally, the dentist checks your gums, measuring the depth of the pocket between your gums and your teeth with a metal probe.

Signs of Trouble

At each visit, a good dentist looks for and asks you if you have noticed any of the following signs of disease:

- Bleeding, swollen, or inflamed gums
- Loose teeth
- Continual bad breath
- Bad taste in your mouth
- Pain when eating sweets or drinking hot or cold liquids, *and*
- Pain when chewing

X Rays

Your dentist should take a full set of X rays (fourteen to twenty films) or a panoramic film every three to five years. X rays help reveal cavities, some remote deposits of calculus, bone loss around the teeth, abscesses of the tooth tip, impacted teeth, retained roots, cysts, and jawbone tumors. A more limited set of X rays called *bitewings* (two to four films) should be taken more frequently to reveal cavities. Always protect yourself during X rays with a lead apron.

Explaining Your Choices

If the exam reveals disease, you may have a choice among several alternatives. For example, a dentist might treat a large cavity in a tooth with a filling, a crown, extraction, or root-canal therapy. You want a dentist who explains the pros and cons of a wide range of old and new approaches.

To help you decide on a treatment, ask the dentist to fully describe the condition of your mouth and the corrections needed. It's a good idea to ask for a written treatment plan. Almost all dentists will do this, although some charge an extra fee for it and the written explanations of diagnosis and treatment might be less than clear.

Unfortunately, diagnosis is replete with conflicts of interest. A specialist has an interest in recommending complex treatment that only he or she can provide. A general practitioner may favor a simplistic approach rather than pass up the opportunity to treat you. Bear in mind that different treatments require more or less of the dentist's time, affecting your bill. Although extensive treatment may be appropriate, be especially cautious if a new dentist recommends far more work than other dentists have suggested in the past.

If a dentist proposes extensive treatment, consider getting a second opinion, perhaps from a specialist. Good dentists often refer patients to an *endodontist* for difficult root-canal treatment, a *periodontist* for gum surgery, an *orthodontist* for moving multiple teeth, or an *oral surgeon* to remove impacted teeth. Discussing treatments with the specialist as well as your general practitioner might give you a balanced view.

Get the second opinion from someone who is independent of your own dentist. Tell this dentist in advance that you won't be using him or her for treatment. Your dentist should be willing to forward X rays and exam results for review.

Deciding What's Right for You

Treatments for the same condition differ in cost, comfort, convenience, and implications for your long-term health. Only you, with the advice of your dentist, can decide what is right for you. You would expect an auto body shop to fully explain the pros and cons of hammer-

- Has a pleasant, clean office and a pleasant staff
- Doesn't keep you waiting long when you arrive
- Doesn't keep you waiting long in the dental chair, *and*
- Arranges appointments quickly when needed

17

ing out dents versus replacing fenders. Demand as much from a dentist—
in language you can understand.

Obtaining Quality Treatment

Once you and your dentist agree on a plan, the dentist sets to
work—with greater or lesser care. Don't assume that any governmental or professional body holds dentists accountable for the quality of
their work. The vast majority of dentists practice in their own offices
with poor accountability and little or no peer review.

Even if a dentist's peers observe low-quality work, they're unlikely to
tell you about it. As recently as two decades ago, the dental code of ethics
prohibited dentists from "referring disparagingly, orally or in writing, to
the services of another dentist, to a member of the public." The code now
states that a "dentist has an obligation to report to the appropriate agency
of his component or constituent dental society instances of gross and
continual faulty treatment by another dentist." Local dental societies
have established patient-relations and peer-review systems, but few dentists are ever disciplined.

Look . . . and Look Again

Credentials don't indicate much about a dentist's skill either. All practicing dentists must be licensed, but that's no guarantee a dentist will practice good dentistry over the years. Renewing the license every few years
requires only paying a nominal fee, and most states grant licenses to
practice for life. Nor should a dentist's membership in professional societies and associations impress you. Generally, these groups only require
a dentist to have a license and pay dues, although membership does give
a dentist a chance to share up-to-date information with colleagues.

However, several factors might suggest a commitment to high-quality
dental care:

Membership or fellowship in the Academy of General Dentistry.
This indicates a dentist's commitment to continual learning. The academy requires seventy-five hours of courses every three years for membership and even more training for fellowship.

Membership in a dental school's faculty. Teaching experience proves
nothing about skill, but a teaching dentist is likely to be up-to-date on scientific developments.

Membership on a hospital staff. Being a staff member exposes a dentist to the knowledge of other dentists and physicians.

Certification. Certification indicates that a dentist once took advanced training and passed a difficult exam. A dental specialist should be certified by the appropriate body, such as the American Board of Endodontics for root-canal therapy.

At least as important as any data you can collect on a dentist's skills is your own judgment or that of friends. Here are a few points to check after receiving treatment:

■ How does your bite feel?

■ Is the tissue around the tooth healthy? Bleeding may signal gum disease or indicate that a crown or other restoration is irritating your gum.

■ Does a treated tooth look like a tooth?

■ Does dental floss or your tongue catch on the tooth? If dental floss catches, so will food particles.

■ Did the dentist take the time to polish your fillings? This improves the appearance *and* extends the life of the filling.

■ Do you feel pain when drinking hot or cold liquids? Some temporary discomfort may be normal after treatment; continuing pain or extreme sensitivity may indicate remaining decay or an improperly sealed filling.

■ Did the dentist leave debris in your mouth?

■ How long does your dental work last? Silver fillings generally last ten years or more, and crowns at least that long.

■ Does the dentist use a water spray to cool your teeth while drilling? Keeping the tooth cool helps avoid possible nerve death.

Referral Source

One indicator of quality is the judgment of another dentist. If possible, ask other dentists where they send their own children. For recommendations that at least help you avoid poor practitioners, call dental schools and hospital dental programs, both of which will recommend their faculty or affiliated staff. You can also call the oral-health program of your state or local health department, and a dental society will recommend its members.

TIP
Four-Handed Dentistry

The less time in the dental chair, the better. One common timesaver is a chairside dental assistant, allowing for "four-handed dentistry." The assistant hands the dentist the proper instruments and tends to the patient's needs. Ask a prospective dentist whether he or she uses a dental assistant.

TIP
X-ray Safety

By far the most important and easiest X-ray protection comes from leaded aprons and collars. When you get an X ray, always ask for a lead apron.

Your Safety

Like any medical procedure, dental care carries a risk of complications or medical emergency. Your dentist should be ready and equipped to handle such situations. In addition, the dentist should expose you to as few risks as possible during treatment.

To protect both you and the dentist from infection, especially from hepatitis B and AIDS, a good dentist wears rubber gloves and a mask when treating you and puts on new gloves for each patient. For the dentist's protection, goggles are also recommended for procedures that spray particles or fluid. In any case, the possibility of contracting HIV/AIDS from a dentist is extremely small.

X rays present another safety concern. Although the exact extent of X-ray risk is uncertain, the benefits almost surely greatly outweigh the risk in most cases. Nonetheless, you want a dentist who takes reasonable steps to minimize any risk, such as offering you a lead apron. This is particularly important because the harmful effects of low doses of X rays, such as those you receive in the dental chair, are now considered greater than was once thought.

A dentist can also minimize other risks of dental treatment, such as anesthesia mishaps and complications related to infections. The best prevention in these cases is the dentist's taking a careful medical history that notes allergies, any history of rheumatic fever, and other danger signals.

Cleanliness is critical. A dentist who cares about the cleanliness of his or her office, especially the lab, will most likely show the same care with his or her instruments and hands. Proper sterilization of equipment will kill all organisms that can cause serious medical problems. An excellent sterilization technique is the use of a stream autoclave. For instruments that can't go in the autoclave, the usual alternative is dry heat, which kills living organisms much more slowly.

Fixing the Damage

The standard procedures for repairing and replacing teeth have changed little for many years: root-canal therapy, crowns, drilling and filling cavities, inserting fixed bridges or partial dentures, and complete dentures. But advances continue on most of these fronts.

Although your regular dentist will handle routine tasks such as cleanings and most restorations, consider a specialist for complex bridges and dentures, oral surgery, periodontal therapy, implants, difficult root-canal therapy, and other extensive procedures. If your dentist offers these services, consider her or him in addition to the specialists. What's key is how often a dentist has performed the procedure in question.

Get names of specialists by asking your general-care dentist or other dentists for suggestions. Ask specialists about their training and how frequently they perform the procedure you need. Ask for the names of patients you can call for references. To ensure that dentists don't simply refer you to their most enthusiastic clients, specify that you want to talk with people who fit in a fairly narrow category, such as patients who are similar to you in age, sex, and required treatment.

The Eight Dental Specialties

Dental specialists typically receive two to four years training in their field beyond the normal training for all dentists. The American Dental Association recognizes eight specialties:

- *Endodontists* perform root canals and treat diseases of the pulp and nerves on the inside of teeth.
- *Oral and maxillofacial surgeons* treat injuries and defects of the mouth and jaw.
- *Oral pathologists* examine, identify, and diagnose diseases of the mouth.
- *Orthodontists* straighten teeth and correct the position of jaws.
- *Pediatric dentists* provide comprehensive dental care for children and adolescents, as well as for special patients who have mental, physical, or emotional problems.
- *Periodontists* treat diseases of the gums and the underlying bone that holds teeth.
- *Prosthodontists* replace missing teeth by designing and fitting dentures and bridgework.
- *Public health dentists* design and administer public or private education, treatment, and prevention programs for entire communities or organizations.

Dental Implants

As a treatment of last resort, dental implants are an alternative to complicated dentures or failed bridgework. In this procedure, a dentist inserts a fixed device below the gum. From this device, one or more posts extend

The Pain Factor

From 10 percent to 14 percent of Americans shun dental treatment because of fear, often living with discomfort because they feel that the cure is worse than the disease. Avoiding the dentist's chair for this reason is silly. Modern anesthetics and equipment can minimize discomfort for even the most sensitive people.

Your dentist should offer you a choice of anesthesia and explain the effects of each one. A person who is extremely sensitive may request nitrous oxide ("laughing gas") or use premedication. For others, a local painkiller such as lydocaine or xylocaine suffices. Still others may want no painkiller. In any case, a dentist concerned about your comfort will arrange a way for you to signal if pain becomes severe.

Some dentists use stereo headphones to help patients relax. Patients can listen to their choice of music rather than the sound of a drill. Waiting-room distractions, including video games and videotaped movies, also make the trip to the dentist less frightening.

17

TIP

Don't Pull That Tooth

Not if you can help it. Extracting a tooth is generally one of several remedies—and almost always the least desirable.

TIP

Consider the Options

Before getting an implant, thoroughly consider whether conventional dentures or a bridge might satisfy your needs.

Also, ask any dentist you approach about an implant how many procedures he or she has done. Get references from dentists and other clients. Discuss the particular technique the dentist plans to use. Has the American Dental Association approved it? And consult your regular dentist.

up through the gum. A bridge or other prosthetic device attaches to the posts. Implants are generally made of titanium, often with a ceramic coating. Bone heals directly to a proper implant, and gum tissue forms a biological seal around the posts.

Implants overcome some disadvantages of dentures. Dentures can move when you speak, eat, or yawn. Also, pressure on the gums when you chew and food particles that sometimes lodge between dentures and gums can make dentures uncomfortable. And the bone supports may shrink, making dentures difficult to wear.

However, implants are expensive—$10,000 or more. And success depends heavily on the type of implant, the patient's health, the skill of the person who performs the implant, the patient's motivation for follow-up self-care, and other factors.

If you want to pursue an implant, carefully select a dentist or dentists to perform the procedure. Implants have increased dramatically in popularity, from just a few thousand per year in the late 1970s to several hundred thousand per year today. They represent a lucrative opportunity for dentists whose income may be suffering from stiff competition and reduced demand for treatment of cavities. As a result, thousands of dentists now do implants, and some may lack adequate training. Implant rejection, stress from the attached appliance, and other problems require specific knowledge and experience.

Get more than one opinion on whether you are a good candidate for an implant and on the plan that best suits your case. A single dentist with good experience might suffice, but a team represents the safest approach. You can have a periodontist certified by the American Board of Periodontology or an oral surgeon certified by the American Board of Oral and Maxillofacial Surgery place the implant. Next, a specialist in dentures and other restorations certified by the American Board of Prosthodontics can prepare and mount the artificial teeth.

Bonding

Bonding places veneers on cracked, chipped, or stained front teeth. It's an alternative to traditional capping, but, unlike capping, it doesn't significantly alter the natural tooth.

Bonding generally costs about one-third less than a conventional crown. And the process is quicker and less painful. For example, a dentist might treat four front teeth with bonding in a single visit, while one crown might require several trips. In addition, some bonding procedures are reversible: If the result is unsatisfactory, the dentist can remove bonded material. Ask about this.

Bonding can also secure bridgework. In the traditional approach to holding a false tooth, the dentist files down the natural teeth around the gap and places a device over them, with the replacement tooth built into the middle of this device. The bonding alternative extends "wings" at each side of a false tooth and bonds the wings to the surrounding teeth. This requires no grinding of the natural teeth, but it only works if the adjacent teeth are relatively strong and there's no biting force to withstand.

Still another application of bonding is to secure orthodontic appliances to teeth. Bonding makes for braces that are less conspicuous.

The Dentist's Portfolio

If you are interested in bonding, ask about the dentist's training and experience. Review pictures of the dentist's past work so you can judge his or her sense of style.

Root-Canal Therapy

In root-canal therapy, a dentist removes the infected nerve and blood supply of a tooth and replaces it with filling material. Success rates are very high, and techniques have changed little in recent years. Some dentists now use lasers to prepare roots for filling.

One debate is whether materials that contain paraformaldehyde, specifically a material called Sargenti paste, should be the root filler. Sargenti paste kills bacteria, so infection is less likely. But Sargenti paste is poisonous and can damage nerves and other tissues in the unlikely event that it leaks out of the root. Dental schools in the United States don't teach use of the paste, and associations of root-canal specialists oppose its use.

If you are concerned, ask for a written treatment plan specifying that Sargenti paste won't be used.

Should You Agree to Gum Surgery?

You should agree to gum surgery only after thoroughly examining alternatives and perhaps by seeking a second opinion. In most cases, nonsurgical approaches cost less, hurt less, and are less likely to disfigure the gum line.

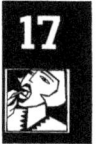

TIP

Seal Those Teeth

Although sealants are an extraordinarily valuable preventive measure, a 1986 survey indicated that fewer than 10 percent of children had them. Parents should insist that a dentist apply sealants unless there are compelling arguments to the contrary.

Dental Tips for Parents and Children

Teeth are susceptible to decay as soon as they appear in the mouth. Take steps to protect your infants' and toddlers' teeth from the start.

From birth to six months:

- Clean the child's mouth with gauze after feedings and at bedtime.
- Ask your pediatrician or dentist about fluoride supplements.
- Regulate feeding habits.

Between six months and one year:

- The first tooth should appear, signaling the time to see the pediatric dentist for an exam.
- Begin to brush the child's teeth after each feeding and at bedtime with a small, soft-bristled brush. Don't use a fluoride toothpaste that the baby can swallow, which could cause tooth discoloration later on.
- As the baby begins to walk, be alert to dental injuries.
- By the first birthday, wean the baby from breast or bottle feeding.

From one to two years:

- Follow schedule of exams and cleanings recommended by pediatric dentist.
- Start using pea-size portions of fluoridated toothpaste when a child can rinse, but make sure he or she doesn't eat the toothpaste.

Babies are susceptible to what is known as "baby-bottle tooth decay." You and others who take care of your baby must know about proper bottle-feeding practices. The National Institute of Dental Research recommends two preventive measures:

1. If your baby needs a bottle at bedtime for comfort, use only plain water. Don't fill the bottle with milk, formula, fruit juice, soft drinks, or any other sweetened liquids. All these liquids contain sugar.

2. Close to your child's first birthday, teach your child to drink directly from a cup.

For older children, ask your dentist about topical-fluoride treatment to prevent tooth decay. Many dentists apply this with a cleaning. The charge tends to be small, only about $15 per treatment. The value of treatment is less clear for adults, especially those with no recent decay.

Plastic sealants are also an excellent option. Placed on the chewing surfaces of your child's teeth, they prevent caries in any permanent teeth that have no perceptible decay or fillings. Plastic sealants can protect the pits and fissures of the chewing surfaces of molars, where most decay occurs. It's surprising and disappointing that sealants aren't applied as standard practice. The best time to do sealants is just after new teeth emerge, requiring two applications—first at six to eight years and then again at twelve to fourteen years.

Presumably, sealants protect adults' teeth as well. On the other hand, a cavity-free adult probably runs little risk of incurring decay even without sealants.

Sealant Service

If you're searching for a dentist for your son or daughter, ask the ones you are considering if they do sealants for children.

Money Matters

A dentist who helps you maintain the health of your mouth has a strong claim to your patronage—but not if the cost is excessive. In fact, some dentists charge more than twice as much as others.

As you select a dentist, ask the candidates about their fees for a few common procedures, such as an initial exam, cleaning, X rays, a topical-fluoride treatment, and a simple extraction. In particular, ask specialists about their charges. Most dentists readily provide such information, but don't be surprised if you find big differences. You may also want to ask if the dentist accepts credit cards or offers senior-citizen discounts.

By far, good preventive care is the best way to save money. Regular brushing with a fluoride toothpaste, proper flossing, and professional cleanings will help you avoid expensive treatments.

If you do require treatment, ask dentists to describe alternatives. For example, you might be just as well off with a nonprecious metal instead of gold in a restoration.

You can hold down dental-care costs in several other ways as well:

■ Get a written estimate before beginning an expensive treatment. Some dentists charge for estimates, but many provide them free. Even a modest fee is worthwhile if a written estimate helps prevent surprises after the work is done.

TIP

Second Opinions

A second opin-
ion, probably the
most underused con-
sumer tool in dentistry,
can help you get appro-
priate, reasonably priced
care. Getting a second
opinion before agreeing
to costly treatment can
also provide some lever-
age if a dispute arises
later.

■ Check out discounts, special offers, and lower-priced packages that include exams, cleaning, and X rays.

■ Some dentists offer discounts for cash up front because it saves them time and money in collecting unpaid bills.

■ Some dentists offer discounts to special groups, such as senior citizens, certain types of professionals, students, people on limited incomes even newly engaged couples.

Prevailing Charges for General Dentists

The American Dental Association collects price data from its members every three to five years. The most recent survey of average fees is for 1993:

- $25.43 for an initial diagnostic oral examination
- $19.54 for a periodic oral examination
- $43.21 for an adult's preventive visit plus a topical application of fluoride
- $36.00 for a child's preventive visit plus a topical application of fluoride
- $17.60 for an adult's topical application of fluoride
- $17.08 for a child's topical application of fluoride

Cost and Quality

What a dentist charges doesn't necessarily correlate with the results of patient surveys on satisfaction or with any credentials that might indicate service quality, such as membership in the Academy of General Dentistry.

In other words, you can pay relatively low fees and still get the very best care.

It's Your Record

You can save money if a new dentist or a dental specialist gets records and X rays from your previous or regular dentist. Unless the new dentist has reason to take new ones, full-mouth X rays are usually good for three to five years.

Your former dentist is ethically bound to pass along copies of X rays and other records. Check with your state department of health on the legal obligation to do so. You might be charged for the copies.

Overtreatment

A written treatment plan and consultation with an independent dentist will safeguard your wallet as well as your mouth. Regardless of a dentist's charges, the cost is too high if you are overtreated.

Both the treatment plan and your bill should itemize costs. A dentist shouldn't make you uncomfortable discussing money and should be willing to work out a payment plan or an alternative treatment if the costs exceed your means.

Warranties

Ask dentists about warranties for restorations. For example, some dentists may guarantee a porcelain crown with nonprecious metal or a silver filling for a certain length of time. Don't expect this, however.

A warranty should describe your needs, the proposed treatment, expected costs, expected results, and a specified period during which the dentist will replace defective work free of charge.

It won't be easy to find a dentist who'll offer such a warranty, especially in writing. But even if a dentist won't give you a written warranty, ask for a free replacement if a restoration doesn't last as it should.

Insurance, Prepaid Dental Plans, and Dental HMOs

You might want to find out whether a dentist participates in an insurance or HMO plan. Participation could mean that a dentist accepts as payment in full an amount set in the insurer's fee schedule. If you have insurance, be sure the dentist will help you get proper reimbursement. And if you are eligible for Medicaid, you will want a dentist who participates in that program.

Insurance benefits vary greatly from policy to policy, so learn about your dental benefits—and their limitations. You may decide to spread out expensive treatment over several years to bypass an annual maximum benefit. Or your plan may tie you to a group of participating dentists who agree to accept a specified fee schedule.

In some areas, a number of prepaid dental plans are available. Typically these plans cover you completely for routine exams and cleanings and give you lower-than-average fees for more expensive treatments—if you use participating dentists.

Whether these plans are appropriate for you depends on how much dentistry you expect to use. Consider the average local fees for services, how much you'd have to pay under a prepaid plan, the annual premium

TIP

Hygiene Schools

For routine dental care—
X rays, cleanings, and
exams—consider a
dental-hygiene school.
They offer a combination
of low cost and high
quality.

for the plan, and the gain (or loss) to your family as a result of enrolling in the plan.

You'll want to be sure a dentist doesn't treat you hastily because your case pays less than a regular fee-for-service case. Also, if your employer provides dental insurance, you almost certainly won't want a separate prepaid plan.

Dental School Clinics

Many dental schools have clinics where students treat patients under faculty supervision. The fees are invariably low for the local area. Schools also offer more comprehensive treatment and care during a routine visit so that students receive more training.

These clinics have drawbacks. Because students are learning, your visits will be longer—and your mouth will be open longer. This means some additional discomfort. And you run a small risk if a new student treats you. For more complicated problems, you might prefer a more advanced student—but then your dentist might graduate before you get follow-up care. In sum, they are a good resource for a person with a limited income and the time to spend at the clinic.

Resources

American Academy of Pediatric Dentistry
211 E. Chicago Avenue, #700
Chicago, IL 60611
(312) 337-2169
Call or write for a free pamphlet, "The Pediatric Dentist."

American Association of Orthodontists
401 North Lindbergh Boulevard
St. Louis, MO 63141
(800) 424-2841
Call or write for a free orthodontics planning kit and several pamphlets, including "Facts About Orthodontics: A Special Kind of Dentistry," "Adult Orthodontics: The Best Smile for Your Best Years," and "Good Beginnings: A Head Start for Healthy Smiles." For information on orthodontics and a list of local orthodontists, call (800) 222-9969.

American Association of Public Health Dentistry
10619 Jousting Lane
Richmond, VA 23235
(804) 272-8344
Call or write for a free pamphlet on fluoridation.

American Dental Association
211 E. Chicago Avenue
Chicago, IL 60611
(312) 440-2593
Provides consumer information on how often you need dental procedures. Call or write for free pamphlets, including "Pregnancy and Oral Health" and "Dental Decisions: Making the Right Choices."

Centers for Disease Control and Prevention
Division on Oral Health

4770 Buford Highway
Mail Stop F-10
Chamblee, GA 30341
(770) 488-3031
Call for information on infection control in dentistry, fluoridation, oral cancer, sealants, and baby-bottle tooth decay.

National Institute of Dental Research
P.O. Box 54793
Washington, DC 20032
Write for free pamphlets and posters in English and Spanish on such topics as fluoride for children and adults, tooth decay, gum diseases, and plaque removal.

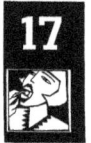

17

Buying Eyeglasses and Contact Lenses

Robert Krughoff

Robert Krughoff directs the Center for the Study of Services, based in Washington, D.C., and San Francisco. The center publishes *Checkbook* magazine, from which this chapter is adapted.

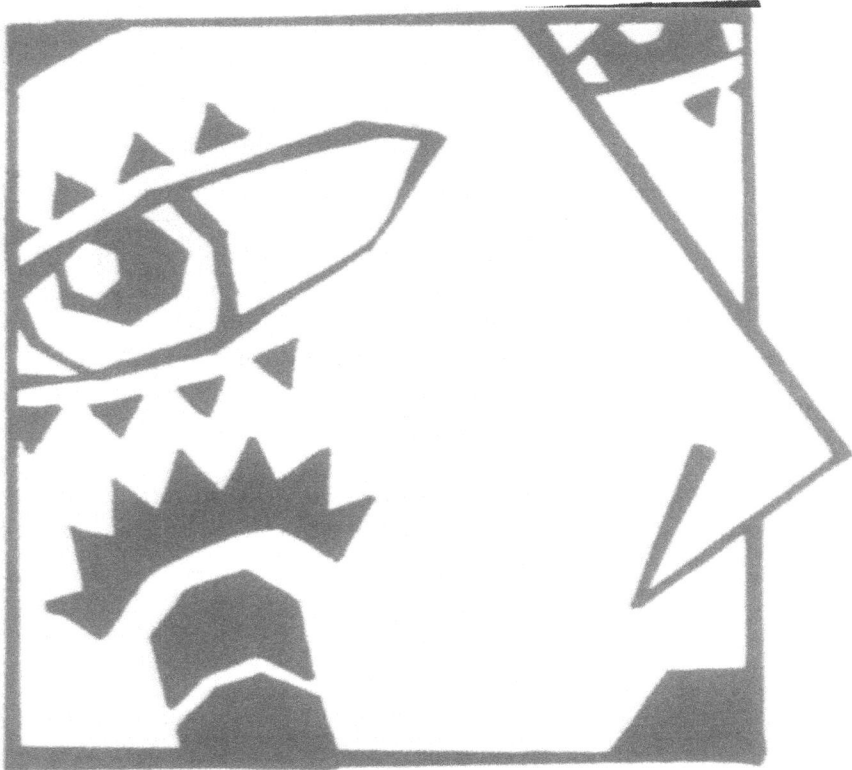

TIP

**Certification
Check**

Many ophthalmol-
ogists are certi-
fied, although this isn't
required. To determine if
an ophthalmologist is
certified, call the American Board of Medical
Specialties Certification
Line at (800) 776-2378.

Over half the people in the United States wear eyeglasses or contact lenses, and all Americans should get their eyes checked regularly. For these basic medical needs, you can choose from a multitude of excellent individual and group practitioners and a variety of national and local chains.

In general, you can seek routine care from ophthalmologists, optometrists, and opticians.

Ophthalmologists are physicians who specialize in eye disorders. They check eyes for vision problems, diseases, abnormalities, and symptoms of such general bodily disorders as diabetes and hypertension. They treat eyes with drugs, surgery, and other means, and they prescribe corrective glasses and contact lenses. Most ophthalmologists expect you to get eyeglasses elsewhere, but quite a few dispense contacts.

Optometrists are not medical doctors but are properly called doctors. Like ophthalmologists, they give eye exams, looking for a wide range of eye problems and symptoms of general health problems. They can prescribe a limited range of drugs. Some use visual therapy to counter certain eye problems, and most prescribe and dispense eyeglasses and contact lenses.

Opticians have less training than ophthalmologists or optometrists, with the exact amount depending on state regulations. Opticians can't write prescriptions. Using a prescription from an ophthalmologist or optometrist, they fit, supply, and adjust glasses and sometimes contacts. A few opticians grind eyeglass lenses to the correct prescription, but most buy the lenses from a wholesaler and fit them into a frame.

Unfortunately, many forms of medical insurance don't cover eyeglasses or contact lenses, so price is critical. Moreover, differences in quality and cost among the types of eye-care providers—let alone the providers of a single variety—are difficult to determine. To a large extent, you must invest time as you seek the best place to buy eyeglasses or contact lenses.

The Eye Exam

Get your eyes checked every one to two years; less often if you have no eye problems. A thorough vision exam takes thirty to sixty minutes.

The examiner should:

- Take a complete health history at the start of the examination.
- Inspect the inside and outside of your eyes for signs of diseases.
- Test your eye's ability to see sharply and clearly at all distances.
- Test your eye's ability to focus light rays exactly on the retina.
- Check eye coordination and eye muscle control.
- Test your eyes' ability to change focus, *and*
- Test for glaucoma.

The exam may also include special tests for color perception, depth perception, field of vision, and other vision skills.

Free Exams

Once each year, the American Optometric Association's Vision USA program provides free eye exams to low-income families.

- At least one person in the household must be employed.
- Recipients must be completely uninsured, including private or public health care coverage, *and*
- Recipients may not have had an eye exam in the last two years.

To arrange a screening for eligibility, call (800) 766-4466 in January to arrange a screening in March.

The Choice: Glasses or Contacts

If you have a recent prescription from an ophthalmologist or optometrist, your preference may largely determine your next step: Do you want eyeglasses or contact lenses?

If you prefer glasses, you can go to any optician or optometrist. Many opticians and optometrists dispense contact lenses as well, as do many ophthalmologists.

Although most practitioners dispense contact lenses based on any recent prescription, some insist on doing their own exam. They argue that the exam, the supplying of lenses, and follow-up care must go together to produce a consistently safe and satisfactory result. Other practitioners dispute this view—especially opticians, who can't do exams.

When you get your exam and buy your lenses at the same office, you receive benefits from accountability as well as convenience: If the lenses don't work out—and many times contact lenses don't—it's clear who is responsible.

Common Vision Problems

Astigmatism: Objects appear blurry or distorted at all distances because the front part of your eye, the cornea, is slightly irregular in shape.

Cataracts: A clouding of the clear lens of your eye, causing blurred or hazy vision. Can lead to blindness if not treated.

Farsightedness (hyperopia): You see far objects more clearly than close ones.

Glaucoma: A buildup of pressure in your eye. Can result in severe vision loss and even blindness.

Nearsightedness (myopia): You see close objects more clearly than distant ones.

Presbyopia: A natural part of aging that begins to blur your reading and near vision about age forty or forty-five and gradually worsens.

18

If you do take a prescription to a different location to be filled, a prescription from the past year is usually new enough; some practitioners let you go back further, particularly for glasses, depending on your age and eye-care history.

If you don't have a current prescription, you can get one at many places. While opticians can't give an exam, you can get one at some optician practices and chain outlets if an optometrist works in the office or an affiliated office nearby. Even in states that prohibit optician firms from employing an optometrist, one can be a door away.

Consumer Alert: Medications

Certain drugs or combinations of drugs can impair your vision and affect the results of diagnostic tests. Tell your eye-care provider the names of any medications you are taking.

Eyeglasses vs. Contacts

Eyeglasses are usually cheaper than contact lenses. They don't irritate the eye's surface and can require less care. Eyeglasses are also harder to lose. You can get them in special frames that protect your eyes against many industrial accidents. Some people even wear eyeglasses as a fashion accessory.

Contact lenses have several major advantages of their own. In the first place, they are virtually invisible. They also provide a wider field of vision, and they don't irritate the nose bridge and ears. Contacts are relatively secure and safe to wear during sports. And they distort your vision less than glasses because they are closer to, and move with, your eyes. Contacts can be a godsend if you are extremely nearsighted or farsighted or have had cataracts removed.

Some people who have preferred glasses may want to reconsider. Because of recent improvements, contacts can now provide a better combination of comfort, safety, and visual acuity than was possible in the past.

Buying Eyeglasses

An important aspect of buying glasses is the selection of a frame. In picking a frame, consider positioning, comfort, durability, appearance, and price.

Also take advantage of professional advice. Opticians and optom-etrists can be a valuable source of information when selecting frames. They can suggest models that might eliminate comfort or positioning problems you have previously experienced, and they can steer you away from models that might cause other problems. But always ask the professionals to explain their recommendations. Be suspicious if all of the suggestions are for higher-priced frames.

Positioning. Eyeglass frames should position the lenses to give you the sharpest vision. Some frames may position the lenses too far from your eyes or too high or low. If the frames slide down your nose, you won't get the full benefit from the lenses.

The stronger your prescription, the more critical positioning becomes. If you use glasses for driving, sports, or other activities requiring peripheral vision, make sure the sides of the frame are located above or below your eye level.

Comfort. The key comfort points are your ears and the bridge of your nose, the places where glasses rest. Unfortunately, trying on a frame for a minute or two doesn't always reveal discomfort that might occur with extended wear. Getting new glasses similar to your old ones helps limit your risk. All else being equal, lighter glasses are more comfortable than heavier ones. Lightweight glasses usually have optyl-plastic or thin metal frames with smallish plastic lenses.

If you are considering metal frames, keep several points in mind. Metal frames usually have a nosepiece of rocking pads. These small adjustable plastic pads are easily adjusted and unlikely to slip. This is an advantage over plastic frames, which usually have a rigid nose support that varies in shape among different manufacturers. On the other hand, rocking pads concentrate the weight on a small surface of the nose. This makes them uncomfortable for some people. If this is a problem for you, consider a model with an inserted molded plastic nosepiece instead of rocking pads. Metal frames are also more likely than plastic ones to irritate your ears. Many models avoid this problem by covering the ends of the temples with plastic or rubber pads.

Durability. Handled with care, most glasses last three or four years, and many people want to change style at least that often. Strength and durability are especially important if you plan to keep the frames longer, or if you knock the frames around a lot in sports, bar fights, or other vigorous

TIP

Chain Stores and Quality

When *Checkbook* magazine surveyed Washington, D.C., consumers, chains and franchise operations generally received fewer "superior" ratings than traditional eye-care practices on "doing service properly." But there was substantial variation among the chain and franchise operations.

activities. The durability of frames depends on the materials used, the thickness of the materials, and the craftsmanship.

The strongest metal frames are usually moderately thick, with a double bar or a single wide bar above the nose. They have smooth welding wherever two pieces of metal join, and they have heavy hinges. The strongest plastic frames are made of nylon, but these tend to be thick, heavy, and plain. Among other plastics, the strongest are usually at least moderately thick and have metal reinforcing for the full length of the temple (unnecessary in nylon or optyl-plastic frames), heavy hinges, and hinges that are secured to the temple with a backing plate of metal on the outside of the temple. However, these are general guidelines. Some frames of other types may be quite durable, and some meeting these standards may be rather frail.

Appearance. Most eyeglasses wearers are concerned about style. Indeed, some frames are sold with clear, nonprescription lenses and worn solely for effect.

The popular concern about fashion and brand names gives optometrists and opticians extra leverage if they wish to guide you to high-priced frames. Your best approach is to try on a variety of frame styles to decide for yourself which few look best. Then look at the price tags. Chances are some will be relatively inexpensive. If not, ask if there is another cheaper frame that looks similar to one you like.

What looks good on someone else—or in an ad—might not look good on you. To look right, frames must accommodate the shape of your eyebrows and cheekbones, the spacing of your eyes, the height of your nose bridge, and the size of your head.

Conventional wisdom says that a person looks best in frames that are shaped differently from his or her face—square or oblong rims for round faces, round rims for square faces, and wide, shallow, oblong rims for narrow faces.

Price. The prices of frames vary tremendously. Decent quality frames range in price from less than $40 to more than $400.

Judging Quality

The quality of eyeglass care can reveal itself in:

- The kind of advice the provider gives you on selecting frames and lens materials to fit your face and your prescription

- The fitting of lenses in frames and the positioning of lenses to match the position of your eyes
- The adjustment of frames to fit your face, nose, and ears, *and*
- The quality of lenses and frames supplied

Choosing Eyeglass Lenses and Features

As with frames, you face many decisions in choosing eyeglass lenses.

One choice is glass or plastic. The lighter weight of plastic is a particular plus when the lenses are for large frames or a strong prescription that requires a thick lens. The scratch resistance of glass is important if you remove your glasses frequently, slipping them into your pocket, purse, or briefcase. Federal regulations require both glass and plastic lenses to resist breakage from moderate impacts, but no lens is unbreakable.

An increasingly popular choice for people who need bifocals or trifocals and don't want others to be aware of this sign of aging is a "progressive," or "no-line," lens. However, such lenses are much more expensive than regular bifocals or trifocals and require special care in fitting.

Several types of lens treatments have grown in popularity in recent years. One of the most popular options treats the lens to filter out the ultraviolet light that may contribute to cataracts or retina damage. This treatment may interest you if you expose your eyes heavily to ultraviolet radiation—for example, by working outdoors or spending a lot of time mountain climbing or at the beach.

Antireflective coatings are rapidly gaining in popularity. This option reduces reflection from your side—an especially helpful feature if you do a lot of night driving. It also reduces the reflection others see when they look at or photograph you.

If you are very nearsighted, you may want lenses made of materials that have a strong capacity to refract light. Such materials permit a thinner, lighter lens but cost extra.

Eyeglass Prices

In a *Checkbook* magazine survey in Washington, D.C., For Eyes outlets stood out for lower prices, with quotes on several types of glasses about 60 percent of the average. However, not all chains and franchise operations had low prices. And prices differed from outlet to outlet for all the major chains, although most tended to relatively uniform pricing.

Many independents charged low prices—substantially below the average for any of the chains except For Eyes. Outlets that offered exams in the office (and therefore had optometrists available) were neither more nor less expensive, on average, than other places. Even practices identified as optometrists' offices (with "Dr." in the name) had roughly average prices. And some optometrists beat the all-outlet average handily.

In other words, prices vary a great deal from one place to another. If you have time, call or shop around.

Optometric Management magazine reports annually on optometrist charges for eyeglass lenses. In 1993 the price for lenses made of glass averaged $54.93 nationally for single-vision lenses and $83.55 for bifocals. For plastic lenses, the national average was $51.31 for single-vision lenses and $80.54 for bifocals.

Sunglasses

When choosing sunglasses, seek lenses that meet your eyes' needs for comfort and protection. All sunglasses screen out or absorb some harmful ultraviolet radiation, but the amount varies considerably. For maximum protection, look for those absorbing from 290 to 380 nanometers (nm), if that information is on the label. Lightly tinted lenses and plastic light-sensitive lenses screen out too little light to be considered sunglasses.

There are four types of sun lenses:

■ *Standard tinted* lenses are made of glass or plastic. Dark gray is best; it doesn't affect your ability to see colors. However, some people prefer green or brown.

■ *Polarizing* lenses reduce reflected glare.

■ *Light-sensitive (photochromic) glass* lenses darken and lighten with the amount of light exposure.

■ *Mirror* lenses, designed to wear under intense glare from snow or water, have a thin metallic coating over a tinted lens.

Choosing Options: If It's Not Broken . . .

When you buy eyeglasses, you can opt for tints, scratch-resistant coating, and antireflective coatings. There are photochromic lenses that darken as the sun gets brighter and polarizing lenses that are especially effective at reducing glare.

With all the possible features and add-ons, buying glasses can resemble car buying. What's more, some firms push options with more force than a high-pressure car dealer.

Although add-ons can be legitimate, treat each one skeptically. If you haven't scratched your glasses in the past or if reflection has never troubled you, don't be pushed into paying to fix something that isn't broken.

Buying Contact Lenses

Most outlets supply two basic types of contacts—soft lenses and gas-permeable rigid lenses. In addition, some contact wearers still have old-fashioned hard lenses.

First introduced in 1971, soft contact lenses are made of a gelatinlike substance containing a great deal of water. Most people adapt to soft contacts quickly and easily. The high water content lets oxygen pass through the lenses to the cornea, the tissue covering the eye. This oxygen supply is crucial.

Rigid gas-permeable lenses, which appeared in 1978, also allow oxygen to pass through easily. This means the lenses can be larger than old-fashioned hard contact lenses, which had to be small enough for oxygen to pass around them. The larger size makes for relative comfort because your eyelid doesn't have to pass over the edge of the lens with each blink. The newest gas-permeable lenses are made with special plastics that are very slick, allowing comfortable movement under the eyelid and minimizing the buildup of various deposits.

Soft lenses have several advantages over rigid lenses:

■ You can wear soft lenses comfortably almost immediately, and you can stop wearing them for days or months and restart without an extended period to readapt.

■ They are easy to fit. Opticians and optometrists generally have many soft lenses in stock and can send you home with a pair in one visit. The softness permits some tolerance of variations in a cornea's shape, making skilled fitting less critical.

■ Because soft lenses cover a large part of the eye's surface, they prevent dust from getting to the eye.

■ Soft lenses are hard to dislodge, making them ideal for contact sports.

On the other hand, rigid gas-permeable lenses have important pluses:

18

TIP

Backups

If you get contacts, it's a good idea to have glasses available as a backup. You'll be glad you did if you lose a contact or must contend with eye infections, allergies, or other problems.

- They provide clearer vision. Their rigidity allows precise shaping. Until recently, that also meant they could help with serious astigmatism beyond the scope of conventional soft lenses.

- They tend to be easier than soft lenses to clean because they are less prone to collect protein deposits.

- Because rigid gas-permeable lenses can be kept clean, they're less likely than soft lenses to scrape the eye surface or to harbor microorganisms that can infect the eye.

- Since they don't absorb moisture, people with relatively dry eyes can wear rigid gas-permeable lenses.

- They last longer than soft lenses. While soft lenses typically are good for a year or less, rigid lenses generally last twice that long.

Insurance and Eye Care

Insurance benefits for eye wear vary from nothing at all to comprehensive coverage. If you have health insurance through your work, your coverage depends on the options your employer chose. In almost every case, eye surgery is covered under the medical part of your health insurance. Insurance often covers annual eye exams as well. It may also include discounts of varying amounts on eyeglasses and contact lenses.

To receive coverage for any eye-care services, you may have to use plan-affiliated providers. And if further care is in order, even for covered services, find out from the insurer who needs to make the referral so you qualify for reimbursement. You might need a referral from your primary care physician, an ophthalmologist, or another physician rather than an optometrist.

Contact Lens Options

There are many variants on the two basic types of contact lenses. Two of the most important are extended-wear lenses and disposable lenses.

Extended-wear lenses. While you remove regular lenses each night, you can wear extended-wear lenses for longer periods of time. Both soft and rigid gas-permeable extended-wear lenses are available.

However, wearing any soft lenses for a long period may weaken and scratch the cornea's surface, as the oxygen supply is restricted and protein deposits develop. This weakened, scratched cornea surface, in turn, is more likely to contract an infection called ulcerative keratitis than is the cornea of someone who removes contacts daily. If not treated immediately, this infection can result in partial or complete loss of sight. Although one study indicates that individuals who use extended-wear lenses have only about one chance in five hundred of getting corneal ulcers, that possibility may be reason enough for you to steer clear of this option.

If you do decide on extended-wear lenses, don't leave them in for longer than seven days at a time. And conscientiously follow the instructions for care and cleaning.

Disposable lenses. These are simply soft lenses that are produced at low-enough cost that you can afford to throw them away. The most widespread plan costs $300 per year for soft lenses that you get in six-packs and wear for two weeks before throwing them away. Disposables spare you the trouble of cleaning your lenses and reduce the risk that you'll damage your cornea with built-up deposits.

Since they eliminate the need for cleaning chemicals, disposable lenses might not cost much more per year than regular extended-wear lenses. But wearing lenses for a week still involves risks, even if they are new each week, because your eyes get less oxygen than they otherwise would. If you decide on disposable lenses, don't assume you can cheat and keep them in a few extra days. That might save you money but cost you the health of your eyes.

More Contact Options

Contact-lens options include bifocal lenses, lenses for astigmatism, tinted lenses, and ultraviolet filtering lenses. New lenses coming on the market have a soft perimeter for comfort and a gas-permeable rigid center to allow oxygen transfer and sharp vision. You can expect all these options to cost more than basic single-correction lenses.

The Cost of Contact Lenses

Comparing prices for contact lenses can be a puzzling experience. Since most people who buy contact lenses pay a package price that includes an exam and some amount of follow-up care, the lens price is only part of the picture. And differences in the amount of service firms include in a package add to the confusion.

TIP

Medicare Coverage

Medicare covers some eye-care services. These include the eye-health part of an eye examination and the necessary treatment if you have a problem. Medicare doesn't cover eye wear itself or checking your vision for changes in your prescription. However, for people who have had cataract surgery, it covers an examination and post-operative eye care when provided by optometrists.

Sometimes the stated price for contacts includes a thorough eye exam. Sometimes it includes just a quick exam with a refraction test and measurements of the size and shape of the eyeball. Sometimes no exam is included. At some firms, the price covers as many follow-up visits as you wish within a stated period of time (such as three months or a year), but at others it covers only one or two visits.

Refund policies and warranties also vary. Most dispensers will give you some or all of your money back if your eyes do not adapt to the contacts within a specified time. A few have no refund policy but promise to make many adjustments to get a satisfactory fit.

Neither arrangement provides you with foolproof protection. Dispensers with refund policies may give up quickly if you are hard to fit and then give you only a partial refund. On the other hand, promises to make extensive adjustments are worth little if the work isn't skillful. Remember, each adjustment requires your time.

A final element of variation arises with replacement policies for lost contacts. Some dispensers promise to replace lost contacts at prespecified prices for a year or two after the initial purchase. With others, you are on your own.

While all the variations in contact-lens service packages mean that prices aren't exactly comparable from firm to firm, you can determine the main elements of cost by getting prices that include at least a basic exam and prescription as well as a follow-up visit. You'll find that some places may charge more than three times as much as others.

Save Now or Later

Soft contact lenses tend to represent a smaller *initial* investment than gas-permeable lenses, but the long-term price may be higher. In *Checkbook*'s Washington, D.C., price survey, soft-lens package prices ranged from about $80 to $260 for exam, lens, and follow-up care, with an average of about $140. Prices for a rigid gas-permeable package ranged from $160 to $340, averaging about $240.

The ease of cleaning and relatively long life of rigid gas-permeable contact lenses mean that the long-range cost is likely to be lower than the cost of soft lenses. You might save from $75 to $350 per year on cleaning chemicals alone.

Picking Up Your Glasses or Contacts

You will rarely get your glasses or contacts on the day you select them. Usually you'll return two to ten days later. This second visit is as important as the first. Check the glasses or contacts carefully when you come to pick them up.

New glasses may have to be adjusted to fit your face or to allow for a difference in the height of your ears. After the adjustment, check positioning and comfort. Be sure there isn't too much pressure on your ears or nose, that the frames don't slip down your nose, and that both lenses are the same height and an equal distance from your eyes.

When you pick up new contact lenses, the practitioner should carefully check their fit on your eyes using a slitlamp biomicroscope. He or she should also use a standard eye chart to test how well you see. If these checks indicate no problems, do your own tests of fit: Look left, right, up, and down several times while holding your head in different positions. And try blinking, squinting, and closing your eyes several times. If contacts don't fit perfectly, you may need new lenses, or a rigid lens may need alterations.

Proper follow-up is an important part of buying contacts and choosing a practitioner. Once contacts seem to fit, most practitioners will ask you to return at least once for an additional check. You may have to make several visits before the fit is perfect, and sometimes a good fit requires a change in basic lens design or material.

When you get the lenses, you should receive thorough instructions on how to insert and remove them, on adaptation (how long to wear them each day during the first few weeks), and on care and cleaning. Listen carefully. Get written instructions, and read them right away. Remember, all contacts can cause permanent eye damage if mishandled.

After You Go Home

If new eyeglass frames feel uncomfortable after a few hours, return to your optician or optometrist and ask for further adjustments. This service should be free.

Wait a few days if discomfort seems to be from lenses—either glasses or contacts—and is in the form of mild eyestrain or things appearing closer than before. Often your eyes and brain need time to adjust to new lenses.

The practitioner should check the lenses to determine if their actual correction coincides with your prescription. For glasses, he or she should check the positioning of the lenses in the frame and the positioning of the frame on your face. In the case of contacts, expect a little discomfort as you adapt to them, particularly to rigid lenses, but there should be no real pain. If there is, remove the lenses immediately and return to the practitioner as soon as possible.

TIP

Check the Fit

Check new eyeglasses realistically. Turn your head sideways, up, and down several times. Turn sideways while looking down. Chew for fifteen seconds. Do the glasses work for their intended purposes? If they are for general use, can you see clearly at a distance and read comfortably? Do they stay in place as you walk?

Practice putting your new contact lenses in and taking them out while the practitioner watches. *Before* leaving the office, make sure you know how to do it.

18

If someone who has sold you uncomfortable glasses checks the lenses and then claims that the refractive power and positioning match the prescription, ask for an explanation of the cause for your complaints. If the explanation doesn't satisfy you, it could be that the seller is right and the original prescription was wrong, or perhaps the seller is wrong and doesn't recognize his or her mistake.

As a first step toward resolving such a problem, take the prescription and the glasses to an optician. Explain your problem and offer to pay to have the refractive power and (in the case of glasses) positioning of the lenses measured. Compare these new measurements to your prescription. The measurements will take only a minute or two. If refractive power and positioning match the prescription, go back to the optometrist or ophthalmologist who wrote the prescription and explain the problem. Your practitioner should check the glasses and might retest your eyes. Sometimes this is free, but check.

As an alternative, you may decide to get another eye examination from a different optometrist or ophthalmologist, explaining your recent difficulties. This will always cost you an additional examination fee. Do it as a last resort.

Go Back

Return to your practitioner if you experience:

- Substantial discomfort with glasses
- Mild discomfort for more than a few days
- Dizziness
- Blurred vision
- A tendency to tilt your head when driving or working, *or*
- Any other unusual reaction

Getting Satisfaction

Will an optometrist or ophthalmologist who wrote an erroneous prescription pay for a new set of lenses? Will an optician who incorrectly filled a proper prescription pay for the second visit you made to an optometrist or ophthalmologist? If the party at fault refuses a fair settlement, explain that you will file a complaint.

File complaints against optometrists at the board of optometry of the state in which the practitioner's office is located. File complaints against ophthalmologists at the state board of medical examiners.

Resources

American Academy of Ophthalmology
P.O. Box 7424
San Francisco, CA 94120
(415) 561-8500
Write for free patient-information brochures on various eye diseases and disorders. Send a self-addressed, stamped envelope and state the eye topic on which you desire information.

American Academy of Pediatrics
141 N.W. Point Boulevard
Elk Grove, IL 60007
Send a self-addressed, stamped envelope for a free pamphlet, "Your Child's Eyes."

American Optometric Association
243 N. Lindbergh Boulevard
St. Louis, MO 63141
(314) 991-4100
Write for free pamphlets on "Family Guide to Vision Care," "Your Baby's Eyes," "Your Preschool Child's Eyes," "Your School-Age Child's Eyes," "Do Vision Problems Cause Adult Reading Problems?" and others. To receive a copy of any of these pamphlets, send a stamped, self-addressed business envelope.

National Eye Care Project
P.O. Box 429098
San Francisco, CA 94142
(800) 222-EYES
Operated by the American Academy of Ophthalmology, the NECP is a nationwide outreach program to provide medical eye care to disadvantaged senior citizens. The project provides referrals for people sixty-five or older to participating ophthalmologists for diagnosis and follow-up care for eye problems. Qualified patients receive treatment at no out-of-pocket expense. Ophthalmologists accept insurance reimbursement as payment in full. Uninsured patients receive care at no charge.

National Eye Health Education Program
2020 Vision Place
Bethesda, MD 20892-3655
(301) 496-5248
(800) 869-2020
Call or write for educational materials on preventing and treating various eye disorders.

18

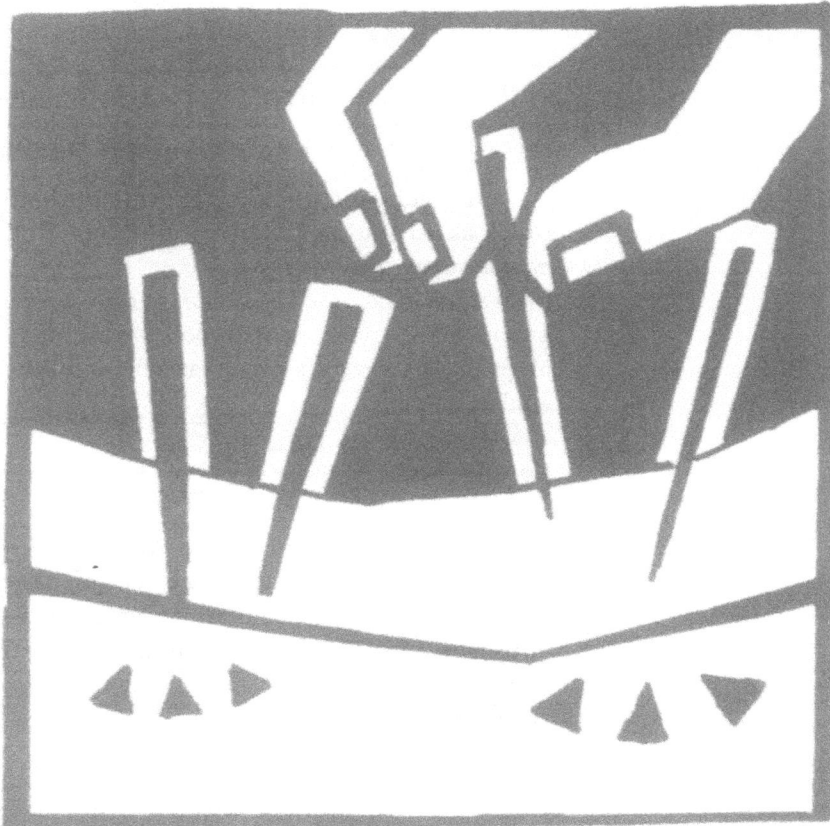

Alternative Health Care

Nicolás P. Carballeira

Nicolás P. Carballeira directs the Latino Health Institute of Massachusetts. He is a doctor of Ayurvedic medicine and a member of the faculties of the New England Institute of Ayurveda and the Boston University School of Public Health.

A growing number of people in the United States are seeking alternative ways to address their health concerns. The prestigious *New England Journal of Medicine* reports that as many as one-third of all American health care consumers try alternative healing practices in a given year—sometimes exclusively, although more often at the same time as they seek conventional care. Moreover, under a mandate from Congress, the National Institutes of Health has begun to study alternative medicines. And many Americans continue to utilize the Asian, African, Native American, and Middle Eastern traditional medicines that are part of their own culture's history, even as these same approaches to health and healing attract other Americans as well.

In fact, if you hesitate to depend totally on conventional medicine, you'll find a bewildering abundance of choices, and they'll have names as exotic as those in mainstream health care practice: Ayurveda, naturopathy, Chinese medicine, chiropractic, Tibb Unani. . . . How can you make informed decisions amid this veritable jumble of probably unfamiliar healing practices? And just as important, why should you explore them at all?

Consumer Reports on Alternative Health Care Providers

"Anyone venturing into the world of alternative medicine . . . is likely to find it as frustrating to explore as it is enticing. This is a field that encompasses vastly different treatments. It's a field whose practitioners range from sober academic physicians to entrepreneurial faith healers. And it's a field where there are still too few careful scientific studies, and where investigators haven't even agreed on what rules of evidence should apply."

Consumer Alert: Time to Walk

When it comes to health care, no one—neither conventional nor alternative providers—can guarantee the result you seek. If anyone does, start walking. You want practitioners who recognize the limitations, as well as the strengths, of their respective systems.

A Short History

Despite the growing popularity of alternatives in health care, many Americans still approach the terrain with ambivalence, confusion, or fear. Thus, it's well to begin at the beginning, with a capsule history of the divergence of conventional and alternative care.

Conventional medicine's dominance over health care in the United States is actually a fairly recent phenomenon. Into the early twentieth century, U.S. medicine was quite pluralistic. Conventional medical doctors—also known as allopaths—outnumbered other types of trained medical providers, yet homeopaths, herbalists, and others comprised about 20 percent of all practitioners.

It was the 1910 *Flexner Report,* commissioned by the Carnegie Foundation and backed by the Rockefeller Institute for Medical Research, that transformed U.S. medicine into a research-oriented, hospital-based science practiced almost exclusively by those who had the means to undertake eight years of university study. Upon publishing his report, Abraham Flexner visited 155 medical schools, recommending funding for those that agreed to pattern themselves on German laboratory-based medical education. By 1922 more than a third of the medical schools in existence in 1900 had closed—including over 70 percent of the schools primarily training minorities and 100 percent of those primarily training women.

While some aspects of the quality of conventional medical education undoubtedly improved as a result of the *Flexner Report,* such training became virtually out of reach for anyone other than upper-middle-class white men. This fed the shortage of conventional medical care for the poor, women, and minorities. Moreover, mainstream funding bypassed alternative medical systems, making training and credentialing of these approaches less reliable. In short, alternative healing retreated from the public eye into the status of marginal knowledge.

Today, many Americans regard alternative healers with suspicion even as they have learned to doubt the infallibility of conventional medicine and its practitioners. And their suspicion is probably often justified, given the fragmentation and minimal opportunities for clinical training in alternative healing. As a result, the consumer's task of finding trustworthy, well-trained practitioners is especially important—and challenging.

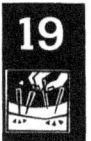

What Is Holistic Medicine?

Holistic medicine, a broad term, encompasses a range of healing philosophies that view a patient as a whole person, not just as a disease or a collection of symptoms. Holistic practitioners often address

Official Recognition

In 1991 the National Institutes of Health, the federal agency funding medical research, established the Office of Alternative Medicine (OAM). The office is an information clearinghouse on alternative medicine, and it awards grants for evaluating alternative approaches to medical care.

With a growing budget ($2 million in 1992; $7.4 million in 1996), the OAM is the government's first institutional foray into complementary and alternative medicine (CAM). While the office doesn't advocate particular treatments, its existence has added to the credibility of alternatives. And its congressional support reflects in part the public's frustration with rising medical costs and the growing awareness that conventional medicine is itself far from a precise science.

their clients' emotional and spiritual dimensions, as well as nutritional, environmental, and lifestyle factors that may contribute to illness. Many holistic practitioners combine natural or alternative techniques with conventional ones such as medication and surgery.

Entering the Mainstream

A 1993 *New England Journal of Medicine* article woke up the mainstream medical profession to the widespread use of alternative practices in the United States—and to the need to recognize this fact. Entitled "Unconventional Medicine in the United States," the article was based on a survey of 1,539 adults: 34 percent had used at least one unconventional therapy in the past year.

According to the article, American consumers spent $10.3 billion out of their pockets on unconventional treatments in 1990, compared to $12.8 billion for out-of-pocket hospitalization costs and $23.5 billion out of pocket for all physician services.

The average person seeking unconventional therapy spent $27.60 for each of nineteen visits over the year. The people most likely to use unconventional care had relatively more education and higher income than the average American—as is true of health care in general.

People tended to seek alternative care and an allopathic physician for the same condition. However, most consumers didn't tell their allopathic doctor about the unconventional treatment. Thus, the article suggests that medical doctors routinely ask patients about their use of unconventional therapy.

A Question of Balance

Even as conventional and alternative medicine have followed separate paths, they have continued to influence each other. Indeed, along with alternative practitioners, some conventional providers today understand health as a proper balance, specific to each individual, that changes with the seasons and time of life. Health isn't just the absence of symptoms of disease. Rather, it's the normal, natural state that enables a person to thrive in, or adapt to, a wide range of environments and stresses. Illness is an imbalance or disharmony arising from stresses that inordinately tax the organism's vital force.

The predominant alternative practitioner's view on healthy behavior is best summarized in Hippocrates' dictum *primum, non nocere*—first, do no harm. When illness arises, the alternative practitioner seeks to determine how and why the patient is out of balance and then prescribe dietary and gentle intervention measures to help the whole person return to the natural state of health. This moves the emphasis away from treatments that encourage long-term dependence on strong external measures and medications and toward prevention and mild corrective measures in opposition to the cause of the disease.

Central to the strength of alternative practices is that they relate health and healing to a person's whole social environment, especially his or her spiritual or religious beliefs. A common critique of conventional medicine is that it ignores connections between the individual and the surrounding environment. In contrast, most systems of alternative medicine claim to treat the body and mind as indivisible.

Who Does What

It's impossible in a single chapter to do justice to every system of alternative medicine, or even to any one approach. Both the depth and the variety of the field are tremendous. Some techniques are geared to the long term and others to a few office visits. Some might form your primary medical care; others you'd consider if you had a specific need, such as a chronic headache. Some people seek all their health care from alternative providers, but, just as often, conventional and alternative practices can complement each other beneficially.

Start by reviewing the following capsule descriptions of a few major systems and techniques that are considered alternative. Then consult a number of publications on those that appeal to you the most. You can also contact the organizations listed at the end of this chapter. Most of them can supply more information on their approach to health care, as well as the names of practitioners in your area.

Ayurveda

Ayurveda, or traditional Indian medicine, is the oldest continuously practiced system of health care in the world, preceding and influencing both Chinese and Western medicines. Endorsed by the World Health Organization as a cost-effective system of care, Ayurveda is the medicine of choice in many countries of the Indian subcontinent. It's also rapidly gaining popularity in the United States, Europe, and Asia because of its sensible, straightforward, and comprehensive approach to health promotion, disease prevention, and treatment.

The Office of Alternative Medicine has placed a priority on research in several specific areas, including:

- Who uses complementary and alternative medicine and how much?

- What specific effects do complementary and alternative medicine practices have on illness? To what degree can conventional medicine address the condition?

- To what extent can complementary and alternative medicine cure an illness, improve quality of life or the emotional well-being of a patient, or stimulate the autoregulatory system?

- How much of complementary and alternative medicine can be incorporated into a self-care program for patients?

- What is the value of complementary and alternative medicine as part of a prevention and wellness health care package?

19

Ayurvedic physicians provide primary care, including internal medicine, surgery and acupuncture, ophthalmology, pediatrics, toxicology, psychiatry, rejuvenation, fertility, and eye, ear, nose, and throat care. In the United States, as well as in India, most Ayurvedic physicians restrict the scope of their surgical practices to minor and throat surgery. However, Ayurvedic medicine is renowned for its surgical procedures, pioneering limb and organ transplants and plastic surgery as early as five thousand years ago.

Ayurvedic medicine holds that health is a state of balance among the physical, emotional, and spiritual components of the person. Illness is viewed as a state of imbalance that can be detected through such diagnostic procedures as reading the pulse, palpation, listening, observation, and inquiry. Through the eight traditional branches of Ayurvedic medicine, practitioners address a broad spectrum of ailments, from allergies to AIDS.

Ayurvedic physicians undertake a minimum of four years of graduate study and clinical internship, and most practitioners in the United States are also trained in conventional medicine, naturopathy, or Chinese medicine. The American Council on Ayurveda establishes standards for the profession, certifies practitioners, and accredits Ayurvedic educational institutions and clinical programs.

Naturopathy

Naturopathic physicians provide primary care, including handling natural childbirth. They treat disease and restore health using nutrition, herbal medicine, homeopathy, physical medicine, exercise therapy, lifestyle counseling, acupuncture, and psychotherapy. Naturopathic physicians cooperate with all branches of medical science, referring patients to other practitioners for diagnosis or treatment when appropriate. A major component of naturopathic medicine is a detailed patient history that provides a comprehensive background. In addition, when appropriate, naturopathic physicians use diagnostic tests, such as blood tests, X rays, and examining by touch.

Naturopathic physicians study conventional medical sciences, although they don't receive a degree as an allopathic medical doctor (MD). To become a naturopathic physician (ND), a person must complete at least four years of graduate study, with courses in traditional naturopathic philosophy, medical science, and natural therapeutics.

Naturopathic Licensing and Registration

Alaska, Arizona, Connecticut, Florida, Hawaii, Montana, Oregon, Rhode Island, Utah, and Washington license naturopathic physicians. The District of Columbia's Occupational and Professional Licensing Administration also registers naturopaths.

Chinese Medicine and Acupuncture

Encompassing a variety of practices, Chinese medicine is based on understanding the relationship between *yin* and *yang* and the five elements. According to this approach, illness results when these forces don't balance. Chinese medical practitioners treat a broad range of both chronic and acute illnesses with a variety of ancient and modern therapeutic methods—including herbal medicine, massage and manipulation, heat therapy, and counseling on nutrition and lifestyle. They rely heavily on basic diagnostic methods: looking, listening, smelling, asking, and touching.

Acupuncture is perhaps the best known and most popular Chinese healing technique. Acupuncturists insert very thin needles into the patient's skin. Often recognized in the United States as a way to relieve pain, acupuncture is also used to improve patients' overall well-being and to treat acute, chronic, and degenerative conditions. Acupressure involves the same concepts as acupuncture but replaces the needles with finger pressure.

Twenty-two states restrict the practice of acupuncture to physicians or people operating under the strict supervision of a physician. In general, there are no restrictions on acupressure, but some states require a massage license.

Consumer Reports recommends a list of points to consider if you are thinking about acupuncture:

■ Consult your doctor before you visit an acupuncturist. Your primary care physician should know about, and cooperate with, *all* your health care providers.

■ Insist that an acupuncturist use sterile, disposable needles to lessen the risk of infection.

■ Discuss fees and any possibility of insurance coverage before treatment.

■ Discuss your expectations with the practitioner.

19

■ Evaluate your progress. If six to eight treatments don't produce some benefit, either the treatment or the practitioner isn't right for you.

Acupuncture Credentials

All states allow physicians to practice acupuncture; fourteen require them to have formal training. Physician acupuncturists often belong to the American Academy of Medical Acupuncture. The National Commission for the Certification of Acupuncturists certifies nonphysician acupuncturists. Twenty-four states and the District of Columbia license nonphysicians to practice acupuncture.

Consumer Alert: Warning Sign

Be wary if an acupuncturist tells you to leave your current doctor or stop taking prescribed medications. Consult your doctor or another primary care provider first.

Homeopathy

Homeopaths address illness by administering infinitesimal amounts of natural substances that in larger amounts would cause the same illness to occur in a healthy person. They commonly treat infant and childhood diseases, infections, fatigue, allergies, arthritis, and other chronic illnesses.

Homeopaths claim to enhance a body's natural defense mechanisms and stimulate a person's own healing process while avoiding harmful side effects. The remedies are available from homeopaths, health food stores, and drugstores, as well as by mail. Homeopathic remedies appeal to some people who are afraid of more potent drugs.

By law, homeopathic remedies can contain *no detectable amount of any active ingredient*. As a result, federal regulations don't apply to these remedies. However, they are also exempt from FDA requirements for scientific proof that a drug is effective against disease.

Homeopathic remedies, because they are so diluted, are safe in themselves. The danger lies in the possibility that you might forgo other necessary treatments or fall victim to excessive claims or insufficient warnings on labels.

Homeopathy Licensing

Only health care professionals who are licensed to prescribe—medical doctors and naturopaths, for example—can legally practice homeopathy.

Despite the law, however, the profession includes many people with no formal medical training. Ask a homeopathic physician for credentials as a licensed health care practitioner before following his or her directions or taking any medications.

Don't replace your regular primary care provider with a homeopath who doesn't also have clinical training. A homeopathic practitioner without clinical training may ignore or misdiagnose early symptoms of a serious disease that may need medical or surgical treatment.

Chiropractic

Chiropractic rests on the premise that the spine is a fundamental conduit and support: misaligned vertebrae press on the spinal cord and lead to illness or otherwise diminish a person's ability to function. A chiropractic doctor (DC) seeks to analyze and correct these misalignments. Most people consult chiropractors for pain. Spinal manipulation is generally recognized to help some people with lower back pain. Chiropractors also prescribe diet modification and exercise to promote wellness. Some chiropractors incorporate other alternative therapies into their practice as well.

All fifty states and the District of Columbia license chiropractors, and the Council on Chiropractic Education accredits schools that teach chiropractic.

Chiropractors don't provide primary care. As with all specialists, consult the person from whom you get your primary care before working with a chiropractor. And make sure the chiropractor you select will work with your primary care provider and keep that person informed about your care.

Biofeedback

Biofeedback is a painless method with which people learn to improve their health and to control such involuntary functions as respiration, heartbeat, and body temperature by using signals from their own bodies.

Biofeedback is a technique rather than a system of medicine. Both conventional and alternative practitioners—psychologists, medical doctors, physical therapists, counselors, nurses, and others—use or prescribe biofeedback. According to the National Institute of Mental Health, biofeedback can be used to address to an ever-lengthening list of conditions, including migraine headaches and tension headaches, many other types of pain, digestive disorders, high and low blood pressure, abnormal heartbeat rhythms, Raynaud's disease (a circulatory disorder that causes

A Few More Alternative Medical Approaches

■ *Clinical hypnotherapy* induces a relaxed or altered state of awareness, consciousness, or perception to focus the mind and make it receptive to therapeutic suggestion. Hypnotherapy is used for both physical and psychological problems. There is no formal licensing for hypnotists, but you might check about membership in the American Society for Clinical Hypnosis or the Society for Clinical and Experimental Hypnosis. And seek therapy from a hypnotist who is also licensed in another field as a health care practitioner.

■ *Herbal medicine* uses natural herbs and plants to prevent and cure illnesses. Herbalists claim that their remedies avoid the harmful side effects so common in modern medicines.

For more information on herbal medicines, turn to chapter 7.

■ *Massage therapy* is an art in which hand manipulation of the body and its muscles eases muscle tension, produces relaxation, alleviates aches and pains, and aids in blood circulation. There are several types of massage

uncomfortably cold hands), epilepsy, and paralysis and other movement disorders.

Your primary care provider can help you decide if biofeedback might help you. If the answer is yes, work only with a professional biofeedback trainer. You might want to talk with several trainers before choosing one with whom you feel comfortable.

Biofeedback Questions

Before beginning biofeedback training, ask:

■ What will biofeedback training cost per session?
■ How many sessions will my treatment take?
■ How many patients have you treated with biofeedback?
■ How long have you trained people in biofeedback?
■ How did you learn the technique?
■ What are your other medical qualifications?
■ What conditions do you treat with biofeedback?

In addition, ask the trainer for professional references from physicians and other health care providers.

Making a Choice

Given the array of techniques and systems that fall under the rubric of "alternative health care," how do you select one?

You might start by looking into practices that are more familiar to you. For example, if you find it difficult to deal with terms and concepts from other cultures, you might feel more comfortable with naturopathy or another broad-based, eclectic Western approach. If you have an affinity for Indian, Chinese, or Arabic culture, you could explore, respectively, Ayurveda, Chinese medicine, or Tibb Unani.

You can also ask relatives, friends, and your current health care providers about their experiences and recommendations. Study each system that appeals to you in more depth to narrow down the field; then really concentrate your research and ask more questions.

Your choice will be influenced by the scope of care you are seeking. For example, if you want an alternative practitioner who is licensed in primary care, look into Ayurveda or naturopathy. For specialized needs, other licensed health care practitioners include chiropractors and acupuncturists. In addition, a growing number of conventional medical doctors, registered nurses, and dentists practice forms of holistic medicine and dentistry.

The Rules of the Game

Finding alternative health care requires research, probably in more depth than for conventional types of health care. As the term *alternative* implies, many of these approaches lie outside the medical mainstream. As a result, getting solid information about proper care—and related dangers—is less straightforward than researching the conventional medical literature.

Fortunately, the more you examine alternative healing practices, the more you'll find that nothing is particularly strange or mysterious about many of the most popular options. Indeed, as in any practice that potentially affects your health, you'll find good practitioners—and some to avoid. Some will treat you with respect—and others will use jargon instead of plain English to explain what they're doing to your body. In other words, approach alternative healing respectfully and cautiously, just as you would in the case of all your health care:

■ Remember the old adage *If it sounds too good to be true, it probably is.* No system provides a cure in every case.

■ Do your research thoroughly. Libraries and reputable organizations can provide you with information on different approaches to health care, including those listed at the end of this chapter. Keep in mind, however, that alternative approaches don't easily lend themselves to clinical trials because they encompass a wide variety of treatments that tend to differ for each individual, based on his or her circumstances.

■ Give the practitioner and the system you choose a fair try. Stick to a system if you respond well on any level: physical, spiritual, or mental. But discontinue care if you have reason to believe that a treatment is hurting you and the explanations you receive aren't satisfactory.

Before you begin treatment, make sure you understand what the practitioner says will happen. Learn your treatment plan. Discuss what to expect in terms of best-case and worst-case scenarios.

Once you locate a practitioner, ask specific questions. Investigate credentials. And don't be surprised that most of the questions match those you'd ask a "regular" doctor:

■ What did your training entail?
■ What clinical experience did your training include?
■ If applicable, what board certifications and licenses do you have?
■ What did you have to do to receive your certifications and licenses?
■ What does your training qualify you to treat?

therapy, including Swedish, Ayurvedic, shiatsu, rolfing, polarity, and bioenergetics.

■ *Metabolic therapy* emphasizes ways to strengthen the body's immune system and ward off illness by ridding the body of toxic substances, adjusting diet and nutrition, prescribing vitamins and supplements, and changing the person's lifestyle.

■ *Orthomolecular therapy* emphasizes the use of very large doses of vitamins to treat illness. It also emphasizes dietary changes to improve the body's nutrient intake.

■ *Tibb Unani,* another name for Greek-Arabic medicine, is a system of healing that relies on reestablishing balance among the body's qualities, such as heat and cold, dryness and moisture. Tibb is the base on which European medicine rested for centuries. It is practiced today in Arabic countries and by many Muslims in the United States.

19

- What clinical studies support your diagnosis and recommended treatments?

If you think you are seriously ill, consult your primary care provider first if at all possible. No matter whom you go to for treatment, someone with a thorough clinical training should diagnose your symptoms.

And always remember that you are in charge of your medical care. At any time in the process, you have the right to stop any treatment for any reason. And no treatment can be done without your *informed consent*.

Get Answers

Honest health care practitioners don't hesitate to provide clear, direct answers to questions about their training and your needs. If answers don't make sense to you, or if you are still doubtful, ask a practitioner to give you references from other clients and health care providers—or move on.

Finding Local Alternative Providers

The best way to locate providers of alternative health services is through the recommendation of relatives, friends, and neighbors who may have relationships with serious, qualified practitioners. However, should you not have access to this source of information, call a reputable national organization. Ask for the names of two or three local practitioners.

If you are looking for alternative primary care, call the American Council on Ayurveda, the American Association of Naturopathic Physicians, or the American Holistic Medical Association. They can refer you to qualified primary care Ayurvedic physicians, naturopaths, or holistic allopaths in your vicinity.

There are also some excellent guides that may be available at health food stores and at comprehensive bookstores that carry alternative health publications.

For more information, turn to the Resources at the end of this chapter.

Money Matters

Alternative medicine, with its relatively low reliance on high technology and pharmaceutical drugs, should prove less expensive than allopathic care in most cases. One limited study compares the cost-effectiveness of naturopathic and allopathic conventional care and clearly shows the medical and economic advantages of naturopathic care. Contact the American Association of Naturopathic Physicians for a copy of this study. In addition, government-sponsored research in this country and Canada demonstrates that chiropractic care is less expensive and more effective in alleviating back pain than conventional medical treatment.

Depending on where you reside and the licensing laws of your state, your insurance may or may not cover particular alternative health services. Be sure to ask providers and your insurers before making an appointment. If the alternative care you seek isn't covered, you'll have to pay out of your own pocket.

Work with your alternative provider to reduce your out-of-pocket costs by exploring all options for reimbursement. A responsible alternative practitioner should be able to guide you in this matter. A cooperative conventional doctor may increase the likelihood of reimbursement by making appropriate referrals.

Two plans specifically cover alternative therapies:

1. The American Western Life Insurance Company's *Wellness Plan* is currently available to residents of California, Utah, Colorado, New Mexico, and Arizona. It covers alternative care as well as major medical expenses, hospitalization, prescription drugs, laboratories, and surgery. Its cost is competitive with more conventional policies.

2. Subscribers to the *Alternative Health Plan,* available nationwide, can receive treatment from licensed physicians acting within the scope of their license to treat any illness or injury or to provide preventive services. This includes providers of acupuncture, Ayurvedic medicine, homeopathy, naturopathy, chiropractic, and Chinese medicine.

For more information on the Wellness Plan, call (800) 925-5223; for the Alternative Health Plan, call (800) 966-8467.

You might also be able to get coverage for alternative treatment if your conventional insurance doesn't restrict you to a list of providers and your state licenses alternative practitioners. Because the laws of each state and the various health insurance plans differ so widely, make sure to research the exact situation in your locality before incurring alternative-medicine expenses. Alternative practitioners usually aren't included in state-sponsored free-care pools. On the other hand, at least eighty private insurers and Medicaid programs in some states cover acupuncture for certain conditions.

TIP

The Rules Apply . . . and Then Some

The questions to ask and the rules to follow as you seek care from alternative providers are essentially the same as for any health care practitioner.

For more on these guidelines, see chapter 5 on primary care and chapter 13 on physician specialists.

However, given the wide variation in the background and training of alternative practitioners, take your research task especially seriously. Licensing regulations outside the medical mainstream vary in effectiveness and scope from state to state and field to field—if they exist at all.

19

TIP

Insurance Source

Call or write the American Association of Naturopathic Physicians for a brochure that assists patients who wish to obtain insurance coverage for alternative providers. AANP, 2366 Eastlake Avenue East, Suite 322, Seattle, WA 98102; tel. (206) 323-7610.

✓ Selected Typical Fees

	Initial Visit	Follow-Ups
Acupuncture*	$ 75–$300	$45–$150
Ayurveda	$ 50–$175	$30–$ 75
Biofeedback	$ 75–$200	$75–$200
Chiropractic†	$ 50–$170	$25–$ 70
Homeopathic, M.D.	$125–$200	$50–$ 75
Naturopathy	$ 50–$150	$40–$ 70

*The higher costs apply when the practitioner is an M.D.
†Add $75 to $120 for X rays.
Source: On Ayurveda, the American Council on Ayurveda; for all others, Health Awareness Resource Center

Resources
Organizations

American Association of Acupuncture and Oriental Medicine
433 Front Street
Catasauqua, PA 18032-2506
(610) 433-2448
Call or write for referrals and general information.

American Association of Naturopathic Physicians
2366 Eastlake Avenue East, #322
Seattle, WA 98102
(206) 323-7610
Send a stamped, self-addressed envelope for general information about naturopathic physicians. Send $5 for a listing of NPs in your area. Call or write for referrals to primary care naturopaths in your area and for information on insurance.

American Chiropractic Association
1701 Clarendon Boulevard
Arlington, VA 22209
(703) 276-8800
Call or write for general information about chiropractic.

American Council on Ayurveda
111 Elm Street, Suites 103–105
Worcester, MA 01609
(508) 755-3744
Call or write for general information about Ayurveda.

American Foundation of Traditional Chinese Medicine
505 Beach Street
San Francisco, CA 94133
(415) 776-0502
Call or write for information.

American Herbalists Guild
P.O. Box 1683
Soquel, CA 95073
(408) 464-2441
Send $2 for a recommended-reading list; send $2 for a directory of schools and resources.

American Holistic Medical Association
4101 Lake Boone Trail
Raleigh, NC 27607
(919) 787-5181
Call or write for general information, including referrals to conventional medical doctors who take a holistic

approach. Send $8 for a directory list-
ing association members.

American Massage Therapy Association
820 Davis Street
Evanston, IL 60201
(708) 864-0123
Call or write for references and referrals.

American Oriental Bodywork Therapy
    Association
6801 Jericho Turnpike
Syosset, NY 11791
(516) 364-5533
Call or write for referrals and membership information.

American Osteopathic Association
142 E. Ontario Street
Chicago, IL 60611
(312) 280-5800
Call or write for referrals.

American Society of Clinical Hypnosis
22000 E. Deven Avenue
Des Plaines, IL 60018-4534
(708) 297-3317
Send a self-addressed, stamped envelope for listings of local providers.

Association for Applied Psychophysiol-
    ogy and Biofeedback
10200 W. 44th Avenue
Wheat Ridge, CO 80033
(303) 422-8436
Send a self-addressed, stamped envelope to receive listings of local providers.
Send $20 for a national directory.

Cancer Control Society
Alternative Therapies
2043 N. Berendo Street
Los Angeles 90027
(213) 663-7801
Call or write for information and referrals to clinic and individual doctors
who treat cancer and other diseases
with alternative therapies.

Commonweal
P.O. Box 316
Bolinas, CA 94924
(415) 868-0970
Call for information about alternative
cancer therapies.

Health Awareness, Inc.
18 Old Padonia Road
Cockeysville, MD 21030
(410) 560-6864
This nonprofit service organization
provides educational resources on
many holistic practices. Call or write
for information on naturopathy, oste-
opathy, acupressure, food additives,
and other topics. No charge for services, but donations are suggested.
Publishes "Awareness Update" quarterly; subscriptions are $20 per year.

Health Information Network Interna-
    tional
4213 Montgomery Drive
Santa Rosa, CA 95405
(800) 743-6996
(707) 539-3967
Call or write for information and
research on natural health substances
and treatment alternatives.

Holistic Dental Association
P.O. Box 5007
Durango, CO 81301
(303) 259-1091
Send a self-addressed, stamped envelope for a listing of local holistic dental
practitioners.

Homeopathic Education Services
2124 Kittredge Street
Berkeley, CA 94704
(510) 649-0294
Call or write for educational materials,
including books, tapes, videos, medicine, and resource information.

National Center for Homeopathy
801 N. Fairfax Street
Alexandria, VA 22314

19

(703) 548-7790
Send $5 for a directory of homeopathic doctors, pharmacists, and other resources.

Office of Alternative Medicine Information Center
National Institutes of Health
6120 Executive Boulevard, EPS #450
Rockville, MD 20892-9904
(301) 402-2467
Contact the OAM for information packages on alternative medicine regarding general information, research, cancer, HIV/AIDS, and online research. For information on a wide variety of specific diseases, call (301) 496-4000 and ask the operator to direct you to the proper office. The OAM report on the uses of alternative medicine, *Alternative Medicine: Expanding Medical Horizons* ($25), cites many cost-effective uses of alternative therapies; to order a copy, contact your nearest Government Printing Office or call the U.S. Superintendent of Documents at (202) 512-1800.

Planetree Health Resources
2034 Fillmore Street
San Francisco, CA 94115
(415) 673-4964
Call or visit for information on health-related matters, including alternative health. The resource library is open to the public.

Society for Clinical and Experimental Hypnosis
6728 Old McLean Village Drive
McLean, VA 22101-3906
(703) 556-9222
Call or write for general information and referrals to local organizations.

Publications

Alternative Medicine Yellow Pages: The Comprehensive Guide to the New World of Health (1994, $12.95) and *Alternative Medicine: The Definitive Guide* ($48 plus

$5.50 for shipping and handling). Both available from Health Awareness, Inc., 18 Old Padonia Road, Cockeysville, MD 21030; tel. (410) 560-6864.

Consumer Reports, January, March, and June 1994. A series of three in-depth articles covering acupuncture, homeopathy, and chiropractic. To order, send $5 per issue to Consumer Reports Back Issues, P.O. Box 53016, Boulder, CO 80322.

Family Guide to Natural Medicine: How to Stay Healthy the Natural Way (Reader's Digest Association, 1993), $32.95.

Full Catastrophe Living: Using the Wisdom of Your Body and Mind to Face Stress, Pain, and Illness, by Jon Kabat-Zinn (Delta/Dell, 1990), $12.95.

"Holistic Health Directory." Lists 7,000 alternative providers in the United States and Canada. Order from *New Age Journal,* 42 Pleasant Street, Watertown, MA 02172; tel. (617) 926-0200. $5.95.

Mind/Body Medicine: How to Use Your Mind for Better Health, edited by Daniel Goleman and Joel Gurin (Consumer Reports Books, 1995), $14.95.

The Natural Family Doctor: The Comprehensive Self-Help Guide to Health and Natural Medicine, by Andrew Stanway and Richard Grossman (Simon and Schuster, 1987), $12.95.

Natural Health, Natural Medicine: A Comprehensive Manual for Wellness and Self-Care, by Andrew Weil (Houghton Mifflin, 1991), $10.95.

"Options in Health Care: Understanding Traditional and Alternative Methods." Order from People's Medical Society, 14 East Minor Street, Emmaus, PA 18049; tel. (800) 624-8773. $4 ($3 for members).

Death with Dignity

George J. Annas

George J. Annas is the
Edward R. Utley
Professor of Health
Law at the Boston
University School of
Medicine and head of
the Health Law
Department at the
Boston University
School of Public Health.
He is the author of
many books, including
The Rights of Patients
(Southern Illinois
University Press, 1989)
and *Standard of Care:
The Law of American
Bioethics* (Oxford
University Press, 1993).
He writes a regular
feature on law in the
*New England Journal of
Medicine.*

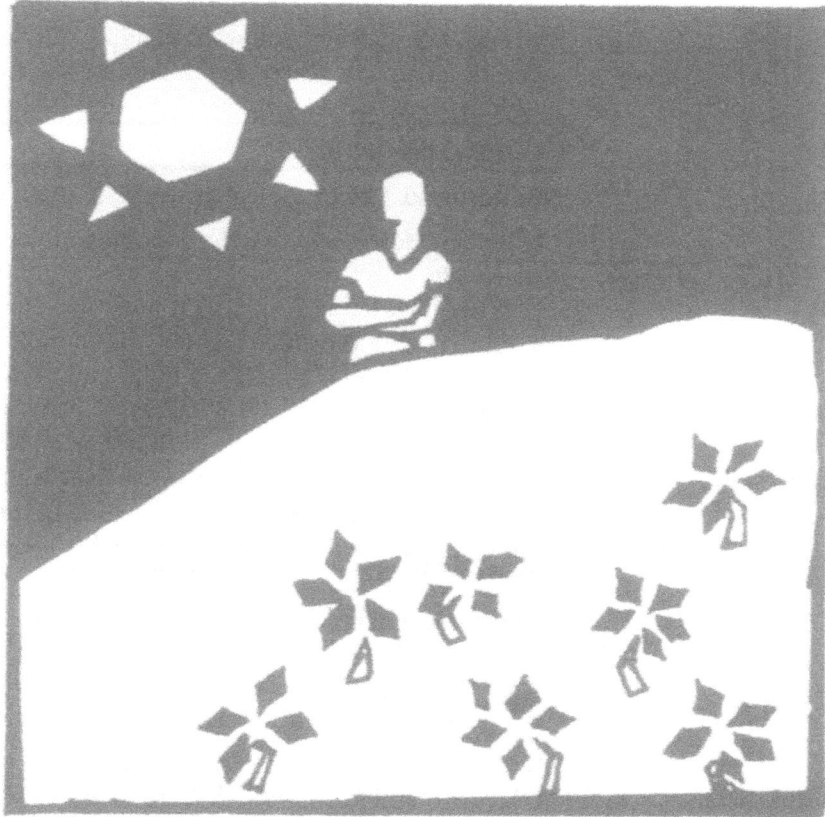

At any given time, millions of Americans are either facing the last stages of their own fatal illness or caring for dying relatives. Almost 2 million Americans die each year, and a million more have a terminal diagnosis.

Nonetheless, as a culture, we persist in denying death. Dying patients often know better. Even more than death, they fear isolation and pain. We can make our deaths a bit easier—for our families and ourselves—by planning and by requiring health care professionals to take our humanity and our needs seriously.

Probably our first and foremost need, and right, is to know the truth about our situation. When people lack the opportunity to discuss their own impending deaths, they simultaneously lose their dignity as adults. The "survivor knows best" attitude is illustrated by the words of a woman who described the death of her uncle as beautiful: "John died happy, never even realizing he was seriously ill."

This "ignorance is bliss" attitude deprives dying people of their last opportunity to accomplish goals and say things they would want to. For example, a father who knows he's dying of cancer might want to put his business affairs in better order now rather than leave his family with problems later. He might also want to tell his children that he loves them.

Silence and Death

Leo Tolstoy describes the dehumanizing effect of silence in *The Death of Ivan Ilyich:*

"What tormented Ivan Ilyich most was the deception, the lie, which for some reason they all accepted, that he was not dying but was simply ill, and that he only need keep quiet and undergo a treatment and then something very good would result. . . . This deception tortured him—their not wishing him to admit what they all knew and what he knew. . . . Those lies—lies enacted over him on the eve of his death and destined to degrade this awful, solemn act to the level of their visiting, their curtains, their sturgeon for dinner—were a terrible agony for Ivan Ilyich."

Hospice Care

Hospice care is designed for people with a terminal illness who will probably die within six months. The hospice movement is built around the principle that people should be able to die at home, free from pain and without complex medical invasions of their bodies. Over 2,000 hospice programs across the United States help make this a reality.

Almost all of these have been established since 1974, and the number has increased by about one-third since 1989 alone.

According to the National Hospice Organization, hospice is a special kind of care for dying people and their families that:

- Treats the physical *and* emotional and spiritual needs of the patient
- Takes place in his or her home or in a homelike setting
- Concentrates on making the patient as free from pain and as comfortable as possible
- Supports family members as an essential part of the mission, *and*
- Believes quality of life to be as important as length of life.

Hospice programs serve more than a quarter million patients and families each year in the United States, and three-quarters of hospice patients die in their own homes. About 80 percent of hospice patients suffer from cancer, 10 percent have heart-related illnesses, and a growing proportion have AIDS, with various other diagnoses making up the remainder. About 40 percent of all cancer deaths and 30 percent of all AIDS deaths occur in hospice programs.

Physicians and other primary care providers are usually the ones who refer patients to hospice programs, but family members, friends, and clergy can do this as well. Hospital discharge planners, nurses, and social workers also refer people to hospice programs, and all these people can help you find one for yourself or a family member.

Hospices provide care through a team of professionals and volunteers. The members of the team range from physicians and nurses to counselors, therapists, and home-health aides. Volunteers are at the heart of hospice care. Each year, about 100,000 volunteers donate over 5 million hours. Staff members and volunteers receive specific training to work with people in the last months of life. They also cooperate with the patient's own health care providers.

The members of a hospice team help keep the patient's environment as free and open as possible. Team members can also help the patient with back rubs and foot massages, matters of personal cleanliness, "being there," open discussions about feelings, assistance with household chores, financial matters, favorite foods or music, and pastimes.

Hospice team members administer drugs only to ease pain and provide comfort. Because the focus of hospice is on dying with dignity, treatments to extend life, such as chemotherapy, are not used. On the other hand, a person in hospice care doesn't forfeit all access to medical technology: About half of U.S. hospice programs admit patients requiring

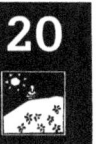

TIP

Hospice Hotline

For referrals to local hospice programs, contact the National Hospice Organization Helpline at (800) 658-8898.

"high-tech" therapies, and almost all will consider such patients on a case-by-case basis. Hospice patients, of course, have the right to change their minds and be admitted to a hospital for high-tech treatment.

Beyond direct service to patients and families, many hospice programs also offer services to the community at large. These activities range from support groups and memorial services to educational programs, individual and family counseling, crisis counseling, and specific children's services.

The Semi-Right to Die at Home

In theory, you have the right to die in your own home. As a practical matter, it's often difficult to arrange. Fewer than 20 percent of all Americans die at home. To do so requires not only the strong resolve of the dying person but also the cooperation of his or her family and anyone with whom the patient lives.

The cooperation of health care providers also matters a great deal. Without it, a person can't get prescriptions for pain-relieving drugs and other medication.

Finding the Right Hospice

Look for a Medicare-certified hospice program, advises "Harvard Health Letter." In the absence of any national organization that regulates hospices, the procedures required to qualify for Medicare payment indicate that a program meets basic standards of quality.

Once you are ready to check out the quality and suitability of a particular hospice program, talk with its staff. "Harvard Health Letter" recommends that you ask about:

- Hospital affiliations
- Procedures for assuring twenty-four-hour access to staff
- Protocol for managing pain
- Criteria for enrolling
- Payment options, *and*
- Arrangements for residential care, if and when it's needed

In particular, try to get a sense of the willingness of staff members to help patients and their families. Do they sound caring and competent? Or do they use lots of jargon or lead you to expect that the program involves a great deal of bureaucracy?

Money Matters

When a Medicare-eligible patient receives care from a Medicare-approved hospice, Medicare pays almost the entire cost for all services and supplies. In general, this coverage includes physician services, nursing care, medical equipment and supplies, drugs for managing symptoms and relieving pain, short-term inpatient and respite care, homemaker services and home-health aides, physical and other therapy, and counseling. Hospice coverage replaces your usual hospital coverage under Medicare Part A. You can revoke the hospice benefit at any time to revert to the usual Part A benefits.

About three-quarters of U.S. hospice programs are either Medicare-certified or have certification pending. To receive Medicare certification, a hospice program must provide:

- Twenty-four-hour staffing
- Medical and nursing care
- Home-health services
- Access to patient care
- Social-work services
- Counseling, including bereavement counseling
- Medications, medical supplies, and durable medical equipment, *and*
- Physical, occupational, and speech therapy

If a person's need for hospice care extends beyond the expected six-month limit, Medicare may still cover the bills. If a person is recertified as needing hospice care, the benefit can be extended indefinitely, and a hospice can't discharge a person without good cause. If private insurance is paying for hospice care, the coverage for extended periods varies. Some plans define a dollar limit, whereas others follow the Medicare rules. If you are paying for hospice care yourself, the admission criteria and other policies and procedures of the hospice govern the situation.

Insured Benefit

The health insurance of more than 80 percent of employees in medium and large companies covers hospice care. It's also covered under Medicare nationally and under thirty-three state Medicaid plans. Three-fifths of all hospice patients receive their care under Medicare or Medicaid.

Hospices will assist families lacking insurance to explore other options for coverage. And most hospices will provide for anyone who can't pay, using money raised from the community or other donations.

Pain and Medication

One reason for the growing availability and acceptance of hospice programs is the failure of the U.S. health care system to alleviate the pain of dying people. Perhaps more than half of terminally ill patients don't receive proper relief from pain. This is a major medical scandal.

Even if you refuse medical care that might lengthen your life, physicians can't withhold needed and appropriate pain medications. Physicians have a legal and ethical obligation to give you all the medication you need to be comfortable, even if it shortens your life. Both you and your advocate should demand that your providers meet this obligation. To alleviate pain, doses often need not be so high as to distort reality. And terminally ill people have no reason to fear drug addiction.

The right to pain-and-comfort medicines doesn't yet extend to marijuana or heroin, although these drugs are used for pain and discomfort in other countries. Some states have decriminalized marijuana for medical purposes.

Your Pain

When he was dying of cancer, columnist Stewart Alsop wrote eloquently of the experience. He suggested allowing patients *"to decide for themselves how much pain-killing drug they will take—it is, after all, they, not the doctors, who are suffering the agonies."*

Saying No

The decision about what treatment options exist is a medical one, but the decision to undergo any particular treatment isn't. It's a personal choice that only you can legitimately make. Specific court cases about refusing treatment have dealt with blood transfusions, mechanical ventilators, kidney dialysis, fluids and nutrition, and chemotherapy, among other things. The point is, you can refuse *any* medical intervention, including lifesaving and life-sustaining treatment and artificial feeding. This even includes cardiopulmonary resuscitation (CPR), which some health care personnel treat differently from other medical procedures because they administer it under emergency conditions.

Physicians *can* treat patients in emergencies without consent. After all, time is of the essence, and it's often impossible to obtain informed consent in these situations. However, if the emergency can be anticipated and the patient refuses to consent in advance, no one has the legal or ethical right to impose any procedure, even CPR. In a hospital, a person who has refused CPR is designated DNR (do not resuscitate) or DNAR (do not attempt resuscitation). All other measures to care for you and ensure your comfort are still available unless you specifically refuse them.

Technology, Life, and Death

Some people wrongly claim that the mere existence of medical technology creates an obligation on the part of patients to submit to its use. Such an attitude would make the right to refuse treatment irrelevant: Patients have rights to decide to use or refuse technology; technologies have no "right" to be used.

Children and Parents

Usually, parents can't refuse potentially life-sustaining care for their children, even for religious reasons. As the U.S. Supreme Court stated in another context, "Parents may be free to become martyrs themselves. But it does not follow they are free . . . to make martyrs of their children."

Parents are legally obligated to provide their children with "necessary medical care." When alternative treatments are available, parents can choose among those that are consistent with generally accepted medical practice. But parents can't legally choose to forgo treatment unless that's consistent with the best interests of the child. To deny a child beneficial treatment may make a parent guilty of child neglect, in which case a physician or hospital can obtain a court order to treat the child.

Planning Ahead

While few of us look forward to our own death, we should all take responsibility for making at least some provision for it.

Rather than leave it to chance, designate someone *now* to make health care decisions for you when you can't decide for yourself. When you are no longer able to give informed consent, your guardian or next of kin can make treatment decisions for you if you haven't designated a

Physicians and Assisted Suicide

In 1996 two U.S. Circuit Courts of Appeals, with jurisdiction over almost half of the population of the United States (including New York and California), ruled that individuals have a constitutional right to "hasten death." According to these courts, this right is strong enough to prevent states from prosecuting physicians who prescribe lethal drugs to competent, terminally ill patients who are suffering severely and who request such a prescription for the crime of assisted suicide. These two rulings have been appealed to the U.S. Supreme Court and will likely be reversed. No matter what the U.S. Supreme Court decides, however, this issue will remain the subject of heated debate.

If a family member or friend expresses a desire to commit suicide, be sure to explore the reasons for this desire, especially depression. Make sure all efforts to deal with these reasons are addressed directly and competently.

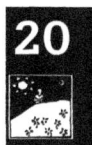

20

proxy. If you don't express your wishes beforehand, the next of kin or guardian must decide what is in your best interest.

The document through which you designate someone to speak for you is called an *advance directive.* The term generally applies to two kinds of legal documents: a living will and a durable power of attorney for health care, also called a health care proxy. These documents let you instruct your family, friends, guardians, health care providers, and others about your medical care in the event that serious illness or some other incapacity prevents you from speaking for yourself.

Forty-five states and the District of Columbia authorize both living wills and the appointment of a health care agent.

Some state laws restrict the applicability of living wills and health care proxies so that, for example, they can't be used to authorize the termination of artificial nutrition and hydration, or the refusal of treatment during pregnancy. However, these restrictions simply mean that you can't use the living will or health care proxy method to attain these ends in these states. Individuals have a *constitutional* right to refuse treatment, and the state can't take this away by statute. There is no constitutional authority for the proposition that women lose their right to refuse treatment when they become pregnant.

Take the time to think carefully about your beliefs and express them fully as you prepare an advance directive. Make sure that it truly reflects your opinions. "Talk openly about your wishes with your family, your friends, and your doctor," advises Choice in Dying, a nonprofit organization that advocates for people's end-of-life rights. "Don't assume that they know what you would want. . . . Family's and physicians' guesses about a patient's preferences are often mistaken. Talking with the people who may have to act on your behalf ensures that they understand your wishes, gives them a chance to ask questions, and also lets you determine whether they will follow your wishes, even if your choices differ from theirs."

Emergencies and Advance Directives

In any emergency, physicians are privileged to treat you. However, emergency medical technicians in most states can't decide whether your written advance directive applies. Instead, technicians do what is necessary to stabilize you for transfer to a hospital.

If you call 911 for another person, expect that person to receive emergency treatment regardless of an advance directive. Thus, the family must be prepared to contact a different person, such as a hospice nurse, when death is expected and emergency treatment is not wanted.

If You Don't Say Otherwise

Without clear evidence about a person's wishes, health care providers often continue to treat patients. Even if your family believes you'd reject treatment, the medical staff may ask for proof of your wishes before agreeing to stop treatment.

Living Wills

A living will is an advance directive in which you set forth in writing your wishes concerning medical treatment in the event you are incapacitated and not able to speak for yourself. A living will is much like a regular will, but it's termed *living* because it takes effect before you die. Living wills usually address only decisions at the end of life, specifying the kinds of treatment you refuse and the conditions under which this refusal applies.

Most people simply don't want to stay alive in a permanent coma. Even this general request, included in a living will, is extremely helpful to physicians and families. If you have strong, specific wishes, tell your physician and family how you want to be treated in various situations. In addition, designate one or more people to act on your behalf to decide about your medical care when you can't do so yourself. You may wish to tell this person verbally how you want to be treated, but it's best to write down directions in a letter that your agent can use to document your wishes should the need arise.

The movement to write living wills received a major boost from the case of Karen Ann Quinlan, a young woman who became permanently unconscious after an accident. Her parents had to go to court to get her medical ventilator removed. They argued that she wouldn't have wanted to live like that. Almost everyone who heard about the case reacted by thinking, "I'd never want to be like Karen Ann Quinlan"—meaning kept alive, in a permanent coma, on a ventilator. To help prevent this from happening, many wrote their wishes down for their relatives.

Lawyers and Advance Directives

You may want a lawyer's help as you prepare a living will or a health care proxy, but this isn't necessary. For advice and state-specific forms and laws at no charge, contact *Choice in Dying, 200 Varick Street, New York, NY 10014-4810 (212) 366-5540 or (800) 989-WILL.*

TIP

Exercise Your Rights

Almost all Americans approve of living wills— yet only 20 percent actually sign them.

20

TIP

Keep It Handy

Advance directives are meant to be read, so keep them handy. Make copies, which can have the same legal authority as the original if the original so specifies. Give copies to your agent and alternative agent.

Durable Power of Attorney

More important than preparing a living will is to formally designate a friend or relative to make decisions on your behalf through a document called a durable power of attorney or health care proxy. A durable power of attorney is valid in every state, and some states have specific documents just for health care decisions. Use this mechanism to designate someone you trust to make health care decisions for you when you can't make them for yourself.

With any power of attorney, you give someone else the authority to perform certain acts as your agent, consistent with your directions. Ordinarily, powers of attorney cease to be effective when you become incompetent, but a *durable* power of attorney continues in effect. In fact, a durable power of attorney for health care usually goes into effect *only* when and if you become incompetent. It's important that you talk to your agent about what you want and make sure your agent is willing to do it.

A health care proxy is better than a living will because it's impossible to anticipate every circumstance in advance. Moreover, a health care proxy generally applies in a wider range of situations than those involving the end of your life. For example, an unforeseen decision might be needed while you are unconscious from an accident, even though you are expected to recover and live for many more years. If specific eventualities worry you, write a detailed letter to your designated agent. But if you don't have someone you trust implicitly, a living will may still be useful.

If You Don't Designate an Agent

You can best protect your wishes by designating a health care agent and providing that person with specific written instructions.

If you don't name someone to make decisions for you, most states have statutes that designate which family member has this authority. Thus, appointing a trusted person as your proxy is especially important if you are estranged from your family or just want someone outside your family to make decisions for you.

Enforcing Your Rights

In the increasingly rare event that physicians or a health care facility doesn't honor your right to refuse treatment—as expressed by you or by your health care agent on your behalf—first determine the specific basis of the action. Then:

- Report the situation to that person's immediate supervisor.
- Report the situation to the administrator of the facility.
- Find out if the facility has a patient representative or a patient-rights advocate. If so, see if that person will help.
- Threaten to hire a lawyer or go to the local newspapers—and act on this threat if necessary.

Donating Your Organs

Under the Uniform Anatomical Gift Act, which every state has enacted in some form, anyone eighteen years or older and of sound mind may donate all or any part of his or her body at death to:

- Any hospital, physician, surgeon, or procurement organization for transplantation, therapy, medical education, dental education, research, or the advancement of medical or dental science
- Any accredited medical or dental school, college, or university for education, research, therapy, or the advancement of medical or dental science, *and*
- Any specified individual for therapy or transplantation needed by that individual

To make your intention to donate your organs more effective:

- Obtain a donor card through the United Network of Organ Sharing, the Organ Donation Living Bank, any hospital, or, in most states, the Registry of Motor Vehicles. Fill out the card in the presence of two witnesses and carry it with you at all times.

- Participate in the organ/tissue donor registry in addition to carrying the card. Your intentions to donate will be on file in a database.

- Carry the donor card in your wallet or purse; your driver's license may note your status as a donor as well.

In most states, you can revoke the gift either by destroying the card or by saying you revoke it in the presence of two witnesses. Write "VOID" on the donor card and contact any organization with which you've signed up as a donor.

After you die, your next of kin can donate your organs even if you didn't sign a donor card. If a family member dies and you would like to donate his or her organs, discuss it with the family member's physician.

Virtually no physician or hospital will take organs from your corpse without your next of kin's consent—even if you sign a donor card. This isn't for legal reasons. It simply doesn't seem proper. Thus, it's especially important to discuss your wishes with your family now if you want to be an organ donor.

For more information about organ donation or to receive forms to register as a donor, call the Organ Donation Living Bank at (800) 528-2971, the United Network for Organ Sharing Organ Donor Hotline at (800) 24-DONOR, or, in most states, the Registry of Motor Vehicles.

A Sample Donor Card

The donor should sign this card in the presence of two witnesses.

Uniform Donor Card

Of _____
(name of donor)

In the hope that I may help others, I hereby make this anatomical gift, if medically acceptable, to take effect upon my death. The words and marks below indicate my desires. I give:

(a) _____ any needed organs or parts

(b) _____ only the following organs or parts:

_____
(specify the organ[s] or part[s])

for the purposes of transplantation, therapy, medical research or education;

(c) _____ my body for anatomical study if needed.

Limitations or special wishes, if any:

_____

What Is Death?

The determination that a person is dead is a medical decision, and physicians have the legal authority to "declare" a person dead. Traditionally, physicians did so when a person's heart stopped irreversibly *and* the person stopped breathing.

However, cardiopulmonary resuscitation can often restart a heart, and since CPR's introduction in the early 1960s, a stopped heart hasn't necessarily meant irreversible destruction of the brain. However, brain destruction always means death. When CPR either fails or isn't tried, and a person's heart stops beating, the person is dead.

Families and the Determination of Death

A family with reason to doubt that a determination of death accords with accepted medical standards can insist that a qualified neurosurgeon or neurologist confirm the judgment before a respirator is disconnected.

If the determination is confirmed, the family has no right to insist on further medical care. All treatment should end upon the pronouncement of death, and unless organ donation or autopsy is planned, the body should be released to the family for burial.

Brain Death

Mechanical respirators that take over breathing make it feasible to artificially sustain respiration and heartbeat in a body that would otherwise stop functioning because the brain is destroyed. Because of this, brain death is now a widely accepted alternative way to determine death in these circumstances.

Under the current medical and legal definition, an individual is considered dead when he or she has sustained either:

- Irreversible cessation of circulatory and respiratory functions, *or*
- Irreversible cessation of all functions of the entire brain, including the brain stem

In either case, the determination of death must accord with accepted medical standards. Note that a permanently unconscious person—such as Karen Ann Quinlan—isn't dead. Among other things, such people can often breathe without mechanical assistance, and so have at least brain-stem function.

Brain Death

Brain death is a technical term that applies only to a body attached to a mechanical ventilator. The body's whole brain must be totally and irreversibly destroyed, and the body *can't ever* breathe on its own.

Autopsies

An autopsy is a comprehensive study of a corpse performed by a trained physician who employs recognized dissection procedures and techniques. Most commonly, autopsies are used to determine the cause of death, but they also play a valuable role in educating health care students. A public official, called a medical examiner or coroner, may also order an autopsy if homicide or suicide is suspected.

Health care professionals and students can practice on a corpse only if the person signed a written consent before he or she died or the next of kin gives consent after the person is dead. If a hospital doctor requests the autopsy, the hospital almost always absorbs the cost. It shouldn't appear on the hospital bill.

The law protects the personal feelings of the survivors. Unless murder, suicide, or accidental death is suspected, the next of kin must consent before an autopsy can be conducted. While the body isn't "property," the next of kin generally wants to see that the body is treated properly, and if it isn't, a suit for intentional infliction of emotional distress is possible.

Resources
Organizations

Children's Hospice International
700 Princess Street
Alexandria, VA 22314
(703) 684-0330
(800) 242-4453
Call or write for information about counseling regarding hospice care for terminally ill children. CHI makes referrals to hospice programs, self-help groups, and other local agencies.

Choice in Dying
200 Varick Street
New York, NY 10014-4810
(212) 366-5540
(800) 989-WILL
Call or write for sample advance directives for every state. Trained professionals answer the toll-free line and provide personal advice, legal assistance, free advance-directive documents, and the latest information on end-of-life laws and regulations in each state. The organization also maintains a network of volunteers in states and a speakers bureau. Publications include "Questions and Answers: Advance Directive and End-of-Life Decisions" ($5.95), and "Medical Treatments and Your Advance Directive" ($4.95).

Compassionate Friends
P.O. Box 3696
Oak Brook, IL 60522-3696
(708) 990-0010
This mutual assistance self-help organization offers friendship and understanding to bereaved parents and siblings through about 650 local chapters. Pamphlets include "Surviving Your Child's Suicide," "When a Brother or Sister Dies," and "Stillbirth, Miscarriage and Infant Death: Understanding Grief." Call or write for a publications list and information on membership and local organizations.

Hospice Education Institute
P.O. Box 713
Essex, CT 06426-0713

(800) 331-1620 (HospiceLink)
Call or write for information and referrals on hospice and related care.

National Hospice Organization
1901 North Moore Street
Arlington, VA 22209
(703) 243-5900
Hospice Help-line: (800) 658-8898
This clearinghouse of information about hospices publishes a national directory and will provide information and referrals to people who write or call.

Publications

Caring and Coping When Your Loved One Is Seriously Ill (Beacon Press, 1995, $10), *Living When a Loved One Has Died* (Beacon Press, 1995, $10), and *Bereaved Children and Teens: A Support Guide for Parents and Professionals* (Beacon Press, 1995, $25), all by Earl A. Grollman.

"Consumer Guide to Hospice Care." A thirty-two-page booklet available from National Consumers League, 815 15th Street, N.W., Washington, DC 20005; tel. (202) 639-8140. $4.

The Hospice Handbook, by Larry Beresford (Little, Brown, 1993), $12.95.

How We Die, by Sherwin Nuland (Knopf, 1994), $24.

Living Wills and More, by Terry J. Barnett (John Wiley & Sons, 1992), $16.95.

"Medicare Hospice Benefits." Free pamphlet available from Social Security Administration offices and the Health Care Financing Administration, 6325 Security Boulevard, Baltimore, MD 21207; tel. (410) 966-3000.

Part Five

For Everyone's Health

21

Unreformed Health Care

Ron Pollack

Ron Pollack is the
Executive Director of
Families USA.

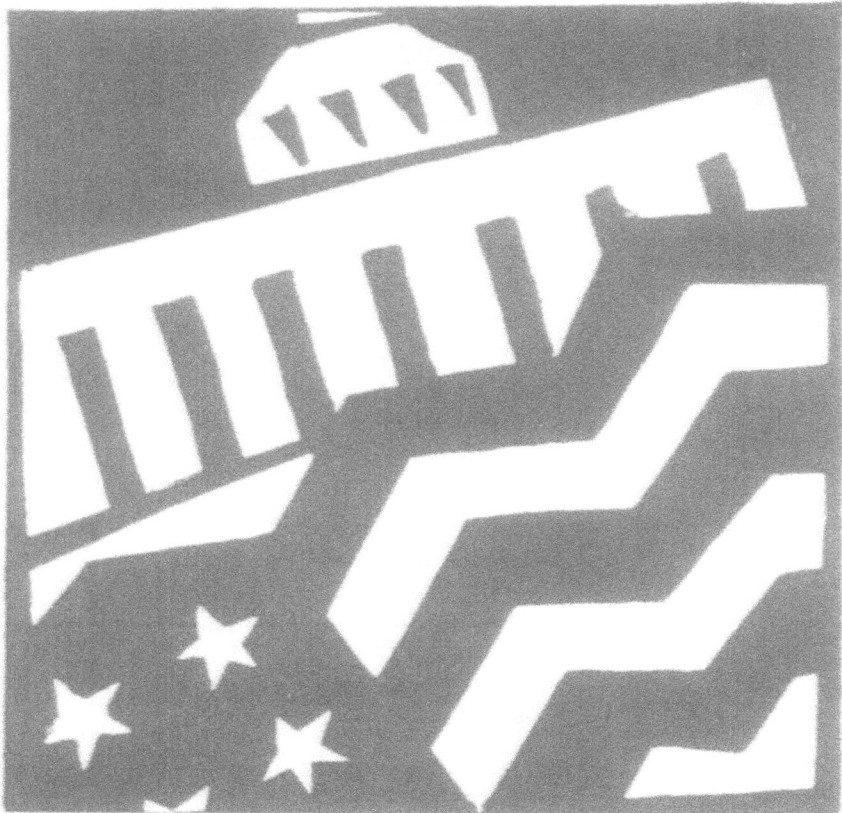

You can benefit from being an active and knowledgeable participant in your health care, as *Health Care Choices* clearly demonstrates. Such participation maximizes the likelihood that you will receive—and can pay for—the care you need. Even so, *systemic* failures limit your ability to achieve the health care security your family deserves. Responding to that situation is one of your greatest challenges as a health care consumer.

In 1995 and 1996 Congress seemed less focused on improving the health system and more interested in slashing Medicare and Medicaid. Although cutbacks in Medicare and Medicaid could reduce federal expenditures, increased bills to the American public would eliminate those cost savings. Either the families of Medicare and Medicaid patients would pay more for health care, or the rest of us would have to bear those costs in some way, such as higher hospital bills, physician bills, and insurance premiums. In any event, cutbacks would not address soaring health bills or the fact that increasing numbers of people are losing their insurance.

What does this mean for the average consumer? What can you expect from the health care system in the years to come? Unfortunately, the probable answers are

- Considerably higher costs for everyone
- Less-comprehensive health insurance for most people, *and*
- Increasing insecurity about your family's future health

Health Insecurity

Health care costs are the driving engine of the growing crisis in health insurance. For many Americans, these costs are often hidden: Some payments do not come *directly* out of your pocket, and others do not *appear* to finance health care. Two methods of paying for health care—employer-paid insurance and taxes—are illustrative. Too few workers fully appreciate that employer-paid health care almost inevitably contributes to stagnant or lower wages, especially when employers face skyrocketing premiums for health insurance. Similarly, rising health care costs help push up the price tags for Medicare and Medicaid, both of which are financed by tax dollars.

Sticker Shock

If you added up all the different ways that you pay for health care, the sum would undoubtedly create "sticker shock." Americans—

directly and indirectly—spent $2,590 per family for health care in 1980. The figure had almost tripled to $7,739 by 1993. Current projections suggest that the average family will spend over $14,500 in the year 2000.

For working families, higher costs for care are almost inevitable. Already, taken together, employers spend more for worker health benefits than U.S. firms receive in profits. Concerned about ever-mounting health care bills, businesses will undoubtedly seek to pass much of the growing burden on to their employees, asking them to pay higher shares of the premiums, higher deductibles, and higher copayments—and they will ask their employees to settle for less coverage.

In addition, more companies will require workers and their families to join managed care plans or specific networks of health care providers, diminishing your opportunities to choose your own doctors and other caregivers. Although the growth of managed care has temporarily decelerated health-cost increases for many employers, most observers believe that such costs will escalate again soon.

The prospects are especially grim for beneficiaries of public programs, especially the tens of millions of elders and lower-income Americans who receive care through Medicare and Medicaid. Because health care is the fastest-growing segment of the federal budget, Congress is considering a variety of ways to cut back these programs and apply the savings to reducing the deficit or to adding tax breaks mainly for the wealthy. These cuts could result in senior citizens' paying more in Medicare premiums and receiving less protection when they need nursing-home or other long term care. The cutbacks could also mean that millions of children and people with disabilities might lose their health coverage.

For more information on Medicare and Medicaid, turn to chapters 4 and 11.

The bottom line? Less security for almost every family. Already, over 50 million people lose or lack health insurance during at least part of each year. Every month, over 2 million Americans lose their health insurance. Although many people lose insurance "only" temporarily, any lapse in coverage places a family in jeopardy—perhaps leading people to defer necessary diagnoses and treatments. As the price of care continues to rise rapidly, and as employers offer fewer and smaller insurance benefits, more and more people will suffer these temporary—and longer term—lapses in coverage.

21

Mutual Assistance and Consumer Advocacy

Several organizations have formed not around one single health care issue but around a variety of concerns that affect many diverse individuals. One of the nation's largest and most effective of these groups is Health Care for All (HCFA) in Massachusetts. Its experience illustrates the benefits that can result when health care consumers unite around a common goal.

HCFA reaches people through problems close to their own lives. For example, one person came to HCFA because he has post–polio syndrome and needs reliable, affordable care; he wanted to know how health care reform would affect him personally. He joined HCFA's Community Leaders Project and met people with similar concerns. Together, they have come to recognize that their health care questions relate to the fragmentation and chaos of the system as a whole. And they are determined to change that system for themselves and others.

In just the past year, HCFA:

- Helped over six thousand callers get needed health care

Delaying Tactics

Inflation in health care has slowed while health care reform remained near the top of the federal agenda, with costs rising at twice, rather than three times, the rate of inflation, but price hikes will likely accelerate once again. During past debates on health reform, insurance companies and health providers moderated their bills to demonstrate that voluntary, private-sector changes could solve runaway costs. Once the "threat" of health reform diminished, prices again soared.

Holes in the Net

Because the health system fails so many citizens, millions of American workers *with* health insurance are locked into jobs they do not want. They fear that a switch in jobs means a loss of health insurance. Some states are responding to this "job-lock" phenomenon with insurance reforms, but the results are mixed at best. In the absence of universal coverage and effective cost controls, it is questionable that such insurance reform will reduce the number of people without health insurance.

Moreover, even insured people face significant gaps in coverage. For example, over 70 million Americans pay the full cost of prescription drugs out of their own pockets. This number includes most senior citizens: Medicare covers prescription drugs only during a hospital stay, and few private Medigap insurance policies offer cost-effective coverage for these medicines. The costs of prescription drugs have risen even faster than those for health care as a whole, and many seniors today forgo filling prescriptions ordered by their doctors.

For more information on prescription drugs, turn to chapter 7.

Similarly, the coverage for long term care is abysmal. Medicare provides no assistance to people with chronic disabilities requiring long term care. Only about 6 percent of America's seniors and 1 percent of the overall population have private insurance for long term care. The only significant protection is Medicaid, but that program will help you only if you spend down your savings to poverty levels—and, even then, the coverage excludes the bulk of home care and community-based care that people want the most. With the costs of a nursing home averaging $40,000 per year—and much more in most urban areas—coverage for long term care remains a major gap in the U.S. health insurance system. The same situation applies to the often major expenses involved with home care.

For more information on long term care and insurance for it, turn to chapter 15.

For more information on home care, turn to chapter 16.

Other serious gaps also persist. For example, private insurers tend to issue "sickness policies" rather than health assurance. That is, they devote far too little attention to preventive care to keep you healthy. The proliferation of managed care—and health maintenance organizations in particular—may improve this situation somewhat and lead to more emphasis on primary care, early screening for diseases, and other preventive measures. But there is far less reason for optimism regarding many other gaps. Consider the prospects for the family of someone who experiences a major sickness or injury or requires care for a mental illness:

■ Most insurance policies "cap" family coverage. Once the family reaches the cap, the insurer will not pay any more bills. A catastrophic illness or serious accident can easily exceed this cap, causing irreparable, severe financial damage to the entire family.

■ Insurance coverage for mental illnesses pales in comparison to the protection that's available to those with a physical malady.

The Active Consumer

The unreformed health care system adds to the costs, and diminishes the security, for consumers. Worsening conditions will only heighten the demand for true health reform. As long as today's many gaps in health insurance persist, consumers will remain insecure.

To hasten the day when the failures of the health care system are history, many consumers are joining with others to achieve reforms that respond to families' needs. While attending to the immediate situation of your own family, you can become active in these efforts in many ways. By actively participating in local, state, and federal debates on health care policy, you can help ensure the creation of a system that meets the needs of your entire family.

How can you play such a larger role? Of course, no answers are uniformly applicable to everyone, but here are a few suggestions:

■ If your state has a health-reform coalition, take part in its activities. These consumer and advocacy organizations provide an opportunity for people from many different backgrounds to work together for better health care.

For more information on statewide health-reform coalitions, turn to page 405.

■ Worked with the Massachusetts Attorney General to establish guidelines requiring nonprofit hospitals and HMOs to invest in the community to maintain a tax-exempt status

■ Developed a network of attorneys who provide free legal assistance to health care consumers

■ Informed over 2,700 people of their rights to free hospital care, *and*

■ Cofounded the Massachusetts Women's Health Care Coalition to ensure that health care reform responds to the needs of women.

HCFA reaches and serves many victims of the health care crisis through an "intake and referral" process that centers on the Health Helpline. Trained volunteers assist people who call about a wide variety of needs—from finding out about low-cost prescription drugs to advice on applying for free health care to keeping their insurance coverage after losing a job.

21

HCFA also produces a variety of materials and publications that explain

(continues)

changes in health care policies and services, translating difficult subjects into language understood by the layperson. These educational and outreach materials keep consumers informed of their rights to health care and help them better understand the issues and contribute to the debate.

For information on contacting Health Care for All and other consumer-advocacy organizations, turn to page 405.

■ Join a national consumer organization—such as the American Association of Retired Persons, Consumer's Union, and the League of Women Voters. Their staffs keep up with the latest developments related to health reform and can help and often involve members—locally and nationally—in efforts to improve the health care system. The same is true of the national headquarters of labor unions, various religious organizations, and groups that serve people with specific diseases, such as the Alzheimer's Association, the Epilepsy Foundation, and the National Mental Health Association.

For a list of national consumer organizations, turn to the resources that begin on page 405.

■ Contact one of the many organizations of health care providers that strongly support a health care system centered on the needs of consumers. A few examples are the American Nurses Association, the American College of Physicians, the American Academy of Family Physicians, the American Academy of Pediatrics, and the Catholic Health Association. These groups can inform you about initiatives in health care policy.

For information on contacting provider organizations, turn to the resources at the end of each chapter, especially chapter 5.

■ Contact Families USA. In particular, Families USA operates *a.s.a.p.*, a network of activists who receive timely information about pending health-reform issues, updates on important policy developments at the federal level, notices of key state-level activities, and action alerts that encourage consumer input on congressional deliberations. This is a free service for people who consistently write letters, send telegrams, or make phone calls to public officials *and* get at least five other people to do likewise.

For more information on a.s.a.p. or on joining Families USA, write to: Families USA, 1334 G Street, N.W., Washington, DC 20005.

Resources
National Organizations

These are a few of the many national organizations involved in health care reform.

AFL-CIO
815 16th Street, N.W.
Washington, DC 20006
(202) 637-5000

Alzheimer's Association
919 Michigan Avenue
Chicago, IL 60611
(800) 272-3900

American Association of Retired Persons
601 E Street, N.W.
Washington, DC 20049
(202) 872-4700

Children's Defense Fund
25 E Street, N.W.
Washington, DC 20001
(202) 662-3548

Citizen Action
1730 Rhode Island Avenue, N.W., #403
Washington, DC 20036
(202) 775-1580

Consumer's Union
101 Truman Avenue
Yonkers, NY 10703
(914) 378-2000

Long-Term-Care Campaign
P.O. Box 27394
Washington, DC 20038
(202) 434-3744

National Council of Senior Citizens
1331 F Street, N.W.
Washington, DC 20004-1107
(202) 347-8800

National Leadership Coalition on Health Care
555 13th Street, N.W.
Washington, DC 20005
(202) 637-6830

Universal Health Care Action Network
2800 Euclid Avenue, #520
Cleveland, OH 44115
(216) 241-8422

Statewide Health Consumer Organizations

Several states and many communities have consumer health organizations. If your state isn't listed here, contact Families USA Foundation/Boston, 30 Winter Street, Boston, MA 02108; tel. (617) 338-6035.

Health Care for All
30 Winter Street
Boston, MA 02108
(617) 350-7279

Health Access
1535 Mission Street
San Francisco, CA 94103
(415) 431-3430

Illinois Campaign for Better Health Care
44 Main Street, #414
Champaign, IL 61920
(217) 352-5600

Louisiana Health Care Campaign
P.O. Box 2228
Baton Rouge, LA 70821
(504) 383-8518

Maine Consumers for Affordable Care
P.O. Box 2490
Augusta, ME 04338
(207) 622-7045

21

Montana People's Action
208 E. Main Street
Missoula, MT 59802
(406) 727-9962

North Carolina Fair Share
530 N. Pearson Street
Raleigh, NC 27604
(919) 832-7130

North Carolina Health Access Coalition
975 Walnut Street
Cary, NC 27511
(919) 469-1116

North Country Institute
P.O. Box 319
Concord, NH 03301
(603) 225-2097

Oregon Health Action Campaign
3886 Beverly Avenue, N.E.
Building 1, #21
Salem, OR 97305
(503) 581-6830

South Carolina Fair Share
P.O. Box 8888
Columbia, SC 29202
(803) 252-9813

Tennessee Health Care Campaign
1103 Chapel Avenue
Nashville, TN 37206
(615) 227-7500

Texas Alliance for Human Needs
2520 Longview, #311
Austin, TX 78705
(512) 474-5019

Vermont Public Interest Research
    Group
43 State Street
Montpelier, VT 05602
(802) 223-5221

Washington Citizen Action
100 S. King Street
Seattle, WA 98104
(206) 389-0050

22 Helping Yourself

A Guide to Self-Help Groups, Going Online, and General Resources for Health Care Consumers

Martha S. Grover

Martha Grover, M.P.H., is an operations coordinator at the Planned Parenthood Clinic of Greater Boston. Formerly, she served as associate editor for the Health Care Choices publications project at Families USA.

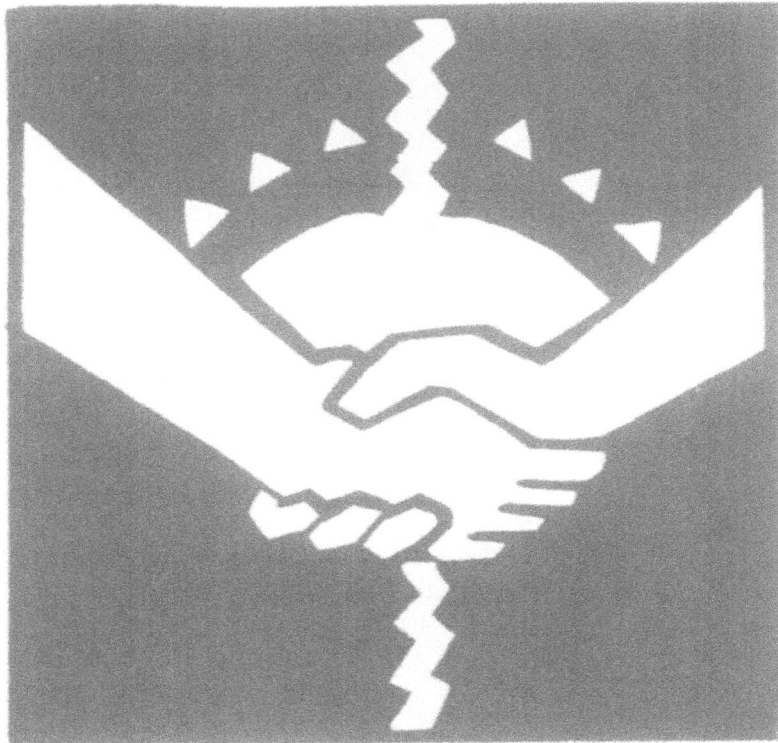

One year ago, the *O'Briens* found out that their son, Christopher, has trachealstenosis, a rare throat disorder that strikes only a few children worldwide. Since then, Christopher, now nine, has been in and out of hospitals and gone through surgery many times. At home, he needs around-the-clock care, sometimes from a visiting nurse but more and more often from his parents. The O'Briens have already fought several battles with their insurance company over Christopher's medical care. And despite everything, Christopher's doctors remain unsure about his case. They recommend that the family travel 1,500 miles from their home in Oklahoma to a New York hospital, where a doctor has treated children like Christopher—with mixed results. The O'Briens are inclined to do what the doctors suggest, but they are unsure. And how can they cope with caring for Christopher for an indefinite amount of time far from home?

Susan Hart had a mastectomy for breast cancer and is beginning to think she can't face another medical procedure. Due to start chemotherapy and radiation, she is having second thoughts. She has heard that chemotherapy is awful and makes people really sick. Whenever she tries to discuss her concerns with her husband, he doesn't seem to understand. After all, Hart's oncologist has recommended and explained these treatments. But she fears dying despite the treatments.

Six months after being diagnosed with genital herpes, *Rob Thompson* is still in shock. The brief relationship with the woman from whom he contracted the virus has ended. The doctor at a clinic for sexually transmitted diseases was comforting and understanding about the initial painful outbreak, but Thompson can't help thinking that he'll have to deal with the virus for the rest of his life. He's had three more outbreaks. The whole experience has paralyzed him, and he can't even talk to his best friend about it.

Lillian Rosenberg's seventy-year-old husband has suffered from Alzheimer's disease for eighteen months. As his primary caregiver, she has taken care of him day and night, making sure he doesn't forget his medication or leave the house without her. She is exhausted—and knows his condition will worsen. Mrs. Rosenberg is overwhelmed by all the tasks her husband once handled—paying bills, doing house repairs, planning their future.

All of these people can improve their situations and relieve some of their stress and isolation. They can take many of the steps on their own—and with other people like themselves.

Mutual Assistance

Every year over 15 million people turn to support groups when faced with their own or their loved ones' health crises. Members of such self-help or mutual-aid groups provide one another with emotional support and practical information far beyond what a physician or professional therapist can offer.

These informal groups are made up of ten to twenty people who face a common problem—such as addiction, illness, or a handicap—or take care of a person with such a problem. Self-help groups don't replace standard medical care, but members do benefit from mutual support and advice based on the vast experiential knowledge and practical coping skills each person has acquired. The groups are voluntary, member-run, and nonprofit, and dues are minimal.

The self-help concept started with Alcoholics Anonymous fifty years ago. Over the past fifteen years, it has spread to support people with a wide variety of problems, and national networks have formed out of many local community groups. Some examples include the Well Spouse Foundation for spouses of people with a chronic illness, Compassionate Friends for parents who have lost a child, Food Addicts Anonymous for overeaters, and Us Too for men with prostate cancer.

Members pool information on the available resources. They also save money as they discover cheaper, more efficient, and more effective ways to treat an illness, get care, buy medical equipment and other supplies, and avoid unnecessary procedures. In many cases, members also benefit from the knowledge of professionals by inviting a physician or specialist to speak to the group, rather than each person paying the expert for an individual consultation.

Almost all self-help groups are controlled by the members themselves rather than professionals or others outside the group. This ensures that the activities of the group address the expressed needs of the members, rather than needs as perceived by others. It also provides members with a sense of ownership, responsibility, community, and power. Often, members become advocates for improved research and health care services, increased state and federal funding of programs, and public education about a specific illness or condition.

Groups use different methods to assist people in need. They may hold educational seminars, one-on-one exchanges, or social gatherings. Many offer hotlines for people with immediate needs, as well as out-

22

reach programs in which members make unsolicited offers of help. Some groups are more formal than others, with written protocols about how meetings are run. The tight structure and approach of Alcoholics Anonymous are favored by certain groups, while others prefer less formal programs. Many groups have a religious or spiritual focus; others are more secular.

Good but Different

Many professional therapists and hospital social-work departments sponsor and convene their own support groups. These aren't technically mutual-help groups, however, because the members don't control the resources or direct the focus of the group. This could make a critical difference in the nature and effect of the information and support provided. According to the *Self-Help Sourcebook,* "The more professionals are involved, the more likely it is to resemble group therapy or another professional service under a different name."

A Remedy That Works

Having someone to turn to for empathy, advice, and assistance can make a big difference in your ability to cope with and survive an illness. People who maintain strong bonds with family and friends have lower death and illness rates, and some researchers believe that social support encourages a positive attitude that helps patients in their fight against illness. This is true for a variety of diseases and health conditions, as a number of studies show:

■ The medical journal *The Lancet* published a study by Dr. David Spiegel of Stanford University. He found that social support might help cancer patients live longer. Eighty-six women with advanced breast cancer received standard medical treatment; of these, fifty also participated in weekly group sessions and learned self-hypnosis for controlling pain. The patients who attended meetings regularly for one year lived an average of eighteen months longer than patients who attended no meetings. They also experienced less pain and depression.

■ Duke University Medical Center researchers found that cardiac patients who lacked a spouse or confidant were three times as likely as patients who were married or had a close friend to die within five years of the diagnosis of heart disease. Writing in the *Journal of the American Medical Association,* the researchers concluded that "a support group may be as effective as costly medical treatment. Simply put, having someone to talk to is very powerful medicine."

■ A UCLA study published in *The Archives of General Psychiatry* found that being part of a support group tripled the chance of survival over a five-year period for patients in the early stages of skin cancer. Patients in the support group experienced fewer deaths and fewer recurrences of the melanoma. The support group met once a week for six sessions to share practical advice about protecting skin from the sun and to learn about coping with anxiety and depression. They also offered one another support during emotional crises. The patients in the comparison group received standard advice from their doctors. All patients were initially treated by surgically removing the cancerous growths. The study also discovered that six months after the group sessions ended, two-thirds of the patients in the support group showed an increase of 25 percent or more of natural cancer-fighting cells in their immune systems. No increase occurred for the members of the comparison group.

Less Depressed, Less Stressed

Older diabetics who learned self-care and attended mutual-support sessions fared better over a two-year study that compared them with diabetics who attended self-care sessions but not the support groups, and with a third group who attended neither. The members of the first group were less depressed and less stressed and rated their quality of life higher than those in the other two groups, according to researchers at the University of Iowa. The study appeared in the *Journal of the American Geriatrics Society*.

Finding a Self-Help Group

You can find a mutual-help group in many ways. Start by investigating some of the more common resources listed at the end of this chapter. Call a national office or hotline to get referrals to the local chapter or affiliate. Look in the phone book. Ask your health care provider for suggestions or contact a hospital social-service department, the local health department, mental health department, or United Way office.

National self-help organizations can also refer you to a regional clearinghouse in your state. Regional clearinghouses serve about half the country and can provide detailed information to patients or physicians about available groups. They can usually give better information about

Self-Help Sources

♥ Two national clearinghouses have information on groups all around the country:

- American Self-Help Clearinghouse, St. Clares–Riverside Medical Center, 25 Pocono Road, Denville, NJ 07834; tel. (201) 625-7101

- National Self-Help Clearinghouse, CUNY Graduate School, 25 W. 43rd Street, #620, New York, NY 10036; tel. (212) 354-8525

Many states also have self-help clearinghouses that can direct you to local groups:

- California: (310) 825-1799 or (800) 222-LINK (in-state only)

- Illinois: (312) 368-9070

- Iowa: (515) 576-5870 or (800) 952-4777 (in-state only)

- Kansas: (800) 445-0116

- Massachusetts: (413) 545-2313

- Michigan: (517) 484-7373 or (800) 777-5556

- Missouri—Kansas City: (816) 472-HELP

- Missouri—St. Louis: (314) 773-1399

smaller, one-of-a-kind community groups than the national clearinghouses can.

Many national, state, and local organizations will assist you in starting a new mutual-help group. These organizations may provide technical support, how-to materials, advice, contacts, and perhaps even some start-up funds. For instance, the American Self-Help Clearinghouse will assist people who want to start a group that isn't already in existence anywhere. Its publication, *The Self-Help Sourcebook: Finding and Forming Mutual Aid Self-Help Groups,* is a good source of advice on organizing groups. The book also identifies many model groups that can be consulted.

Computers and Self-Help

♥ Computers are increasingly valuable as a source of consumer health information in addition to the knowledge and advice you can get from health care providers, health organizations, self-help groups, and books and magazines. Personal computers equipped with a modem and communications software offer a rapidly growing assortment of health information—to those with the basic know-how to log on and the curiosity to experiment.

Once you go online, you'll find many ways to meet other patients, providers, and specialists, share information, and ask and answer questions from home about hundreds of health issues, diseases, and treatments. The challenge is to learn to focus and manage your search so you don't get overwhelmed, spend endless hours, and waste a lot of money just browsing. "Surfing the Internet" *can* turn up some fascinating information—as long as you keep in mind that much of what's online is unfiltered and unedited.

Get the Books

♥ For a comprehensive guide to online health resources and how to use them, consult:

- *Dr. Tom Linden's Guide to Online Medicine,* by Tom Linden and Michelle L. Kienholz (McGraw-Hill, 1995), $18. In addition to advice on how to go online, it lists hundreds of Internet sites and computer bulletin boards organized by health or disease topic.

- *Health Online: How to Find Health Information, Support Groups, and Self-Help Communities in Cyberspace,* by Tom Ferguson (Addison-Wesley,

1996), $17. Dedicated to the concept of online self-help, this book covers the basics of going online as well as the latest on access to discussion groups, mailing lists, health care Web sites, and other starting points.

■ *HealthNet: Your Essential Resource for the Most Up-to-Date Medical Information Online,* by Jeanne C. Ryer (John Wiley & Sons, 1997), $16.95. This book presents hundreds of online sources for timely and comprehensive health information. It covers all major health information services and rates them for reliability, technical level, and price.

Bulletin Board Systems

Free bulletin board systems—BBSs—are popping up daily. To access them, all you need is simple communications software.

Look in computer magazines and local computer papers for listings of BBSs. Already, hundreds are available across the country with only a local call. Usually, you'll leave a computer message or post a question and get an answer within a few days (or up to a week internationally).

Many BBSs carry newsletters, news items, and educational programs, and they also facilitate networking. A few examples are HEX (Handicapped Users of Exchange), Easy-Does-It Recovery, Neuropsychology-Bound Bulletin Board (for head injury and stroke victims), and many bulletin boards for HIV/AIDS.

To get a listing of over three hundred health-related BBS phone numbers, send $5 and a legal-size, stamped, self-addressed envelope to Dr. Ed Del Grosso, P.O. Box 632, Collegeville, PA 19426. Send e-mail to list @ blackbag.com, or contact his Black Bag BBS by modem at (610) 454-7396 to download the list. You can reach Health Online, another comprehensive health care BBS, at (310) 831-6775.

Free Access

If you don't have a computer or can't afford an online service, most large public libraries, all medical school libraries, and some hospital libraries have access to Medline, the largest biomedical journal database in the world. Call the National Network of Libraries of Medicine at (800) 338-7657 to find a library near you.

Although the Medicine terminology can be very technical, you can get information on the latest medical studies and treatments. Many libraries will also have other computer services and resources available to "lay" users.

- Nebraska: (402) 476-9668
- New Jersey: (201) 625-7101, (800) 367-6274 (in-state only), TDD: (201) 625-9053
- New York: (212) 586-5770
- North Carolina: (704) 331-9500
- Ohio—Dayton area: (513) 225-3004
- Ohio—Toledo area: (419) 475-4449
- Oregon and Washington: (503) 222-5555
- Pennsylvania—Pittsburgh area: (412) 261-5363
- Pennsylvania—Scranton area: (717) 961-1234
- South Carolina: (803) 791-9227
- Tennessee—Knoxville area: (615) 584-6736
- Tennessee—Memphis area: (901) 323-0633
- Texas: (512) 454-3706
- Washington, D.C. area: (703) 941-5465

22

Commercial Online Access

A number of companies provide access to the Internet and other online services. Consult friends, staff at computer centers or stores, or computer and consumer magazines for information and advice on which service to purchase.

Most of these companies charge a monthly fee with a per-hour cost after a certain number of base hours. Many will send you a free start-up or trial kit so you can find out how easy the service is to use and what it offers. Each service has its own menu of health and medical resources and search mechanisms.

Some larger self-help organizations have launched their own forums through the commercial services. For example, the American Self-Help Clearinghouse responds to requests for information on CompuServe's "Self-Help Support" Health and Fitness Forum. Also on CompuServe, the National Organization for Rare Disorders maintains the NORD Rare Disease Database. America Online has forums sponsored by the American Diabetes Association, the American Cancer Society, the National Multiple Sclerosis Society, the National Alliance for the Mentally Ill, and the United Cerebral Palsy Association.

Online Services

Here are some of the larger online services:

- America Online (800) 227-6364 or (800) 827-6364
- CompuServe, (800) 848-8199 or (800) 524-3388
- Delphi (800) 695-4005
- Genie (800) 638-9636
- Prodigy (800) 776-3449

Health on the World Wide Web

The World Wide Web, or the Web, makes it easier to search for information on the Internet using software known as a *browser*—for example, Netscape or Mosaic. You click on "word links" to transfer directly to a destination, without opening or closing any documents. You can move from site to site or document to document. Just point and click your computer mouse on the key words or icons, and you're at a new Web site.

Here are just few examples of the many general-health Web sites you'll find as you explore and learn to narrow your search.

■ Begin your quest on the Web with a search mechanism—for example, *Healthseek* (http://www.healthseek.com/). It provides a large list of other health-related Web sites and lets you search the Web for specific topics using a key word or phrase.

■ *Health Link,* an online database of health care resources, lists the names, addresses, and phone numbers of health organizations and providers related to search topics you enter (http://pages.bluecrab.org/hlink/link.htm).

■ *Excite*'s Health & Medicine Web page is a search tool and a good starting point for links to health information sites (http://www.excite.com/subject/health_and_medicine/s-index.h.html).

■ *Yahoo,* a subject catalogue of the Web and Internet, can lead you to many sites (http://www.yahoo.com/health).

Software Packages

You can buy health databases and health encyclopedias on disk or CD-ROM at computer and bookstores. Covering both general health and specific topics, these software packages include:

■ *Grateful Med* software helps you search for in-depth articles on any medical subject. For a free Grateful Med demonstration disk and brochure, call (800) 638-8480 or (301) 496-6308.

■ *CHESS* (Comprehensive Health Enhancement Support System) can put you in touch with other patients and gives you twenty-four-hour access to a library of medical information. CHESS can also help people choose among different treatments for many conditions, including AIDS/HIV infections, breast cancer, adult children of alcoholics, and stress management. For more information, call Health Decisions Plus at (800) 454-4465. CHESS software packages cost $295.

■ *The Directory of Online Health Care Databases* includes databases on a broad range of health issues. It is available for $38. Call (503) 471-1627.

You can "ask" computer-based health encyclopedias to display information about symptoms, procedures, possible diagnoses, and treatments using video clips, text, and anatomical diagrams. Examples of such encyclopedia packages are

22

- *Dr. Schueler's Home Medical Advisor Pro* (Pixel Perfect, CD-ROM: $99.95; diskette: $87.50)
- *Medical HouseCall* (Applied Medical Informatics, $99.95)
- *Mayo Clinic Family Health Book* (IVI Publishing, $59.95)
- *PharmAssist* (Softkey International, CD-ROM: $44.95; diskette: $55.95) —call (800) 323-8088
- *Complete Guide to Drugs* (HealthSoft, $65.55)—call (800) 795-4325

Health Data Brokers

A number of consumer-oriented commercial data brokers will run searches on health topics. Most use *Medline* and other smaller databases. Searches can be costly, ranging from $25 to $275.

- *The Health Resource, Inc.,* 564 Locust Street, Conway, AR 72032, tel. (501) 329-5272, provides in-depth research reports on specific problems. The reports include information on conventional and alternative treatment options, self-help measures, resource organizations, and specialists. Health Resource updates reports annually for a fee, sends out news bulletins on new information, and publishes a newsletter. Reports cost $295 for cancer reports and $195 for all others, plus shipping and handling.

- *Medical Information Service,* Palo Alto Medical Foundation, 400 Channing Avenue, Palo Alto, CA 94301, tel. (800) 999-1999 or (415) 853-6000, has a "Consumer Guide to Medical Information" available for free to assist you in conducting a medical information search. You can also order a search from the service for $89, plus shipping and handling.

- *Medical Data Source,* 5959 W. Century Boulevard, #1000, Los Angeles, CA 90045, tel. (800) 776-4MDS or (310) 641-3111, offers information on medical conditions, prescription drugs, and physician backgrounds, as well as referrals to local health facilities such as nursing homes, rehabilitation centers, and support groups. Subscription rates vary but are usually under $48 per year.

- *Planetree Health Resource Center,* 2040 Webster Street, San Francisco, CA 94115, tel. (415) 923-3681, provides an in-depth packet on a particular illness for $100, a basic packet on common conditions for $20, or a Medline search for $35. It will also put you in touch with other organizations as well as with people who have the same condition as you. The center provides information on conventional and alternative treatments.

■ *Medical Data Exchange,* 4730 Galice Road, Merlin, OR 97532, tel. (503) 471-1627, offers a search on its own consumer-health databases, MDX Health Digest and Personal Medical Advisor, for $25. It also offers a Medline search for $48 and a more extensive customized search for $60 an hour.

Online Sources

Many health-related organizations have their own online information services. Here's a brief sampling:

■ Agency for Health Care Policy and Research: This federal agency offers information to help consumers and providers make health care decisions. http://www.ahcpr.gov/

■ American Medical Association: The AMA's Web page offers article abstracts from the *Journal of the American Medical Association,* and other AMA publications. http://www.ama-assn.org

■ "The Body" offers AIDS information supplied by the federal Centers for Disease Control, the American Psychiatric Association, and Johns Hopkins University AIDS Service. http://www.thebody.com

■ Boston Women's Health Book Collective: e-mail address is bwhbc @ igc.apc.org

■ National Cancer Institute: http://www.nci.nih.gov/

■ National Library of Medicine: By establishing a Medline account, you can conduct your own literature searches. http://www.nlm.nih.gov/

■ National Organization for Rare Disorders: http://www.w2.com/nord1.html

Finding Solutions

Self-help groups, computer services, health databases, and consumer health organizations can improve people's lives and reduce health care bills. Used wisely, these resources can help you find and decide on the most appropriate care based on the most up-to-date information. Good health care information provides a sense of control and empowerment at a time when many people feel confused, out of control, and at the mercy of their health care providers' limitations.

22

How does all this benefit the O'Briens, Susan Hart, Rob Thompson, and Lillian Rosenberg?

■ On the advice of one of Christopher's nurses, *Mrs. O'Brien* called the National Organization for Rare Disorders. She received a packet of information—including a report on current research and the phone number of a national support group for parents of children with trachealstenosis. Soon she talked with parents in Texas who had taken their child to New York for surgery, and they shared their experiences with the O'Briens. They offered advice on traveling with all of Christopher's medical gear, staying cheaply in New York, and knowing what to expect from the surgery and the surgeons. Most important, they assured the O'Briens that they had looked at all their options and were doing the right thing.

■ *Susan Hart* called the local chapter of the American Cancer Society, which referred her to a support group for breast-cancer patients. She went to a meeting and found people who understood her hesitations and concerns; their support helped her work through her depression. The women in the group shared their experiences with chemotherapy and radiation, lessening her fear of the treatment. She learned about various types of chemotherapy drugs and later discussed those options with her oncologist.

■ Tired of feeling sorry for himself, *Rob Thompson* dug out pamphlets he had stuffed in a drawer and started to read about the herpes virus. On the back of one pamphlet was the toll-free number of the American Social Health Association. He called and got the number of a support group nearby. Initially, Thompson hesitated. What if he knew someone there? What would they talk about? He couldn't imagine talking to strangers about something so personal. Finally, Thompson decided to just go. A little uncomfortable at first, he gradually welcomed the opportunity to talk to others coping with herpes. A year later, he attends meetings every few months to get up-to-date information—and to share his experiences with newcomers to the group.

■ Through her computer modem and the local Alzheimer's Association, *Lillian Rosenberg* connected with a caregiver support group. She could reach it at all hours of the day, particularly at night when she would become most frustrated. Through the bulletin-board system, she has found out about respite services that give her a break from the twenty-four-hour care she provides for her husband and has learned what to expect as his disease progresses.

Appendix A

The Short List: Selected National Resources

In addition to these self-help groups and general resources, consult the more comprehensive listings at the end of each chapter.

Self-Help Organizations

Most of these national organizations can refer you to affiliates and support groups in your area. Many are also a good source of information from specialists on prevention, diagnosis, treatment, and current research and clinical trials. Unless otherwise noted, you can call or write to receive information and published materials.

National AIDS Hotline
Centers for Disease Control and Prevention
(800) 342-AIDS
(800) 243-7889 TDD

Alcoholics Anonymous
P.O. Box 459
Grand Central Station
New York, NY 10163
(800) 344-2666
(212) 647-1680
Check the Yellow Pages for a local group.

ALS Associates
20121 Ventura Boulevard, #321
Woodland Hills, CA 91364

(800) 782-4747
Call or write for information on Lou Gehrig's Disease.

Alzheimer's Association
(800) 272-3900

Alzheimer's Disease Education and Referral Center
P.O. Box 8250
Silver Spring, MD 20907
(800) 438-4380
Call or write for a list of publications and referrals to local support groups.

American Academy of Allergy and Immunology
Allergy Information Referral Hotline
(800) 822-ASMA
Call or write for a list of publications and referrals to health care providers.

American Anorexia/Bulimia Association
(212) 501-8351

American Cancer Society
1599 Clifton Road, NE
Atlanta, GA 30329
(404) 320-3333
(800) 227-2345
Call or write for referrals to local chapters.

American Chronic Pain Association
P.O. Box 850

Rocklin, CA 95677
(916) 632-0922
This self-help organization has over five hundred groups internationally and publishes workbooks and a newsletter.

American College of Allergy and Immunology
85 W. Algonquin Road, #550
Arlington Heights, IL 60005
(800) 842-7777

American Council on Alcoholism
5024 Campbell Boulevard
Baltimore, MD 21236
(800) 527-5344
(410) 889-0100

American Diabetes Association
1660 Duke Street
Alexandria, VA 22314
(800) 232-3472

American Dietetic Association
Consumer Nutrition Hotline
(800) 366-1655
Call for pamphlets containing basic dietary guidelines, general health, and maintaining or achieving a healthy weight.

American Foundation for the Blind
15 West 16th Street
New York, NY 10011
(800) AF-BLIND
(212) 620-2000
(212) 620-2158 TDD
(212) 620-2147 (NY residents)

American Foundation for Urologic Disease
(800) 242-2383
(410) 727-2908
Call for information on urologic disorders, prostate cancer, incontinence, infertility, urinary tract infections, and referrals to support groups.

American Heart Association
7372 Greenville Avenue
Dallas, TX 75231
(214) 706-1220
(800) 242-8721

American Institute for Cancer Research
Nutrition Hotline
1759 R Street, N.W.
Washington, DC 20009
(800) 843-8114
Call or write to receive pamphlets on preventing cancer and treatment through diet and nutrition.

American Kidney Fund
62110 Executive Boulevard, #1010
Rockville, MD 20852
(800) 638-8299
Call or write about obtaining assistance in funding the treatment of uninsured dialysis patients.

American Liver Foundation
1425 Pompton Avenue, #1–3
Cedar Grove, NJ 07009-1000
(800) 223-0179
(201) 256-2550
Call or write for information and referrals.

American Lung Association
1740 Broadway
New York, NY 10019-4374
(800) 586-4872
Call or write for referrals and for information on lung cancer and smoking.

American Lyme Disease Foundation
Mill Pond Offices
293 Route 100
Somers, NY 10589
(800) 876-LYME
(914) 277-6970
Call or write for referrals or to receive a copy of the pamphlet, "A Quick Guide to Lyme Disease."

American Pain Society
5700 Old Orchard Road
Skokie, IL 60077-1057
(908) 966-5595

American Paralysis Association
500 Morris Avenue
Springfield, NJ 07081
(800) 225-0292
Call or write for information on research to find cures for paralysis.

American Parkinson's Disease Association
1250 Hyland Boulevard
Staten Island, NY 10305
(800) 223-2732

American Red Cross
430 17th Street, N.W.
Washington, DC 20006
(202) 737-8300
Call or write for information on blood services.

American Self-Help Clearinghouse
St. Clares–Riverside Medical Center
25 Pocono Road
Denville, NJ 07834
(800) 367-6274 (New Jersey only)
(201) 625-7101
(201) 625-9053 TDD
Call to locate local self-help groups or to receive help starting your own self-help group if a similar type doesn't already exist. For a copy of *The Self-Help Sourcebook: Finding and Forming Mutual Aid Self-Help Groups,* a national directory of self-help groups, send $10.

American Social Health Association
P.O. Box 13827
Research Triangle Park, NC 27709
(800) 227-8922
Call or write for comprehensive information on sexually transmitted diseases.

American Trauma Society
8903 Presidential Parkway
Upper Marlboro, MD 20772
(800) 556-7890
(301) 420-4189

Arthritis Foundation
1314 Spring Street, N.W.
Atlanta, GA 30309
(404) 872-7100
(800) 283-7800
Call or write for free brochures, low-cost handbooks and guidebooks, and lists of support groups and arthritis specialists. The foundation also conducts an Arthritis Self-Help Course throughout the country. For information, call your local Arthritis Foundation branch or the national office.

Asthma and Allergy Foundation of America
1125 Fifteenth Street, N.W., #502
Washington, DC 20005
(800) 7-ASTHMA
Call for referrals and information packets.

Autism Society of America
7910 Woodmont Avenue
Bethesda, MD 20814-3015
(301) 565-0433
Call or write for referrals and information.

Better Hearing Institute
P.O. Box 1840
Washington, DC 20073
(800) 327-9355
(703) 642-0580
Call or write for information on hearing loss.

Cancer Information and Counseling Line
American Medical Centers
(800) 525-3777
(303) 233-6501

Cancer Information Service
National Cancer Institute
National Institutes of Health
Building 31, Room 10A24
Bethesda, MD 20892-3100
(800) 4-CANCER (422-6237)
PDQ by fax (301) 402-5874
WWW site: http://www.nci.nih.gov/
Call or write for general information on treatments, services, and provider referrals. A list of treatment centers and about 1,500 experimental programs, physicians, and organizations is available through their Physician Data Query (PDQ). It's set up on a computer bulletin board accessible through Grateful Med software (see page 415), or you can request a free PDQ search from the institute.

Candlelighter Childhood Cancer Foundation
7910 Woodmont Avenue
Bethesda, MD 20814
(301) 657-8401
(800) 366-2223
Call or write for referral to a local support group for families of cancer patients. The foundation will do a search for protocols, treatment options, and literature on childhood cancers. Ask for a publications list.

Cleft Palate Foundation
1218 Grand View Avenue
Pittsburgh, PA 15211
(800) 24-CLEFT
Call or write for information and referrals.

Cooley's Anemia Foundation
129-09 26th Avenue
Flushing, NY 11354
(800) 522-7222
(718) 321-2873
Call or write for information and referrals.

Crohn's and Colitis Foundation of America
386 Park Avenue South
New York, NY 10016
(800) 343-3637
The foundation maintains a list of support groups for inflammatory bowel disease.

Cystic Fibrosis Foundation
(800) FIGHT-CF
(800) 344-4823
(301) 951-4422
Call for referrals to 110 cystic fibrosis centers around the country.

Disability Information Clearinghouse
Office of Special Education and Rehabilitative Services
U.S. Department of Education
330 C Street, S.W., #3132
Washington, DC 20202
(202) 205-8241
Call or write for information about services available through public schools.

Epilepsy Foundation of America
4351 Garden City Drive
Landover, MD 20785
(800) EFA-4050

Foundation Fighting Blindness
11350 McCormick Road
Hunt Valley, MD 21031-1014
(800) 683-5555
Call or write for information on current research and diseases that cause blindness.

Hearing Aid Helpline
20361 Middlebelt
Livonia, MI 48152
(800) 521-5247
Call or write for information on hearing aids, including types and costs.

Huntington's Disease Society of America
140 W. 22nd Street
New York, NY 10011
(800) 345-4372
(212) 242-1968

International Association for the Study
of Pain
909 N.E. 43rd Street
Seattle, WA 98105-6020
(206) 547-6409

International Foundation for Bowel
Dysfunction
P.O. Box 17864
Milwaukee, WI 53217
(414) 964-1799
Contact the foundation for information
on support groups and a newsletter
addressing the concerns of people with
irritable bowel syndrome.

Juvenile Diabetes Foundation
432 Park Avenue South
New York, NY 10016
(212) 889-7575

Leukemia Society of America
600 Third Avenue
New York, NY 10016
(212) 573-8484
(800) 955-4LSA

Lupus Foundation of America
4 Research Plaza
Rockville, MD 20850-3226
(800) 558-0121
(301) 670-9292

March of Dimes Birth Defects Foundation
233 Park Avenue South
New York, NY 10003
(212) 353-8353
Call or write for information on birth
defects, including what causes them.

Multiple Sclerosis Society
733 Third Avenue
New York, NY 10017
(800) LEARN-MS
(212) 986-3240

Myasthenia Gravis Foundation of
America
222 S. Riverside Plaza, #1540
Chicago, IL 60606
(800) 541-5454

National Alliance for Breast Cancer
Organizations
1180 Avenue of the Americas
New York, NY 10036
(212) 719-0154
(212) 719-0394 in emergencies
Call or write for information and for
referrals to medical, support, and advocacy groups.

National Arthritis Foundation Clearinghouse
P.O. Box AMS
9000 Rockville Pike
Bethesda, MD 20892
(301) 495-4484
Call or write for information on arthritis, treatments, and prevention.

National Association of Anorexia Nervosa and Associated Disorders
P.O. Box 271
Highland Park, IL 60035
(312) 831-3438

National Bone Marrow Donor Program
(800) 654-1247
Call for information on transplants, a
directory of bone-marrow donors, and
how to become a donor.

National Chronic Pain Outreach Association
7979 Old Georgetown Road, #100
Bethesda, MD 20814-2429
(301) 652-4948
This information clearinghouse publishes a newsletter and makes referrals.

National Clearinghouse for Alcohol and Drug Information
P.O. Box 3245
Rockville, MD 20852
(301) 468-2600
(800) 729-6686
Call or write for information on counseling, treatments, helping teens, and other matters related to alcohol and drug use.

National Clearinghouse for Infants with Disabilities and Life-Threatening Conditions
Center for Developmental Disabilities
Department of Pediatrics
University of South Carolina
Columbia, SC 29208
(800) 922-9234

National Diabetes Information Clearinghouse
1 Information Way
Bethesda, MD 29892-3560
(301) 654-3327

National Digestive Diseases Information Clearinghouse
2 Information Way
Bethesda, MD 29892-3570
(301) 654-3810

National Down's Syndrome Congress
(800) 232-6372

National Down's Syndrome Society
666 Broadway
New York, NY 10012
(800) 221-4602
(212) 460-9330

National Easter Seal Society
230 W. Monroe, #1800
Chicago, IL 60606
(800) 221-6827
Call or write for information on communication disorders, developmental disorders, and mental and physical disabilities.

National Head Injury Foundation
(800) 444-NHIF
(202) 296-6443

National Headache Foundation
428 W. St. James Place
Chicago, IL 60614
(800) 843-2256
Call or write for information on causes and treatment. The foundation also publishes a newsletter on recent research.

National Hemophilia Foundation
(800) 42-HANDI

National Kidney and Urologic Diseases Information Clearinghouse
P.O. Box NKUDIC
9000 Rockville Pike
Bethesda, MD 20892
(301) 654-4415

National Kidney Foundation
30 E. 33rd Street
New York, NY 10016
(800) 622-9010
Call or write for information on diseases affecting the kidneys and on kidney transplants.

National Library Service for the Blind and Physically Handicapped
Library of Congress
1291 Taylor Street, N.W.
Washington, DC 20542
(800) 424-8567
(202) 707-5100
The service offers a collection of large-print and braille books.

National Mental Health Consumers' Self-Help Clearinghouse
311 South Juniper Street
Philadelphia, PA 19107
(800) 553-4539
(215) 735-6082
Call or write for a publications list on a wide variety of mental health topics.

The clearinghouse handles inquiries from consumers, family members, professionals, and others about locating mental health self-help groups. It also offers technical assistance for developing self-help groups.

National Multiple Sclerosis Society
733 Third Avenue
New York, NY 10017
(800) 344-4867
Call or write for referrals to local chapters and a list of publications.

National Organization for Rare Disorders
100 Route 37
P.O. Box 8923
New Fairfield, CT 06812-8923
(800) 999-NORD or (800) 999-6673
(203) 746-6518
Call for one of 950 reports on lesser-known diseases. NORD reports, written in lay terms, cover symptoms, therapies, current research, and support groups. The first two reports are free, and subsequent reports cost $3.75 each.

National Osteoporosis Foundation
2100 M Street, N.W.
Washington, DC 20037
(800) 223-9994
Call or write for information on causes, treatments, and prevention.

National Parkinson's Foundation
1501 N.W. Ninth Avenue
Miami, FL 33136
(800) 327-4545
(305) 547-6666
Call or write to order pamphlets on outpatient services, research, physician referrals, nutrition, drugs, and help for families.

National Psoriasis Foundation
6600 S.W. 92nd Avenue, #300
Portland, OR 97223

(800) 723-9166
Call or write for referrals and information.

National Reye's Syndrome Foundation
(800) 233-7393

National Self-Help Clearinghouse
CUNY Graduate School
25 West 43rd Street
New York, NY 10036
(212) 354-8525
Call for assistance with starting a self-help group and referrals to regional clearinghouses and groups around the country. Send a stamped, self-addressed envelope for a list of support-group information. The clearinghouse publishes a quarterly newsletter, "The Self-Help Reporter" ($10 for one year).

National Sexually Transmitted Disease Hotline
(800) 227-8922

National Sickle Cell Disease Association of America
200 Corporate Pointe, #495
Culver City, CA 90230-7633
(800) 421-8453
(213) 736-5455

National Spinal Cord Injury Association
545 Concord Avenue, #29
Cambridge, MA 02138
(800) 962-9629
Call or write for information, referrals, and counseling services.

National Stroke Association
8480 E. Orchard Road, #1000
Englewood, CO 80111
(800) 787-6537
Call or write for information on preventing and treating strokes.

National Stuttering Hotline
200 E. 33rd Street

New York, NY 10016
(800) 221-2483
(212) 532-1460
Call or write for information on causes and treatments.

National VD Hotline
(800) 227-8922

Paget Foundation
200 Varick Street, #1004
New York, NY 10014
(800) 23-PAGET
Call for information on hyperparathyroidism and Paget's disease.

SIDS National Headquarters
1314 Bedford Avenue, #210
Baltimore, MD 21208
(800) 638-7437
Call for referrals and information on preventing Sudden Infant Death Syndrome.

Simon Foundation
P.O. Box 835
Willamette, IL 60091
(800) 23-SIMON
Call for information on incontinence and referrals to related organizations.

Spina Bifida Association of America
4590 MacArthur Boulevard, N.W., #250
Washington, DC 20007-4226
(800) 621-3141
(202) 944-3285

Tourette' Syndrome Association
4240 Bell Boulevard, #205
Bayside, NY 11361
(800) 237-0717
To receive information and a referral list for your state, send a self-addressed, stamped ($.75) envelope.

United Cerebral Palsy Association
1660 L Street, N.W.
Washington, DC 20036
(202) 842-1266

(800) USA-5UCP
Call or write for information and referrals.

United Ostomy Association
36 Executive Park, #120
Irvine, CA 92714
(800) 826-0826
Call or write for information on colitis, colostomy, familial polyposis, and so on.

Y-ME Breast Cancer Information and
     Support Hotline
(800) 221-2141

Other National Resources

AIDS Clearinghouse
P.O. Box 6003
Rockville, MD 20850
(800) 458-5231
Call or write for information on AIDS/ HIV.

American Institute for Preventive
     Medicine
30445 Northwestern Highway
Farmington Hills, MI 48334
(800) 345-2476
(810) 539-1800 (in Michigan)
Call or write for free information on stress reduction, weight control, smoking cessation, and health education.

American Medical Radio News
(800) 448-9384
Call for a recorded message on a current health topic or feature story in medicine.

Ask-A-Nurse
Call (800) 535-1111 for the toll-free number of the Ask-A-Nurse closest to you. This advice line sponsored by hospitals and managed care companies provides help and reassurance from nurses on a broad range of questions.

Center for Medical Consumers
237 Thompson Street
New York, NY 10012
(212) 674-7105
The center's medical library is open to the public. Call and ask for a publications list on surgical treatments. A monthly newsletter, "Health Facts," provides clear, in-depth, referenced discussions of key health issues. Write for a subscription ($21 per year).

Center for Science in the Public Interest
1501 16th Street, N.W.
Washington, DC 20036
(202) 332-9110
This resource center on nutrition and health publishes "Nutrition Action" a monthly newsletter on health ($24 per year).

Center for the Study of Services
733 15th Street, N.W.
Washington, DC 20005
(202) 347-9612
(800) 475-7283
A nonprofit organization, the center publishes *Consumers' Checkbook* magazines for the Washington, D.C., and San Francisco metropolitan areas. The magazines include consumer ratings and information on dentists, hospitals, HMOs, physicians, and many on nonmedical consumer services and products. ($30 for a two-year subscription— 4 issues.)

Centers for Disease Control and Prevention
1600 Clifton Road, N.E.
Atlanta, GA 30333
Public Inquiries: (404) 639-3311
Fax Information Service for International Travelers: (404) 639-1733
http://www.cdc.gov/
This federal agency provides free and immediate disease reports on outbreaks, risk, and prevention all over the world.

Consumer Health Information Resource Institute
300 E. Pink Hill Road
Independence, MO 64057
(800) 821-6671
(816) 228-4595
Call or write for referrals to local, regional, and national organizations; information about a patient education library; sources of health information on various conditions, procedures, and medications; and information about health fraud and quackery.

Consumer Nutrition Hotline
American Dietetic Association
(800) 366-1655
Call with questions about nutrition and diet.

Consumer Product Safety Commission Hotline
5401 Westbard Avenue
Bethesda, MD 20207
(800) 638-2772
(301) 504-0580
(800) 638-8270 (TTY)
Call for information on health-related products.

Consumers Union/*Consumer Reports*
P.O. Box 56356
Boulder, CO 80322
(800) 234-1645
Call or write to subscribe to "On Health Newsletter" ($24 per year), a monthly source of practical advice for consumers. *Consumer Reports* magazine ($24 per year for 12 issues) also contains valuable health care information. Recent Consumers Union books include *Complete Drug Reference* (1996, $39.95), *Examining Your Doctor* (1995, $22.50), and *Mind-Body Medicine* (1995, $14.95). Call or write for a complete publications list. Back issues of *Con-*

sumer Reports are available for one year after publication ($5 each). Reprints of selected *Consumer Reports* articles are available in quantities of 10 copies or more ($3 per copy); to order, write CU/Reprints, 101 Truman Avenue, Yonkers, NY 10703.

Environmental Protection Agency
Public Information Center
PM-211B
401 M Street, S.W.
Washington, DC 20460
EPA Pesticide Clearinghouse: (800) 358-7378
EPA Safe Drinking Hotline: (800) 426-4791
Call for referrals and information on EPA programs in nontechnical language.

Harvard Medical School Publications
P.O. Box 420235
Palm Coast, FL 32142
(800) 829-9080
Call or write for an annual subscription to any of the following newsletters: *Harvard Health Letter* ($24), *Harvard Mental Health Letter* ($48), and *Harvard Women's Health Letter* ($24).

International Association for Medical Assistance for Travelers
417 Center Street
Lewiston, NY 14092
(716) 754-4883
Call or write for information on health and travel and for referrals to about 500 physicians in 120 countries, excluding the United States.

Medic Alert Foundation
P.O. Box 1009
Turlock, CA 95381
(209) 668-3333
(800) ID-ALERT
Contact the foundation to order emergency medical identification bracelets

for a one-time fee or at no cost to those who are qualified.

Medical Data Source
5959 W. Century Boulevard, #1000
Los Angeles, CA 90045
(310) 641-3111
(800) 776-4MDS
Call for an annual membership to receive comprehensive, easy-to-use information on medical conditions, prescription drugs, and physician backgrounds, as well as referrals to health facilities in your community, such as nursing homes, rehabilitation centers, and support groups. Subscription rates vary but are usually under $48 per year.

National Consumers League
1701 K Street, N.W.
Washington, DC 20006
(202) 835-3323
(800) 876-7060 National Fraud Information Center
Call or write for a list of consumer-oriented publications, including "When Medications Don't Mix" and "Guide to Warning Labels on Nonprescription Medicine" ($1 each).

National Emergency Medicine Association
(800) 332-6362
Call for referrals for emergency medical services, as well as booklets, brochures, free transcripts of radio programs, and basic information on handling emergencies.

National Health Information Center
U.S. Public Health Service
P.O. Box 1133
Washington, DC 20013-1133
(800) 336-4797
(301) 565-4167 (in Maryland)
This national toll-free service puts people with health questions in touch with

organizations best able to provide answers. Call or write for free literature on such topics as AIDS, cancer, Medicare, Medicaid, health insurance, asthma, allergies, and drug and alcohol abuse. Ask for a publications list and the "Health Finder" list of toll-free numbers.

National Library of Medicine
National Institutes of Health
8600 Rockville Pike
Bethesda, MD 20894
(800) 638-8480
http://www.nlm.nih.gov/
Call or write about medical literature searches on health-related topics. Go online to conduct your own literature searches for free.

Office of Minority Health Resource Center
P.O. Box 37337
Washington, DC 20013-7337
(800) 444-6472
(301) 587-1938
Call for free information on minority health-related topics in Spanish and English.

People's Medical Society
462 Walnut Street
Allentown, PA 18102
(215) 770-1670
(800) 624-8773
Call or write for an extensive catalogue of consumer health books on issues ranging from pediatrics to aging. Among many other things, the society publishes: a monthly newsletter ($20 per year); *Dial 800 for Health* ($5.95) listing toll-free health information numbers nationwide; *Getting the Most for Your Medical Dollar,* by Charles B. Inlander and Karla Morales (1991, $15.95); *Your Medical Rights,* by Charles Inlander (1990, $14.95); *150 Ways to Be a Savvy Medical Consumer* ($4.95); and *Consumers Medical Desk Reference: Information Your Doctor Can't or Won't Tell You,* by Charles B. Inlander and the staff of the People's Medical Society ($24.95).

Planetree Health Resource Center
2034 Fillmore Street
San Francisco, CA 94115
(415) 923-2680
A program of the Institute for Health and Healing, Planetree's library includes professional medical literature, popular health publications, and resources on alternative therapy. Planetree also has a database of medical literature, health-related audiotapes and videotapes, and directories of support groups, health practitioners, and health organizations. If you can't visit the center, Planetree may be able to send you information. Other services include a personalized folder of current medical and consumer-health literature, computer-searched bibliographies, and basic packets of general health information. Contact Planetree for the cost of these services.

Prologue
Consumer Health Services, Inc.
(800) DOCTORS
(800) DENTISTS
Call for free physician and dentist referrals in Chicago, Dallas/Fort Worth, Denver, Houston, Kansas City, Miami/Ft. Lauderdale, Philadelphia, Pittsburgh, and Washington, D.C. Prologue matches patient needs and doctor specifications on over 500 variables.

Public Citizen Health Research Group
2000 P Street, N.W.
Washington, DC 20036
(202) 588-1000
HRG publishes many reports about consumer health issues and rights. "Health Letter," published monthly,

costs $18 per year. Other publications include *Medical Records: Getting Yours* ($10) and *Women's Health Alert,* by Sidney M. Wolfe ($8).

U.S. Dept. of Health and Human Services
Agency for Health Care Policy and
 Research
Publications Clearinghouse
P.O. Box 8547
Silver Spring, MD 20907-8543
(800) 358-9295
Call or write for free booklets on common health problems including pain control after surgery, unstable angina, cancer pain, urinary incontinence, enlarged prostate, pressure ulcers, depression, cataracts, sickle cell anemia, HIV, and others. Pamphlets are available in English and Spanish.

Wheaton Regional Library
Health Information Center
11701 Georgia Avenue
Wheaton, MD 20902
(301) 929-5520
(301) 929-5524 TDD
(301) 929-5485 Senior Health InfoLine
The library is a leading national resource for health information with an extensive walk-in and telephone referral service on a variety of health topics and access to online information.

Publications

American Medical Association Family Medical Guide ($29.95) and the *American Medical Association Encyclopedia of Medicine* ($45). Call the AMA at (800) 621-8335 to order these books.

The Best Medicine: How to Choose the Top Doctors, the Top Hospitals, and the Top Treatments, by Robert Arnot (Addison-Wesley, 1992), $14.95.

Better Health Care for Less, by Neil Shulman and Letitia Schweitzer (Hip-

pocrene Books, 1993), $14.95. A newsletter of the same name is also available for $24 per year. Contact Better Health Care for Less, P.O. Box 15369, Atlanta, GA 30333-0369; tel. (404) 816-6548.

Confronting Life-Threatening Illness. Order from Consumers Index, Pierian Press, P.O. Box 1808, Ann Arbor, MI 48106; tel. (800) 678-2435. $12.95.

Consumer Health Information Source Book, by Alan M. Rees and Catherine Hoffman (Oryx Press, 1990). Consult a library for this collection of information sources, clearinghouses, hotlines, and organizations focusing on health issues.

Consumers Guide to Free Medical Information by Phone and by Mail, by Arthur Winter and Ruth Winter (Prentice-Hall, 1993), $14.95. Call (800) 288-4745 for a copy.

Directory of National Helplines: A Guide to Toll-Free Public Service Numbers, 1995, $9. Order from Consumers Index, Pierian Press, P.O. Box 1808, Ann Arbor, MI 48106; tel. (800) 678-2435.

Dr. Tom Linden's Guide to Online Medicine, by Tom Linden and Michelle L. Kienholz (McGraw Hill, 1995), $18.

A Doctor's Guide to the Best Medical Care, by Michael Oppenheim (Rodale, 1992), $14.95.

Encyclopedia of Health Information Sources, edited by Alan M. Rees (Gale Research). Check your library for the latest edition.

Examining Your Doctor: A Patient's Guide to Avoiding Harmful Medical Care, by Timothy McCall (Carol Publishing Group, 1995), $18.95.

The Gift of Life, $12.95. Order from Consumers Index, Pierian Press, P.O. Box 1808, Ann Arbor, MI 48106; tel. (800) 678-2435. This book covers organ donations.

HealthNews is a consumer newsletter from the Massachusetts Medical Society, which also publishes *The New England Journal of Medicine.* $29 per year (17 issues). P.O. Box 52924, Boulder, CO 80322-2924; tel. (800) 848-9155.

Health Online, by Tom Ferguson (Addison-Wesley, 1995), $17.95.

Health Pages. Consumer-health magazines for the St. Louis, Boston, Atlanta, and Pittsburgh metropolitan areas. $9.95 for three issues per year. To subscribe, contact Health Pages, 36 West 15th Street, 12th Floor, New York, NY 10011; tel. (212) 505-0103.

Healthwise Handbook ($14.95) for children, adolescents and adults to age fifty, and *Healthwise for Life* ($14.95) for adults over age fifty. These self-care manuals contain comprehensive information on a wide range of illnesses and emergencies as well as dental care, nutrition, stress reduction, mental health, and fitness. For copies, contact Healthwise, P.O. Box 1989, Boise, ID 83701; tel. (208) 345-1161.

The Mayo Clinic Family Health Book: The Ultimate Home Medical Reference (William Morrow Co., 1996), $40.

Smart Patient, Good Medicine: Working with Your Doctor to Get the Best Medical Care, by Richard L. Scribnick and Wayne B. Scribnick (Walker and Co., 1994), $8.95.

Take Care of Yourself: The Consumer's Guide to Medical Care, by Donald Vickery and James Fries (Addison-Wesley, 1986), $14.95.

The Wellness Encyclopedia of Food and Nutrition: How to Buy, Store, and Prepare Every Fresh Food, by the editors of the University of California at Berkeley Wellness Letter (Random House, 1992), $29.95.

Wellness Letter, University of California at Berkeley, Subscription Department, P.O. Box 420163, Palm Coast, FL 32142; tel. (904) 445-4662. 12 issues for $24. Features stories and advice on health and wellness, including buying guides on food and exercise programs. Call or write for a one-year subscription.

What to Do When You Can't Afford Health Care, by Matthew Lesko (Info USA, 1993), $24.95.

Your Good Health: How to Stay Well and What to Do When You're Not, by William I. Bennett (Harvard University Press, 1987), $14.95.

Appendix B

Toll-Free Health Help

By calling these toll-free numbers, you can receive information on particular diseases or conditions, assistance during a crisis, referrals to support groups and health care providers, and publications and other resources for health care consumers. For more information on any of these numbers and the specific services available from each, consult the index and turn to the appropriate section in *Health Care Choices for Today's Consumer.*

For information on resources available online by computer, turn to chapter 22.

Abortion/Reproductive Health

National Abortion Federation Hotline: (800) 772-9100
Planned Parenthood Federation of America: (800) 829-7732

Aging

National Institute on Aging Information Center: (800) 222-2225; (800) 222-4225

AIDS/HIV

AIDS Clearinghouse: (800) 458-5231
AIDS National Hotline, Centers for Disease Control and Prevention: (800) 342-AIDS; TDD: (800) 243-7889
Sexually Transmitted Diseases Hotline, National Centers for Disease Control: (800) 227-8922

Alcohol and Drug Abuse

Alcoholics Anonymous: (800) 344-2666
American Council on Alcoholism: (800) 527-5344
National Clearinghouse for Alcohol and Drug Information: (800) 729-6686
National Council on Alcoholism and Drug Dependence: (800) NCA-CALL

Allergies

Allergy Information Referral Hotline, American Academy of Allergy and Immunology: (800) 822-ASMA
Asthma and Allergy Foundation of America: (800) 7-ASTHMA

Alzheimer's Disease

Alzheimer's Association
National Help Line: (800) 272-3900
Alzheimer's Disease Education and Referral Center: (800) 438-4380

Arthritis

Arthritis Foundation: (800) 283-7800

Asthma

Asthma and Allergy Foundation of America: (800) 7-ASTHMA

Breast Implants

FDA Breast Implant Information Line: (800) 532-4440

Breast-feeding

La Leche League International: (800) 525-3243

Cancer

American Cancer Society: (800) 227-2345

Nutrition Hotline, American Institute for Cancer Research: (800) 843-8114

American Medical Centers Cancer Information and Counseling Line: (800) 525-3777

Cancer Information Service, National Cancer Institute: (800) 4-CANCER

Candlelighter Childhood Cancer Foundation: (800) 366-2223

Leukemia Society of America: (800) 955-4LSA

Susan G. Komen Breast Cancer Foundation: (800) IM-AWARE

Y-Me National Association for Breast Cancer: (800) 221-2141

Cerebral Palsy

United Cerebral Palsy Association: (800) USA-5UCP

Child Abuse

National Council on Child Abuse—Referrals: (800) 222-2000
Crisis Hotline: (800) 422-4453

Childbirth

American Academy of Husband-Coached Childbirth: (800) 423-2397

American Society for Psychoprophylaxis in Obstetrics: (800) 368-4404

Children's Health

American Academy of Pediatrics: (800) 433-9016

Candlelighter Childhood Cancer Foundation: (800) 366-2223

Children's Hospice International: (800) 242-4453

Children's Rights Council: (800) 787-KIDS

National Clearinghouse for Infants with Disabilities and Life-Threatening Conditions: (800) 922-9234

National Information Center for Children and Youth with Disabilities: (800) 695-0285

Shriner's Hospital Referral Line: (800) 237-5055

Cleft Palate

Cleft Palate Foundation: (800) 24-CLEFT

Cooley's Anemia

Cooley's Anemia Foundation: (800) 522-7222

Crohn's/Colitis

Crohn's and Colitis Foundation of America: (800) 343-3637

United Ostomy Association: (800) 826-0826

Cystic Fibrosis

Cystic Fibrosis Foundation: (800) FIGHT-CF

Death

Choice in Dying: (800) 989-WILL

Dental Care

American Association of Orthodontists: (800) 424-2841; (800) 222-9969

Depression

National Depressive and Manic Depressive Association: (800) 82-NDMDA

National Foundation for Depressive Illness: (800) 248-4344

Diabetes

American Diabetes Association: (800) 232-3472

Diet/Nutrition

Consumer Nutrition Hotline, American Dietetic Association: (800) 366-1655

Nutrition Hotline, American Institute for Cancer Research: (800) 843-8114

Down's Syndrome

National Down's Syndrome Society: (800) 221-4602

Drug Abuse

National Clearinghouse for Alcohol and Drug Information: (800) 729-6686

National Council on Alcoholism and Drug Dependence: (800) NCA-CALL

Elders

Eldercare Locator, National Association of Area Agencies on Aging: (800) 677-1116

Children of Aging Parents, Inc.: (800) 227-7294

Epilepsy

Epilepsy Foundation of America: (800) EFA-4050

Eyes

American Foundation for the Blind: (800) AF-BLIND

Foundation Fighting Blindness: (800) 683-5555

National Eye Care Project: (800) 222-EYES

National Eye Health Education Program: (800) 869-2020

General Information and Referral Services

Ask-A-Nurse: (800) 535-1111

Center for the Study of Services: (800) 475-7283

Consumer Health Information Resource Institute: (800) 821-6671

Harvard Medical School Publications: (800) 829-9080

National Easter Seal Society: (800) 221-6827

National Health Information Center, U.S. Public Health Service: (800) 336-4797

National Library of Medicine: (800) 638-8480

People's Medical Society: (800) 624-8773

Prologue/Consumer Health Services: (800) DOCTORS; (800) DENTISTS

U.S. Dept. of Health and Human Services, Agency for Health Care Policy and Research: (800) 358-9295

Genetic Illnesses

Alliance of Genetic Support Groups: (800) 336-GENE

Headaches

National Headache Foundation: (800) 843-2256

Head Injuries

National Head Injury Foundation: (800) 444-NHIF

Hearing

Better Hearing Institute: (800) 327-9355
Hearing Aid Help-line: (800) 521-5247

Heart

American Heart Association: (800) 242-8721

Hemophilia

National Hemophilia Foundation: (800) 42-HANDI

Hospice Care

Children's Hospice International: (800) 242-4453
Hospice Help-line, National Hospice Organization: (800) 658-8898
HospiceLink, Hospice Education Institute: (800) 331-1620

Hospitals

Hill-Burton Hospital Free Care: (800) 638-0742

Huntington's Disease

Huntington's Disease Society of America: (800) 345-4372

Impotence

Impotence Institute of America: (800) 669-1603

Kidney

American Kidney Fund: (800) 638-8299
National Kidney Foundation: (800) 622-9010

Liver

American Liver Foundation: (800) 223-0179

Lou Gehrig's Disease

ALS Associates: (800) 782-4747

Lung

American Lung Association: (800) LUNG-USA

Lyme Disease

American Lyme Disease Foundation: (800) 876-LYME

Marriage/Family Counseling

American Association for Marriage and Family Therapy: (800) 374-2638

Medical Records

American Health Information Management Association: (800) 335-5535

Mental Health

Knowledge Exchange Network, Center for Mental Health Services: (800) 789-2647
National Mental Health Association: (800) 969-NMHA
National Mental Health Consumers' Self-Help Clearinghouse: (800) 553-4539

Minority Health

Office of Minority Health Resource Center: (800) 444-6472

Multiple Sclerosis

Multiple Sclerosis Society: (800) LEARN-MS

Myasthenia Gravis

Myasthenia Gravis Foundation of America: (800) 541-5454

Nurses

American Nurses Association: (800) 274-4ANA

Occupational Safety and Health

National Institute for Occupational Safety and Health: (800) 35-NIOSH

Organ Donation

National Bone Marrow Donor Program: (800) 654-1247
Organ Donation Living Bank: (800) 528-2971

Osteopathy

American Osteopathic Association: (800) 621-1773

Osteoporosis

National Osteoporosis Foundation: (800) 223-9994

Ostomy

United Ostomy Association: (800) 826-0826

Paget's Disease

Paget Foundation: (800) 23-PAGET

Paralysis

American Paralysis Association: (800) 225-0292

Parkinson's Disease

American Parkinson's Disease Association: (800) 223-2732
National Parkinson's Foundation: (800) 327-4545

Pregnancy

Birthright: (800) 550-4900

Preventive Medicine

American Institute for Preventative Medicine: (800) 345-2476

Prostate

American Prostate Society: (800) 308-1106

Psoriasis

National Psoriasis Foundation: (800) 723-9166

Rare Disorders

National Organization for Rare Disorders: (800) 999-NORD

Reye's Syndrome

National Reye's Syndrome Foundation: (800) 233-7393

Sexually Transmitted Diseases

STD Hotline, National Centers for Disease Control: (800) 227-8922

Sickle Cell Disease

National Sickle Cell Disease Association of America: (800) 962-9629

Social Security

Social Security Administration, U.S. Department of Health and Human Services: (800) 772-1213

Social Workers

National Association of Social Workers: (800) 638-8799

National Federation for Societies of Clinical Social Work: (800) 270-9739

Speech Impediments

National Stuttering Hotline: (800) 221-2483

Spina Bifida

Spina Bifida Association of America: (800) 621-3141

Stroke

National Stroke Association: (800) 787-6537

Sudden Infant Death Syndrome

SIDS National Headquarters: (800) 638-7437

Suicide

Suicide Crisis Line: (800) 621-4000

Tourette's Syndrome

Tourette Syndrome Association: (800) 237-0717

Trauma

American Trauma Society: (800) 556-7890

Urologic Disease

American Foundation for Urologic Disease: (800) 242-2383

Simon Foundation: (800) 23-SIMON

Women's Health

American College of Obstetricians and Gynecologists: (800) 673-8444

Appendix C

Emergency Health Care Phone Numbers

As a visitor to any of these metropolitan areas, you can go to the hospital listed for emergency health care. You can also call the hospitals for referrals to local doctors and other health care practitioners and for the phone numbers of pharmacies open twenty-four hours a day. One major general medical and surgical hospital is listed for each of the fifty largest metropolitan areas in the United States.

Atlanta, GA: Crawford Long Hospital (404) 686-4411

Austin/San Marcos, TX: St. David's Hospital (512) 476-7111

Boston/Worcester/Lawrence, MA: Massachusetts General Hospital (617) 726-2000

Buffalo/Niagara Falls, NY: Buffalo General Hospital (716) 859-5600

Charlotte/Gastonia/Rock Hill, NC: Carolinas Medical Center (704) 355-2000

Chicago/Gary/Kenosha, IL: Cook County Hospital (312) 633-6000

Cincinnati/Hamilton, OH: University of Cincinnati Hospital (513) 558-1000

Cleveland/Akron, OH: Metrohealth Medical Center (216) 398-6000

Columbus, OH: Riverside Methodist Hospitals (614) 566-5000

Dallas/Fort Worth, TX: Baylor University Medical Center (214) 820-0111

Dayton/Springfield, OH: Miami Valley Hospital (513) 208-8000

Denver/Boulder/Greeley, CO: Saint Joseph Hospital (303) 764-2000

Detroit/Ann Arbor/Flint, MI: Henry Ford Hospital (313) 876-2600

Grand Rapids/Muskegon, MI: Butterworth Hospital (616) 774-1774

Greensboro/Winston-Salem/High Point, NC: Memorial Hospital (919) 574-7000

Hartford, CT: Hartford Hospital (203) 524-3011

Houston/Galveston/Brazoria, TX: Methodist Hospital (713) 790-3311

Indianapolis, IN: Methodist Hospital of Indiana (317) 929-2000

Jacksonville, FL: St. Vincent's Medical Center (904) 387-7300

Kansas City, MO: St. Luke's Hospital (816) 932-2000

Las Vegas, NV: Sunrise Hospital and Medical Center (702) 731-8000

Los Angeles / Riverside / Orange County, CA: Cedars-Sinai Medical Center (310) 855-5000

Louisville, KY: Norton Hospital of Alliant Health System (502) 629-8400

Memphis, TN: Baptist Memorial Hospital (901) 227-2727

Miami/Fort Lauderdale, FL: Jackson Memorial Hospital (305) 325-0234

Milwaukee/Racine, WI: St. Luke's Medical Center (414) 649-6000

Minneapolis/St. Paul, MN: Fairview Riverside Medical Center (612) 672-6000

Nashville, TN: Vanderbilt University Hospital and Clinic (615) 322-5000

New Orleans, LA: Medical Center of Louisiana at New Orleans (504) 568-2856

New York, NY/Northern New Jersey/Long Island: New York Hospital/Cornell Medical Center (212) 746-5454

Norfolk/Virginia Beach/Newport News, VA: Sentara Norfolk General Hospital (804) 668-3000

Oklahoma City, OK: Baptist Medical Center of Oklahoma (405) 949-3011

Orlando, FL: Florida Hospital Medical Center (407) 281-8663

Philadelphia, PA/Wilmington, DE/Atlantic City, NJ: Thomas Jefferson University Hospital (215) 578-3400

Phoenix/Mesa, AZ: Good Samaritan Regional Medical Center (602) 239-2000

Pittsburgh, PA: Allegheny General Hospital (412) 359-3131

Portland/Salem, OR: Providence Medical Center (503) 215-1111

Providence/Fall River/Warwick, RI: Rhode Island Hospital (401) 444-4000

Raleigh/Durham/Chapel Hill, NC: Wake Medical Center (919) 250-8000

Rochester, NY: Strong Memorial Hospital (716) 275-2100

Sacramento/Yolo, CA: University of California Davis Medical Center (916) 734-3096

St. Louis, MO: Barnes Hospital (314) 362-5000

Salt Lake City/Ogden, UT: LDS Hospital (801) 321-1100

San Antonio, TX: Santa Rosa Health Care Corporation (210) 704-2111

San Diego, CA: Mercy Hospital and Medical Center (619) 294-8111

San Francisco/Oakland/San Jose, CA: San Francisco General Hospital Medical Center (415) 206-8000

Seattle/Tacoma/Bremerton, WA: University of Washington Medical Center (206) 548-3300

Tampa/St. Petersburg/Clearwater, FL: Tampa General Hospital (813) 251-7585

Washington, DC/Baltimore, MD: George Washington University Medical School (202) 994-1000

West Palm Beach/Boca Raton, FL: St. Mary's Hospital (407) 844-6300

Glossary

This glossary covers some of the more common terms you'll encounter in health care. While many of these terms have other meanings in the everyday world, these explanations apply to their use in health care.

Activity of daily living (ADL) A basic task such as dressing or eating that can be used as part of a formal measure of the severity of a disability.

Acute illness An illness that has occurred suddenly and may be serious.

Admitting privileges The authorization a hospital gives to a health care provider to admit a patient to that facility.

Adult day care A variety of health, social, and related support services provided on an outpatient basis for adults who have functional impairments and need supervision.

Advance directive A document in which a person designates someone to make health decisions when he or she is no longer able to make those decisions.

Allopathic physician A medical doctor.

Ambulatory care Health services that are provided without an overnight stay in a health care facility.

Ancillary services Miscellaneous tests such as laboratory or radiological exams.

Assignment *See* Medicare assignment.

Assisted-living facility Living quarters in which aides help a disabled person cope with ordinary chores, routines, and responsibilities.

Attending physician The physician who is primarily responsible for the care of a particular patient in a hospital.

Balance billing When health care providers charge and collect more for a medical service than an insurance plan will cover; the individual who received the service pays the additional amount.

Board certified A medical provider who has passed a national examination in a particular field such as anesthesiology, family practice, or surgery.

Board eligible A medical provider who is preparing for a certification exam and has the training to take it.

Capitation A payment system in which the insurer pays a provider a set fee per person signed up with that provider to cover all medical services the person receives from the provider.

Care coordination *See* Case management.

Case management The process of having a person's health care needs coordinated by using an ongoing plan.

Certificate of coverage The document that describes the benefits, providers, and general rules and regulations of an insurance policy.

Certificate of insurance *See* Certificate of coverage.

Certified *See* Board certified.

Certified nurse-midwife A nurse with specialized training to care for pregnant women and deliver babies.

Chronic illness A condition that can't be cured, can last a lifetime, or reoccurs.

Clinic A part of a hospital that deals chiefly with outpatients *or* a health care facility with several collaborating practitioners.

Clinician A health care professional who is directly involved with patient care.

Coinsurance A percentage of the total bill (often 20 percent) that an insured person pays for a hospital stay, a treatment, or a visit to a physician or other health care provider.

Community health center A clinic that serves the surrounding community with accessible and affordable health care, including primary care.

Community hospital A hospital that primarily serves the needs of its local area with general medical and surgical services.

Community rating A method of setting insurance premiums for people in a given geographic area based on the expected use and costs of health care services by all people in that area. An *adjusted* community rating reflects certain characteristics of the people in the area.

Concurrent review A review by an insurer at the time of service to ver-ify that a patient needs continued inpatient care.

Continuity of care Care that is coordinated as a patient moves from one setting or one health care provider to another.

Conversion Process by which a policyholder shifts his or her health insurance to another policy.

Copayment A fixed dollar amount the recipient pays for health care services at the time of receiving the service.

Credentialing The review process for health care providers that examines such items as their license, certification, malpractice insurance, and history.

Custodial care Institutional care for basic physical and emotional needs.

Daily living skills Tasks, such as bathing, eating, and grooming, done each day to meet a person's basic needs.

Deductible The amount of money an insured person pays for services before the insurer starts paying the bill.

Diagnosis Identification of a disease producing a specific condition.

Diagnostic services Procedures to determine the presence of a health condition.

Disability An impaired physical or mental ability.

Discharge planning The planning process before a patient leaves a hospital, nursing home, or other health care facility to determine that person's needs at the time of and following discharge.

Discharge status A person's health condition when leaving a hospital or nursing facility.

Durable medical equipment A long-lasting medical supply, such as a wheelchair.

Durable power of attorney A document in which a person designates someone to make decisions on his or her behalf.

Elective procedure A procedure that isn't an emergency and that a patient and doctor plan in advance.

Emergency An injury or acute medical condition likely to cause death, disability, or serious illness if not attended to very quickly.

Exclusions Health conditions that an insurance policy specifically doesn't cover.

Extended-care facility A nursing home or other institution that provides long term care.

Family practitioner A medical doctor with special training in a variety of fields to handle primary health care for individuals and families.

Fee-for-service plan A policy under which an insurer reimburses hospitals and physicians each time the policyholder receives care; often called an *indemnity plan.*

Gatekeeper The person who controls a patient's access to health care services, whether as a case manager or a primary care provider. Typically, this person must approve all uses of health care services.

Geriatrics The special knowledge and skills applied through medicine, nursing, social work, and other professions to help elders stay independent.

Group insurance Policies offered to an individual through his or her present or past employer or through his or her membership in a union or other organization.

Group model HMO A prepaid health care system that contracts with physicians in an established group practice to provide health services.

Health care power of attorney A document in which a person authorizes someone to control his or her medical care when the person becomes unable to do so.

Health maintenance organization (HMO) An entity that provides, offers, or arranges for coverage of designated health services needed by plan members for a fixed, prepaid premium.

Health plan The set of services in an insurance policy for health care.

History The record of a person's medical background.

Holistic medicine Medical care that considers the physical, social, emotional, and spiritual needs of the patient.

Home care Care, ranging from everyday tasks to advanced medical care, that takes place in a home setting.

Home-health agency An organization that makes skilled nurses and other therapists available to provide services in a patient's home.

Home-health care Home care administered by health care professionals.

Hospice Facility or program for terminally ill people that includes counseling and health care services that comfort a dying patient and his or her family.

Iatrogenic illness An illness caused by a physician or other health care provider.

Indemnity plan *See* Fee-for-service plan.

Independent provider association (IPA) An HMO that contracts directly with physicians in independent practices to provide health services to the HMO's members.

Informed consent A person's agreement to undergo specific medical treatment while understanding what that treatment entails and implies.

Inpatient A patient who stays in a hospital overnight.

Intermediate care facility (ICF) A nursing home that provides supervised care on a twenty-four-hour basis that is less intense than is found in a skilled nursing facility.

Internist A medical doctor who specializes in the nonsurgical diagnosis and treatment of adults.

Licensed practical nurse (LPN) A graduate of a formally approved program of practical nursing who is licensed by the appropriate state authority.

Lifetime maximum The total amount that an insurance policy will pay out for medical care during the life of the policyholder.

Living will An advance directive in which a person sets forth his or her wishes concerning medical treatment in the event he or she is incapacitated.

Long term care Care provided over the long term to people who can't take care of themselves without assistance.

Malpractice The basis for a lawsuit for injuries a patient suffers due to a health care provider's mistake or carelessness.

Managed care A term that describes strategies of health care plans to control costs by monitoring services, providers, or fees.

Mandated benefit A specific benefit that an insurer must offer by law.

Mandated provider A type of health care provider a plan must cover by law.

Maximum out-of-pocket cost The maximum amount of money a member of an insurance plan will have to pay from his or her own funds for deductibles, copayments, or other covered expenses.

Medicaid A federally aided, state-operated program that provides health insurance benefits for certain low-income people.

Medically necessary Services required to prevent harm to the patient or to ensure the patient's quality of life.

Medical record The documentation of a person's medical care.

Medical savings account A savings account for medical expenses. A medical savings account is not health insurance.

Medicare A national health-insurance program for older Americans, the blind, and disabled.

Medicare assignment An agreement between a health care provider and Medicare that he or she will accept the amount Medicare approves as full payment for Medicare-covered services.

Medicare-certified agency A health care provider that Medicare will reimburse for providing Medicare-covered services.

Medicare risk contract An arrangement between a health plan and Medicare in which the plan acts like an HMO for providing Medicare and supplemental benefits.

Medicare supplemental insurance (Medigap insurance) Insurance policies that cover the costs of some health care services not covered by Medicare.

Mortality rate The proportion of deaths within a population in a given period of time.

Mutual-aid group A support group composed of people in a similar situation; also referred to as a *self-help group*.

Network model HMO A prepaid health care system that contracts with more than one independent physician group to provide services.

Nongroup plan Insurance policy sold directly to an individual; also referred to as an individual policy.

Nonparticipating provider A provider who isn't part of a specific health plan.

Nosocomial infection An infection acquired in a hospital.

Nurse practitioner A registered nurse with advanced training to assume many of the responsibilities of physicians, including some primary care.

Nursing home *See* Intermediate care facility and Skilled nursing facility.

Occupational medicine Medicine that focuses on diseases and injuries associated with the workplace.

Ombudsman/ombudsperson A person responsible for investigating and seeking to resolve consumer complaints.

Open-enrollment period A time during which employees of a company can change health plans or during which members of a plan can change coverage.

Outcome The results of treatment.

Out-of-pocket costs All the health expenses that a policyholder pays himself or herself.

Outpatient A patient who visits a hospital or another health care facility for a specific treatment, procedure, or test but doesn't stay overnight.

Participating providers Providers who are under contract with a health plan to provide services to plan members.

Patient-care plan A written program of care for a patient that is based on the assessment of needs and that identifies the role of each service in meeting those needs.

Peer review organization (PRO) A group that assures that patients are getting services they need in the appropriate place and that the services meet professional standards.

Physician assistant (PA) A health care worker with at least three years of college education, additional specialized schooling, and on-the-job training to work under the supervision of a physician. Some PAs deliver parts of primary care.

Point of service plan (POS) A health plan that allows the policyholder to receive a service from either a participating or a nonparticipating provider, with lower benefit levels associated with the use of nonparticipating providers.

Preadmission review A review undertaken by a health plan that happens before a patient enters a hospital to determine if the admission is necessary and appropriate.

Precertification Similar to preadmission review but requires a certificate or authorization from the patient's health plan.

Preexisting condition A health condition that a person has prior to joining a plan. An insurance policy may specifically exclude it from coverage, or it may prevent the person from qualifying for insurance.

Preferred provider organization (PPO) A form of managed care in which medical providers contract with an insurer to provide services at prenegotiated fees. Subscribers may use providers outside this provider network by paying more out of pocket.

Premium The regular charge, usually monthly, that a policyholder or his or her employer pays to an insurer for health coverage, regardless of the policyholder's use of service.

Prepaid health plan A health plan in which the member pays a premium for health care services provided later at minimal additional charge. Many providers are also prepaid for their services.

Preventive care Health care that stresses healthy behavior, regular testing, screening for diseases, and other services that detect diseases early on or prevent them from occurring.

Primary care First-level or generalist care.

Primary care physician/primary care provider The health care provider a person most commonly calls first when a problem arises.

Prior authorization A cost-control procedure in which an insurer requires a service or medication to be approved in advance for coverage.

Prognosis An explanation by a health care provider to a patient of the likely course of an illness.

Provider A person or an institution that delivers a service.

Quality assurance A process that examines the services a provider offers to see that they are provided with high standards.

Reasonable and customary charge The maximum amount an insurer will reimburse a provider for a given service or procedure.

Referral When one health care provider suggests you visit another one for the purpose of further evaluation or treatment.

Registered nurse (RN) A nurse with a degree from a formal program of nursing education and a license from the appropriate state authority.

Rehabilitation Services and facilities a patient uses as a part of recovering from an accident or illness.

Respite care Care that offers temporary relief to a caregiver from some tasks.

Risk factor A characteristic or behavior that entails possible damage to a person's health.

Screening test A procedure to determine if a person has a certain medical condition.

Secondary care Care, often provided in hospitals and long term facilities, that makes more use of caregivers with specialized training than does primary care.

Self-help group *See* Mutual-aid group.

Self-referral When a health care provider stands to benefit financially from referring a patient to another provider for care.

Service area The geographic area a health plan serves.

Skilled nursing facility A long term care facility that offers extensive professional nursing services twenty-four hours a day, but not acute care.

Social HMO (SHMO) An HMO that provides some coverage for long term care, such as for home care.

Specialist A physician whose training focuses on a particular area beyond the general training for all physicians.

Specialty hospital A hospital that treats patients with a specific type of disease or condition.

Staff model HMO A prepaid health care system in which a salaried physician group employed by the HMO delivers health services.

Subspecialist A specialist with additional training in a particular clinical subject.

Supplemental Security Income (SSI) A national program that guarantees a minimum income to older Americans with insufficient resources.

Teaching hospital A hospital that is affiliated with a medical school and has a teaching program for medical students, interns, and residents.

Tertiary care Highly specialized care for severe health problems.

Usual and customary rates (UCR) *See* Reasonable and customary charge.

Utilization management Also called utilization review, the process health plans and insurers use to make sure the treatment and care recommended for a patient is necessary and appropriate.

Veterans Affairs, Department of A division of the federal government that, among other things, offers certain forms of health care to veterans of the armed forces.

Wellness A program to keep a person healthy.

Workers' compensation A program paid by employers and managed by states to provide financial assistance to workers who lose wages or incur health care bills as a result of workplace injuries and work-related health problems.

Index

About the Editor

Marc S. Miller is project director for the Health Care Choices series of consumer guidebooks. An award-winning writer and editor on human rights and social justice, Dr. Miller's books include *State of the Peoples: A Global Human Rights Report on Societies in Danger* (Beacon Press, 1993), *The Irony of Victory: Lowell During World War II* (University of Illinois Press, 1988), and *Working Lives: The* Southern Exposure *History of Labor in the South* (Pantheon, 1981). He has a doctorate in American history and is an actor and theater director in his spare time.

About Families USA

Families USA Foundation is dedicated to the achievement of high-quality, affordable health and long term care for all Americans. A nonprofit, nonpartisan organization, its work at the national, state, and community levels has earned it a reputation as an effective consumer voice for health care.

Families USA acts as a watchdog over government actions affecting health care, alerting consumers to changes and helping them have a say in the development of policy. It provides training and technical assistance to, and collaborates with, state and local organizations as they address critical health care problems in their communities. It produces highly respected reports describing the problems facing health care consumers and outlining steps to solve them. And it serves as a consumer clearinghouse for information about the health care system.

Families USA:
Guiding Your Health Care Choices

"Essential"* guides to health care. Order one for yourself and several for friends and family!

Take charge of your family's health care with these step-by-step sourcebooks!

Bay Area Health Care Choices
Chicago Area Health Care Choices
Seattle-Tacoma Health Care Choices
Health Care Choices in the Boston Area
Health Care Choices in the Washington Area

These companion guides to *Health Care Choices for Today's Consumer* provide local facts, listings, regulations, and resources for consumers.

Order Now! Call (800) 699-6960 or send the order form on the other side to:
Community Catalyst, Health Care Choices, 30 Winter St.,
Boston, MA 02108-9915

* *Library Journal*

Yes! **I want to make the right decisions about health care!**
Please send me:

_____copies of the local *Health Care Choices* companion book at $10.95 each (check city below)

_____ Bay Area   _____ Seattle-Tacoma   _____ Washington, D.C.

_____ Chicago   _____ Boston

Total Enclosed: $ _____

Please enclose a check, payable to Community Catalyst.

Name _____

Mailing Address _____

City _____ State _____ Zip _____

Telephone _____

_____ Please send me information about Families USA Foundation.

Copy or clip this form and mail to: Community Catalyst, Health Care Choices, 30 Winter St., Boston, MA 02108-9915 or call (800) 699-6960
    Allow 3–4 weeks for delivery.

www.ingramcontent.com/pod-product-compliance
Lightning Source LLC
Chambersburg PA
CBHW080224270326
41926CB00020B/4132